Low Back Pain: Recent Advances and Perspectives

Special Issue Editor
Robert J. Gatchel

MDPI • Basel • Beijing • Wuhan • Barcelona • Belgrade

MDPI

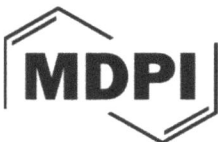

Special Issue Editor
Robert J. Gatchel
University of Texas at Arlington
USA

Editorial Office
MDPI AG
St. Alban-Anlage 66
Basel, Switzerland

This edition is a reprint of the Special Issue published online in the open access journal *Healthcare* (ISSN 2227-9032) from 2015–2016 (available at: http://www.mdpi.com/journal/healthcare/special_issues/Low-Back-Pain).

For citation purposes, cite each article independently as indicated on the article page online and as indicated below:

Author 1; Author 2. Article title. *Journal Name*. **Year**. Article number/page range.

First Edition 2017

ISBN 978-3-03842-657-8 (Pbk)
ISBN 978-3-03842-656-1 (PDF)

Table of Contents

About the Special Issue Editor

Robert J. Gatchel received his BA in Psychology, Summa Cum Laude, from SUNY at Stony Brook, and his Ph.D. in Clinical Psychology in 1973 from the University of Wisconsin. He is also a Diplomate of the American Board of Professional Psychology. At the University of Texas at Arlington, Dr. Gatchel is currently: a Distinguished Professor of the Department of Psychology, College of Science; the Nancy P & John G Penson Endowed Professor of Clinical Health Psychology; and the Director of the Center of Excellence for the Study of Health & Chronic Illnesses. He has conducted extensive clinical research in the area of pain, much of it continuously funded for the past 35 years by grants from the National Institutes of Health (NIH), National Science Foundation, and the Department of Defense. He was also the recipient of a prestigious Senior Scientist Award from NIH. Dr. Gatchel has received numerous national and international awards associated with his research, most recently, the 2017 American Psychological Foundation's Gold Medal Award for Life Achievement in the Application of Psychology.

Preface to "Low Back Pain: Recent Advances and Perspectives"

After evaluating the lack of attention to the problem of pain and pain care in the United States, the Institute of Medicine (IOM; https://www.ncbi.nlm.nih.gov/books/NBK92516/) highlighted the importance of addressing this prevalent and costly issue. In fact, low back pain (LBP) results in greater societal cost than cancer, coronary heart disease, and AIDS combined (Baird & Sheffield, 2016)! In response to these staggering statistics, the National Pain Strategy (NPS; https://iprcc.nih.gov/National-Pain-Strategy/Implementation) was formulated and released in 2016, with the intention to improve pain care in the US. This then stimulated the formation of the Interagency Pain Response Coordinating Committee (IPRCC; https://iprcc.nih.gov/), with the specific charge to develop and prioritize specific research recommendations in order to advance the NPS agenda. Relatedly, a systematic review by Dionne and colleagues (2006) concluded that the prevalence of LBP for those over the age of 60 was approximately 20%. These older Americans also have the highest long-term consumption rates of medications for pain. McFarlane and colleagues (2012) reported that older persons were also more likely to be prescribed pain medications (such as opioids), and less likely to be referred for physical therapy, compared to younger persons. Thus, there is a high prevalence of LBP in older adults, who are more often treated with pharmacotherapy. Reid and colleagues (2016) highlighted the urgent need for non-pharmacologic approaches to manage chronic LBP in older adults, as well as a better understanding of underlying mechanisms. In response to this great need for clinical research on LBP, the present series of articles was developed to include the many clinical research studies that have addressed the various biopsychosocial mechanisms of LBP, ranging from basic functional measures (such as strength, balance, brain activation patterns, and surface EMG), to important psychosocial factors (such as depression and psychiatric comorbidities, as well as demoralization), to interdisciplinary treatment methods. This series is meant to stimulate the extension of these significant clinical research areas. I would like to personally thank all the authors who have contributed to this compilation of articles.

References

Baird, A.; Sheffield, D. The Relationship between Pain Beliefs and Physical and Mental Health Outcome Measures in Chronic Low Back Pain: Direct and Indirect Effects. *Healthcare* **2016**, *4*(3), 58.

Dionne, C.E.; Dunn, K.M.; Croft, P.R. Does back pain prevalence really cecrease with increasing age? A systematic review. *Age and Aging* **2006**, *35*, 229–234.

Macfarlane, G.J.; Beasley, M.; Jones, E.A.; Prescott, G.J.; Docking, R.; Keeley, P.; McBeth, J.; Jones, G.T.; MUSICIAN Study Team. The prevalence and management of low back pain across adulthood: results from a population-based cross-sectional study (the MUSICIAN study). *Pain* **2012**, *1*, 27–32, doi:10.1016/j.pain.2011.08.005.

Reid, M.; Ong, A.D.; Henderson, C.R., Jr. WHy we need nonpharmacologic approaches to manage chronic low back pain in older adults. *JAMA Internal Medicine* **2016**, *176*(3), 338–339, doi:10.1001/jamainternmed.2015.8348.

Robert J. Gatchel

Special Issue Editor

healthcare

MDPI

Review

The Continuing and Growing Epidemic of Chronic Low Back Pain

Robert J. Gatchel

The University of Texas at Arlington, Arlington, TX 76019, USA; gatchel@uta.edu

Academic Editor: Sampath Parthasarathy

Received: 7 July 2015; Accepted: 6 September 2015; Published: 15 September 2015

Abstract: Because of the great prevalence of chronic pain, it is not surprising that there have been a number of influential reports by the Institute of Medicine, National Institutes of Health, and the World Health Organization that have documented the medical, social and economic problems caused by it, and the need for better pain-management programs. The present article briefly reviews these reports, and then focuses on three important areas that need to be considered when addressing the continuing and growing epidemic of one of the most prevalent types of chronic pain [chronic low back pain (CLBP)]: the biopsychosocial model of chronic pain; the paradigm shift in medicine from a disease model to an illness model of CLBP; and a review of the treatment- and cost-effectiveness of interdisciplinary chronic pain management programs. This overview will serve as an important prelude to other topics related to low back pain included in this Special Issue of *Healthcare*. Topics covered will range from assessment and treatment approaches, to important psychosocial mediators/moderators such as coping and pain beliefs.

Keywords: chronic pain prevalence; low back pain; biopsychosocial model; interdisciplinary chronic pain management; illness *versus* disease

1. Introduction

The very influential Institute of Medicine (IOM) Report, *"Relieving Pain in America"* [1], has highlighted the urgent need for the development of better methods for pain management because the ever-increasing costs associated with current treatment approaches cannot be sustained. This urgency has been further emphasized by the National Institutes of Health's recent *National Pain Strategy: A Comprehensive Population Health Level Strategy for Pain* [2]. The Strategy also highlighted the use of a *biopsychosocial model of pain* (to be reviewed in the next section). This was stimulated by the initial IOM Report [1], which estimated that the total direct and indirect costs of chronic pain to the U.S. economy ranges between $ 560 to $ 630 billion annually. This amount excludes those adults in the military, VA Health Care System, incarcerated individuals, and those hospitalized in psychiatric facilities [3]. Moreover, 100 million American adults have some form of chronic pain, and it is also common among children and adolescents. Overall, this makes chronic pain more common than the total number of individuals in the U.S. with diabetes, heart disease, and cancer combined [4]! However, because most people with chronic pain do not die, it does not get the public attention it greatly deserves, and is often overlooked by federal and philanthropic funding agencies. However, as will be reviewed below, it affects a tremendous number of individuals around the world.

The IOM Report also documented that musculoskeletal pain is the most common single type of chronic pain; chronic low back pain is the most prevalent in this category. A recent article in the *Journal of the American Medical Association* reported that low back pain is one of the major health problems in the U.S., and is associated with the largest number of years lived with disability [5]. Moreover, as noted by Turk [3] in 2008, there were more than 7.3 million emergency hospital room visits, and more than

2.3 million hospital inpatient stays, that were related to back problems [6]. Globally, similar findings have been published in recent reviews in the *New England Journal of Medicine* [7] and *The Lancet* [8]. These reviews were based on the World Bank and World Health Organization's Study of the Global Burden of Disease (GBD). As a follow-up to the previous GBD Study 2010, a more recent GBD Study 2013 [9] reported that years lived with disability (YLDs) are increasing due to population growth and aging in most countries around the world. As noted: "Leading causes of YLDs included low back pain and major depressive disorder among the top ten causes of YLDs in every country." (p. 1) [9]. Again, the economic burden of low back pain is quite large, and continues to grow in the U.S., as well as internationally [1,9].

It should also be kept in mind that, with the "graying of America," this low back pain problem will significantly increase in the future. In 2010, there were approximately 40.3 million Americans, age 65 years or older, accounting for 13% of the total population [10]. By the year 2030, it is projected that about 20% of the population will be 65 years of age or older [11]. Awareness of these population trends, both nationally and internationally, contributes to increased concern about healthcare issues among older adults, including pain problems, their psychiatric sequelae, and the associated increased and potentially dangerous opioid medication use.

With the above staggering statistics in mind, it was felt that a Special Issue of the Journal *Healthcare* was warranted in order to update many of the recent advances and perspectives in this growing area of clinical and economic importance. Besides the now most widely accepted and heuristic approach to chronic low back pain—*the biopsychosocial perspective*—to be reviewed next, a host of biopsychosocial-related topics will be presented. They range from medical evaluations and other assessment techniques, to low back pain management approaches, including surgery and opioid medication, as well as important psychosocial mediators/moderators such as coping and pain beliefs. An earlier review by Gatchel, Peng *et al.* [12], delineated a number of such moderators and mediators (e.g., emotional distress, catastrophizing, fear avoidance). This Special Issue is meant to provide readers with the most updated information on these important topics related to low back pain.

2. The Biopsychosocial Model of Chronic Pain

George Engel [13] first introduced the term "biopsychosocial" to medicine in the context of chronic physical illnesses. He initially highlighted the fact that many chronic illnesses were not solely caused by some specific underlying pathophysiology. Rather, lifestyle/psychosocial factors were important contributors to the maintenance and/or exacerbation of the illness process. This perspective started to replace the outdated *biomedical reductionism*, or "dualistic" perspective that mind and body function separately and independently, to the more comprehensive biopsychosocial approach to medicine (e.g., [4,14]). This biopsychosocial perspective began to be adopted by many clinical researchers in the area of pain, now viewing pain as the result of a dynamic interaction among biological, psychological and social factors that can perpetuate and even worsen the clinical presentation. The reader is referred to many relevant publications on this topic (e.g., [4,12,14–20]).

A major outgrowth of this biopsychosocial model of pain was the development of more comprehensive and effective interdisciplinary interventions for chronic pain in order to address both the physical and psychosocial factors involved (e.g., [4,16]). Indeed, as reviewed by Gatchel and Okifuji [17], traditional interventions for chronic pain had predominantly involved monotherapies, such as surgery, injections, and a wide array of pharmacotherapeutic approaches. However, as Turk and Gatchel [21] began to highlight, more comprehensive interdisciplinary approaches, based on the biopsychosocial model, were needed to address both the physical and psychosocial factors involved in chronic pain. This model has become very influential in the area of pain, especially with the resultant development of treatment- and cost-effective interdisciplinary pain management programs in this country [12,17], as well as other countries such as Canada [22], Denmark [23,24], France [25], Germany [26], and Japan [27]. Such programs (to be discussed next), based upon the biopsychosocial model, have been found to be the most heuristic approach to understanding and assessing chronic pain [12]. Indeed, the earlier reviewed influential IOM Report [1]; p. 35 states that: "Today, most researchers and clinicians who specialize in pain issues use the "biopsychosocial model" (denoting the combination of biological, psychological and social/family/cultural contexts of pain to understand and treat chronic pain [12])." Further support for the use of interdisciplinary pain management as an evidence-based clinical guideline for the treatment of low back pain is the fact that Chou and colleagues [28] concluded that " ... it is strongly recommended that clinicians consider intensive interdisciplinary rehabilitation with a cognitive/behavioral emphasis (strong recommendation, high-quality evidence)" (p. 1070).

3. Disease *versus* Illness

It should also be noted that, as originally summarized by Turk and Monarch [19], the biopsychosocial model focuses on both disease and illness, with illness being viewed as the complex interaction among biological, psychological and social factors. As they note:

> *"The distinction between "disease" and "illness" is crucial to understanding chronic pain. Disease is generally defined as an "objective biological event" that involves disruption of specific body structures or organ systems caused by pathological, anatomical, or physiological changes ... In contrast to this customary view of physical disease, illness is defined as a "subjective experience or self-attribution" that a disease is present; it yields physical discomfort, emotional distress, behavioral limitations, and psychosocial disruption. In other words, illness refers to how the sick person and members of his or her family and wider social network perceive, live with, and respond to symptoms and disability ... The distinction between disease and illness is analogous to the distinction between "pain" and "nociception." Nociception entails stimulation of nerves that convey information about tissue damage to the brain. Pain is subjective perception that results from the transduction, transmission, and modulation of sensory input filtered through a person's genetic composition and prior learning history and modulated further by the person's current physiological status, idiosyncratic appraisals, expectations, current mood state, and sociocultural environment."*

(pp. 6–7) [19]

Because the biopsychosocial model of chronic pain views each individual as experiencing pain uniquely, it is important to evaluate the different dimensions of this interactive process [16]. Also, chronic pain should be generally viewed as an illness, which can be successfully managed (using comprehensive interdisciplinary pain management programs to be discussed next), but cannot often be completely cured by traditional surgical procedures or solely by medication. Indeed, this represents a significant paradigm shift from the older biomedical reductionist curative model of medical disorders, to a more pragmatic and effective biopsychosocial management model of medical disorders such as chronic pain.

4. Interdisciplinary Pain Management

Intensive interdisciplinary pain management programs, such as functional restoration (first developed by Mayer and Gatchel [29]), were established for patients who were experiencing the effects of significant physical deconditioning, chronic disability, and major psychosocial consequences. As outlined by both Gatchel and Okifuji [17] and Gatchel, McGeary *et al.* [4], the treatment team of such programs consists of a physician, nurse, psychologist or psychiatrist, physical therapist, and an occupational therapist. They interact on a daily basis in order to coordinate the following:

- The objective quantification of physical/functional deficits (at the beginning, during, and at the end of treatment) in order to tailor/individualize, monitor and guide physical and functional progress and gains. Indeed, one of the most frequent barriers to rehabilitation is physical deconditioning. Such deconditioning occurs when inactivity and disuse of the injured body part culminates in a general loss of function, which becomes progressively worse as the degree of disue and immobilization increases [30]. The effects of this deconditioning may result in muscle atrophy, the development of stiff/hypomobile joints, loss of endurance and cardiovascular fitness, and an increase in muscle spasms [29].

- Likewise, psychosocial evaluations are conducted to aid in the tailoring of treatment for each patient, as well as to guide and monitor progress and gains.
- These above psychosocial evaluations are used in a multimodal pain and disability program, using cognitive-behavioral therapy (CBT) approaches. As previously reviewed by Gatchel and colleagues [31], CBT is a major component of interdisciplinary treatment: "The central aims of CBT are to identify and replace maladaptive patient cognitions, emotions, and behaviors with more adaptive ones in the hope of maximizing the benefits of other interdisciplinary care components (e.g., physical therapy) and increasing functional capacity through improved coping . . . CBT has emerged as the psychosocial treatment of choice for chronic pain." (pp. 124–125) [31].
- Psychopharmacological interventions are also often used for detoxification purposes, as well as for psychosocial management purposes.
- Regular, ongoing interdisciplinary, medically-directed formal team staffings are held at least on a weekly basis, as well as frequent team meetings in order to ensure that patients are progressing, and that any potential barriers to improvement are immediately addressed. This regular communication and feedback among the staff is a requisite element for ensuring successful treatment outcomes.

    As noted earlier, this interdisciplinary approach has been found to be both therapeutically- and cost-effective in U.S. studies, as well as studies in other countries. Successful outcomes, such as decreases in pain and opioid medication use, increases in return-to-work and activities of daily living, and decreases in subsequent healthcare visits, are obtained after intervention. This attests to the robustness of the clinical research findings and utility, as well as its fidelity [4,17]. It should also be noted that, for more acute patients, a less intensive interdisciplinary intervention program has also been found to be therapeutically- and cost-effective [31–33].

5. Summary and Conclusions

    As has been reviewed, there have been a number of recent and very influential reports from the IOM, the National Institutes of Health and the World Health Organization that have highlighted the urgent need for the development of better methods for pain and disability management because the ever-increasing costs associated with treatment approaches cannot be sustained. Musculoskeletal pain is the most common single type of chronic pain, with low back pain the most prevalent in this category. Because of this increased problem of chronic pain, there has been a great increase in the number of clinical research studies evaluating aspects of the assessment, treatment and prevention of chronic pain (see [12]). The majority of this clinical research is being guided by the biopsychosocial model of pain, which views pain as a result of a dynamic interaction among biological, psychological and social factors that can perpetuate and even worsen the clinical presentation. A major outgrowth of this biopsychosocial model of pain has been the development of more comprehensive and effective interdisciplinary interventions for chronic pain in order to address both the physical and psychosocial factors involved. Such interdisciplinary approaches to pain management have been found to be more therapeutic- and cost-effective than traditional biomedical approaches on a variety of important outcome measures. Indeed, such findings have resulted in a significant paradigm shift from the outdated biomedical approaches to chronic pain, which try to "cure" the pain by surgical or medication use (often, though, unsuccessfully), to a more comprehensive pain management approach using interdisciplinary pain management programs to help patients better manage and cope with the chronic pain and any remnants of it. Moreover, the distinction between disease and illness is crucial in understanding chronic pain. In contrast to the disease perspective, which is generally defined as looking for an objective biological event involved in the disruption of specific bodily

Healthcare **2015**, *3*, 838–845

structures or chronic systems caused by some type of pathophysiology, illness is defined as a more subjective experience or self-attribution that a disease is present and will yield physical discomfort, emotional distress and psychosocial disruption.

Finally, using this biopsychosocial "illness" approach to interdisciplinary pain management programs, such as functional restoration, have been developed for patients who are experiencing the effects of significant physical deconditioning, chronic disability and major psychosocial consequences. Also, for more acute patients, less intensive interdisciplinary intervention programs have also been found to be therapeutically- and cost-effective. In these programs, a number of psychosocial moderators and mediators (e.g., emotional stress, catastrophizing, fear avoidance) need to be taken into account. Subsequent articles in this Special Issue have been provided to update information on these variables, as well as the overall topic of low back pain.

Conflicts of Interest: The author declares no conflict of interest.

References

1. Institute of Medicine of the National Academy of Science. *Relieving Pain in America: A Blueprint for Transforming Prevention, Care, Education, and Research;* Institute of Medicine: Washington, DC, USA, 2011; p. 5.
2. National Pain Strategy: A Comprehensive Population Health Level Strategy for Pain. Available online: http://iprcc.nih.gov/National_Pain_Strategy/NPS_Main.htm (accessed on 20 August 2015).
3. Turk, D.C. The Biopsychosocial Approach to the Assessment and Intervention for People with Musculoskeletal Disorders. In *Handbook of Musculoskeletal Pain and Disability Disorders in the Workplace;* Gatchel, R.J., Schultz, I.Z., Eds.; Springer: New York, NY, USA, 2014.
4. Gatchel, R.J.; McGeary, D.D.; McGeary, C.A.; Lippe, B. Interdisciplinary chronic pain management: past, present and the future. *Am. Psychol. Spec. Issue Psychol. Chronic Pain* **2014**, *69*, 119–130. [CrossRef] [PubMed]
5. U.S. Burden of disease collaborators. The State of U.S. Health, 1990–2010: Burden of diseases, injuries, and risk factors. *JAMA* **2013**, *310*, 591–608.
6. Agency for Health Research and Quality. Healthcare Cost and Utilization Project. Available online: http://www.hcup-us.ahrq.gov/reports/statbriefs/sb105.jsp (accessed on 12 June 2015).
7. Murray, C.J.L.; Lopez, A.D. Measuring the global burden of disease. *N. Engl. J. Med.* **2013**, *369*, 448–457. [CrossRef] [PubMed]
8. Vos, T.; Flaxman, A.D.; Naghavi, M.; Lozano, R.; Michaud, C.; Ezzati, M.; Shibuya, K.; Salomon, J.A.; Abdalla, S.; Aboyans, V.; *et al.* Years Lived with Disability (YLDs) for 1160 sequelae of 289 diseases and injuries 1990–2010: A systematic analysis for the global burden of disease study 2010. *Lancet* **2012**, *380*, 2163–2196. [CrossRef]
9. Global Burden of Disease Study 2013 Collaborators. Global, Regional, and National Incidence, Prevalence, and Years Lived with Disability for 301 Acute and Chronic Diseases and Injuries in 188 Countries, 1990–2013: A Systematic Analysis for the Global Burden of Disease Study 2013. *The Lancet* **2015**, *386*, 743–800.
10. U.S. Census Bureau. *The Older Population: 2010;* U.S. Department of Commerce Economics and Statistics Administration: Washington, DC, USA, 2011.
11. U.S. Census Bureau. *Population Projections of the United States by Age, Sex, Race, Hispanic Origin, and Nativity: 1999 to 2000;* U.S. Census Bureau: Washington, DC, USA, 2000.
12. Gatchel, R.J.; Peng, Y.; Peters, M.L.; Fuchs, P.N.; Turk, D.C. The biopsychosocial approach to chronic pain: Scientific advances and future directions. *Psychol. Bull.* **2007**, *133*, 581–624. [CrossRef] [PubMed]
13. Engel, G.L. The need for a new medical model: A challenge for biomedicine. *Science* **1977**, *196*, 129–136. [CrossRef] [PubMed]
14. Gatchel, R.J. Comorbidity of chronic mental and physical health disorders: The biopsychosocial perspective. *Am. Psychol.* **2004**, *59*, 792–805. [CrossRef] [PubMed]
15. Feinberg, S.D.; Brigham, C.R. Assessing Disability in the Pain Patien. In *Comprehensive Treatment of Chronic Pain by Medical, Interventional, and Integrative Approaches: The American Academy of Pain Medicine Textbook on Patient Management;* Deer, T.R., Leong, M.S., Buvanendran, A., Gordin, V., Kim, P.S., Panchal, S.J., Ray, A.L., Eds.; Springer: New York, NY, USA, 2013.

16. Gatchel, R.J. *Clinical Essentials of Pain Management*; American Psychological Association: Washington, DC, USA, 2005.
17. Gatchel, R.J.; Okifuji, A. Evidence-based scientific data documenting the treatment and cost-effectiveness of comprehensive pain programs for chronic nonmalignant pain. *J. Pain* **2006**, *7*, 779–793. [CrossRef] [PubMed]
18. Gatchel, R.J.; Turk, D.C. *Psychological Approaches to Pain Management: A Practitioner's Handbook*; Guilford Publications, Inc.: New York, NY, USA, 1996.
19. Turk, D.C.; Monarch, E.S. *Biopsychosocial Approaches on Chronic Pain, in Psychological Approaches to Pain Management: A Practitioner's Handbook*; Gatchel, R.J., Turk, D.C., Eds.; Guilford Press: New York, NY, USA, 2002; pp. 3–29.
20. Dworkin, S.F.; von Korff, M.R.; LeResche, L. Epidemiological studies of chronic pain: A dynamic-ecologic perspective. *Ann. Behav. Med.* **1992**, *14*, 3–11.
21. Turk, D.C.; Gatchel, R.J. *Psychological Approaches to Pain Management: A Practitioner's Handbook*, 2nd ed.; Guilford: New York, NY, USA, 2002.
22. Corey, D.T.; Koepfler, L.E.; Etlin, D.; Day, H.I. A limited functional restoration program for injured workers: A randomized trial. *J. Occup. Rehabil.* **1996**, *6*, 239–249. [CrossRef] [PubMed]
23. Bendix, A.E.; Bendix, T.; Vaegter, K.; Lund, C.; Frølund, L.; Holm, L. Multidisciplinary intensive treatment for chronic low back pain: A randomized, prospective study. *Cleveland Clin. J. Med.* **1996**, *63*, 62–69. [CrossRef]
24. Bendix, T.; Bendix, A. Different training programs for chronic low back pain—A randomized, blinded one-year follow-up study. In Proccedings of International Society for the Study of the Lumbar Spine, Seattle, WA, USA, June 1994; pp. 21–25.
25. Jousset, N.; Fanello, S.; Bontoux, L.; Dubus, V.; Billabert, C.; Vielle, B.; Roquelaure, Y.; Penneau-Fontbonne, D.; Richard, I. Effects of functional restoration *versus* 3 hours per week physical therapy: A randomized controlled study. *Spine* **2004**, *29*, 487–493. [CrossRef] [PubMed]
26. Hildebrandt, J.; Pfingsten, M.; Saur, P.; Jansen, J. Prediction of Success from a Multidisciplinary treatment program for chronic low back pain. *Spine* **1997**, *22*, 990–1001. [CrossRef] [PubMed]
27. Shirado, O.; Ito, T.; Kikumoto, T.; Takeda, N.; Minami, A.; Strax, T.E. A novel back school using a multidisciplinary team approach featuring quantitative functional evaluation and therapeutic exercises for patients with chronic low back pain. *Spine* **2005**, *30*, 1219–1225. [CrossRef] [PubMed]
28. Chou, R.; Shekelle, P. Will this patient develop persistent disabling low back pain? *J. Am. Med. Assoc.* **2010**, *303*, 1295–1302. [CrossRef] [PubMed]
29. Mayer, T.G.; Gatchel, R.J. *Functional Restoration for Spinal Disorders: The Sports Medicine Approach*; Lea & Febiger: Philadelphia, PA, USA, 1988.
30. Mayer, T.G.; Polatin, P.B. Tertiary nonoperative interdisciplinary program: The functional restoration variant of the outpatient chronic pain management program. In *Occupational Musculoskeletal Disorders: Function, Outcomes & Evidence*; Mayer, T.G., Gatchel, R.J., Polatin, P.B., Eds.; Lippincott, Williams & Wilkins: Philadelphia, PA, USA, 2000; pp. 639–649.
31. Gatchel, R.J.; Polatin, P.B.; Noe, C.E.; Gardea, M.A.; Pulliam, C.; Thompson, J. Treatment- and cost-effectiveness of early intervention for acute low back pain patients: A one-year prospective study. *J. Occup. Rehabil.* **2003**, *13*, 1–9. [CrossRef] [PubMed]
32. Rogerson, M.D.; Gatchel, R.J.; Bierner, S.M. Cost utility analysis of interdisciplinary early intervention *versus* treatment as usual for high risk acute low back pain patients. *Pain Pract.* **2010**, *10*, 382–395. [CrossRef] [PubMed]
33. Whitfill, T.; Haggard, R.; Bierner, S.M.; Pransky, G.; Hassett, R.G.; Gatchel, R.J. Early intervention options for acute low back pain patients: A randomized clinical trial with one-year follow-up outcomes. *J. Occup. Rehabil.* **2010**, *20*, 256–263. [CrossRef] [PubMed]

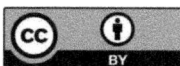

healthcare

MDPI

Review

A Systematic Review of the Effects of Exercise and Physical Activity on Non-Specific Chronic Low Back Pain

Rebecca Gordon * and Saul Bloxham

Department of Sport and Health Sciences, University of St Mark and St John, Plymouth PL6 8BH, UK; sbloxham@marjon.ac.uk
* Correspondence: rgordon@marjon.ac.uk; Tel.: +44-1752-636700 (ext. 6526)

Academic Editor: Robert J. Gatchel
Received: 28 February 2016; Accepted: 19 April 2016; Published: 25 April 2016

Abstract: Back pain is a major health issue in Western countries and 60%–80% of adults are likely to experience low back pain. This paper explores the impact of back pain on society and the role of physical activity for treatment of non-specific low back pain. A review of the literature was carried out using the databases SPORTDiscuss, Medline and Google Scholar. A general exercise programme that combines muscular strength, flexibility and aerobic fitness is beneficial for rehabilitation of non-specific chronic low back pain. Increasing core muscular strength can assist in supporting the lumbar spine. Improving the flexibility of the muscle-tendons and ligaments in the back increases the range of motion and assists with the patient's functional movement. Aerobic exercise increases the blood flow and nutrients to the soft tissues in the back, improving the healing process and reducing stiffness that can result in back pain.

Keywords: aerobic fitness; non-specific chronic low back pain; pedometer; physical activity

1. An Introduction to the Impact of Back Pain on Society and the Importance of Physical Activity

Back pain is a major health issue in Western countries and is associated with increasing medical expenditure, work absence [1,2] and is the most common musculoskeletal condition [3–5]. Sixty to eighty percent of adults will at some point in their lives experience low back pain [6–8], and 16% of adults in the United Kingdom (UK) consult their general practitioner every year [9]. Back pain costs the National Health Service (NHS) £1.3 million every day [10] and results in 12.5% of all work absence in the UK [11]. However, the most appropriate intervention to treat non-specific chronic low back pain (NSCLBP) remains elusive [12].

It is recommended for patients with NSCLBP to remain physically active, as long periods of inactivity will adversely affect recovery [13,14]. A variety of different types of exercise have been explored to treat CLBP, including low-to-moderate intensity aerobic exercise [15,16], high intensity aerobic exercise [17,18], core stabilization and muscular strength exercises [19–24] and flexibility programmes [25–27]. However, the most effective form of exercise as a method of rehabilitation for NSCLBP is unknown [6,28] reflecting its complexity [17] and more research is required [29].

Physical activity (PA) to increase aerobic capacity and muscular strength, especially of the lumbar extensor muscles, is important for patients with CLBP in assisting them to complete activities of daily living [30]. However, different exercises have been found to result in varying levels of effectiveness in reducing lower back pain [31]. In addition, too much or too little PA can be associated with low back pain [32], suggesting that PA as an intervention for low back pain is complex.

Eight-five percent of back pain cases have an unknown cause [33], normally diagnosed after undergoing tests such as X-ray, MRI scan and blood tests [34]. Understanding the cause of back pain is important in order to remove it from the patient's life and not to replicate the movement during therapy [35]. However, when the cause of the back pain is unknown, prescribing targeted therapy can prove difficult, and general exercise is often recommended [36]. Typically intervention programmes have adopted a monodisciplinary approach to rehabilitate NSCLBP [15,21,25]. Although promising findings were reported following a multicomponent exercise programme [37]. Thirty-seven patients with NSCLBP were allocated into control, (who just maintained their current rehabilitation programme), or training groups, which combined an additional functional training programme of aerobic exercise, muscular strength and flexibility. Back pain was found to significantly decrease by 52.5% in the training group compared to no significant change in the control group. In addition, disability significantly decreased by 27.3% in the training group according to the Oswestry Disability Index, compared to no significant change in the control group. The aim of this article is to review the effects of PA and exercise interventions involving aerobic exercise, muscular strength and stabilisation exercises and/or flexibility training on NSCLBP to identify effective strategies for treatment.

2. Method

A systematic review was carried out between 2014 and 2015 using the databases SPORTDiscuss, Medline and Google Scholar. The first author selected intervention programmes published between 2005 and 2015 which investigated the effect of PA or exercise interventions for NSCLBP patients involving aerobic exercise, muscular strength and stabilisation exercises and/or flexibility training on NSCLBP. The first author read and reviewed the articles. Chronic pain was defined as pain remaining for longer than three months and further inclusion criteria was that the participants involved in the studies should be ⩾18 years old. The intervention programmes were identified using the search terms "non-specific chronic low back pain and exercise" which returned 141 results. Other search terms included "chronic low back pain and aerobic exercise" (187 results), "chronic low back pain and muscular strength" (120 results) and "non-specific chronic low back pain" (173 results). A total of 14 studies were included within the final review. The review summarised the effect on NSCLBP within the included intervention programmes.

2.1. Eligibility Criteria

Studies were included within the final review based on the following: population, intervention and the outcome.

2.2. Inclusion Criteria

Population: NSCLBP patients aged 18 years or older.

Intervention: Aerobic exercise, muscular strength or stabilisation exercises and/or flexibility training intervention programmes. There was no restriction on the inclusion of a follow up in the included studies.

Outcome: Investigate effect of the intervention on NSCLBP which was not limited to one specific measure for pain.

2.3. Exclusion Criteria

Literature reviews and any article which did not involve a delivery of an intervention programme to NSCLBP patients.

3. Defining Back Pain and the Impact of Physical Activity and Exercise

Back pain is defined as chronic when the pain remains for longer than three months [38]. CLBP can have a debilitating effect on patients' lives, resulting in disability and reducing their ability to carry out activities of daily living [29]. Acute back pain is pain that remains for less than 6 weeks [39,40] and sub-acute back pain is back pain for between 6 weeks and 3 months. Forty percent of patients with acute low back pain are at an elevated risk of developing CLBP [41].

Back pain is then further categorised into specific or non-specific back pain. Non-specific back pain is diagnosed when the cause of the back pain is unknown [42,43], and specific back pain refers to a specific cause for the pain, for example an infection or a fracture [44]. Non-specific low back pain is the most common type of back pain to occur [45,46], and accounts for 85% of all back pain cases [39,47].

PA increases the blood flow to the back which is important for the healing process of the soft tissues in the back [48]. Being physically active, through activities of daily living, has been highlighted as important in assisting the recovery of acute and NSCLBP [49]. However, following a review of 39 trials into the effects of exercise on non-specific acute low back pain [2], it was suggested there is strong evidence that an exercise programme was not more effective for recovery of non-specific acute low back pain, compared to inactivity. Thus, patients with acute low back pain should not start an exercise programme for rehabilitation [50].

The difference between PA and exercise is that exercise is planned and structured which involves disrupting homeostasis by concentric, eccentric and isometric muscular activity and involves repetitive movements [51]. PA is not structured, and includes any movement that involves contraction of skeletal muscles requiring energy expenditure [52] typified by activities of daily living such as walking and housework [53].

Most people with non-specific acute low back pain recover in 4–6 weeks with or without a treatment [5]. Therefore if acute low back pain patients recover without a treatment in a similar timescale to patients with a treatment, there is no added benefit in completing an exercise programme such as muscle strengthening exercises. Muscle strengthening exercises could potentially cause extra damage to acute back pain due to the additional strain on the ligaments and muscles in the back, which may have swelling [48]. It is important to stop exercise in order to reduce the swelling of the affected area and therefore reduce the back pain [39], suggesting it is a case of waiting for acute low back pain to recover.

Furthermore, a review of six randomised controlled trials researched the effect of exercise programmes on patients with non-specific sub-acute low back pain [54]. The review suggested that there was moderate evidence that a graded-activity exercise programme is effective for improving absenteeism from work for patients with non-specific sub-acute low back pain, however it was unclear if other types of exercise programmes are effective.

4. Results

4.1. Aerobic Exercise

Aerobic exercise can benefit CLBP as it increases the blood flow and nutrients to the soft tissues in the back, improving the healing process and reducing stiffness that results in back pain [55]. In addition 30–40 min of aerobic exercise increases the body's production of endorphins [55], a brain chemical that bind to the opiate receptors in the pain control system in the brain and spinal cord to decrease the perception of pain [56]. Endorphins act in a similar way to pain reducing drugs such as morphine and codeine [57]. However increasing the body's endorphin production is a natural alternative for pain relief for the body [58], and can reduce CLBP [59]. Rehabilitation involving aerobic exercise can be used as a conservative method for reducing CLBP, and could prevent patients relying on medication for pain reduction.

A low aerobic fitness level is associated with CLBP [60,61], and maximum oxygen consumption (VO_{2max}) was significantly lower by 10 mL/kg in men with CLBP compared to men without [62]. VO_{2max} was also significantly lower by 5.6 mL/kg in women with CLBP compared to healthy counterparts.

Aerobic exercise for 20 min on a cycle ergometer at 70% peak oxygen uptake reduced the pain perception for more than 30 min for patients with CLBP [63]. Aerobic exercise also provides additional benefits such as improving functional status [64], and reducing the fear of movement [65]. Fear of movement is a predictor for functional limitations [66] and is associated with disability in patients with CLBP [67]. Aerobic exercise can reduce disability and improve the functional status of patients with CLBP by increasing fitness levels, helping patients conduct activities of daily living.

4.1.1. Impact of Aerobic Exercise Interventions on Chronic Low Back Pain

A 6-week moderate intensity aerobic exercise programme (walking on a treadmill at 50% heart rate reserve) for 52 sedentary NSCLBP patients was compared to a 6-week programme involving specific strengthening exercises for the trunk and upper and lower limbs [16]. CLBP significantly reduced by 20% in the aerobic exercise group and 15% in the muscle strengthening group, although there was no significant difference between the two groups. This suggests that patients could be provided with a choice of which type of exercise programme they would most enjoy. This is important as enjoyment of exercise is an important factor in exercise adherence [68]. However this study involved a 6-week intervention, and an 8-week intervention programme is important to significantly improve aerobic fitness [69], by allowing greater physiological adaptions to occur [15].

An 8-week moderate intensity aerobic exercise intervention at 40%–60% of heart rate reserve combined with conventional physiotherapy, significantly reduced NSCLBP by 47% [15]. This was compared to a significant reduction of 42% in NSCLBP in the control group, involving only conventional physiotherapy. However there was no significant difference between the two groups, suggesting the combination of moderate intensity aerobic exercise and conventional physiotherapy does not provide any additional benefits to CLBP.

The 8-week intervention programme was also found to increase aerobic fitness by 3.3% as measured by VO_{2max}. This increase was not significant, and also suggests that additional factors excluding aerobic fitness levels must have had an influence on reducing CLBP. This was in contrast to previous research which suggested aerobic fitness levels to be associated with CLBP [60,61]. The conventional physiotherapy involved activities such as back mobilisation exercises, core stabilisation exercise and education on back care, suggesting a general programme involving a range of activities may be optimal.

A 12-week high intensity aerobic exercise programme involving running on a treadmill at 85% of heart rate reserve and was compared to passive treatment (ultrasound and did not include any form of PA) [17]. The 12-week high intensity exercise programme significantly reduced NSCLBP by 41% compared to no improvement in the passive treatment group.

The effect of high intensity aerobic exercise on CLBP was further supported by a 12-week high intensity aerobic exercise programme (running on a treadmill at 85% heart rate reserve) which significantly reduced NSCLBP by 30% [18]. This study involved a larger sample size of 64 patients, compared to the previous study [17].

However the study [18] excluded patients with NSCLBP who were obese, classified by a body mass index of 30 or over [70,71]. The researcher stated this was due to possible cardiovascular problems and the risk of injury to the patients, as the study involved high intensity exercise. Therefore the results from this study cannot be generalised to obese NSCLBP patients, despite obesity being associated with NSCLBP [72].

Walking is known to be a safe form of exercise for CLBP patients as it is associated with a low injury rate [73] and does not involve twisting or vigorous forward flexion [74]. Although, exercising at a low intensity at 40% VO_{2max} does not significantly increase cortisol levels [75], and low cortisol levels are associated with CLBP [76].

These studies indicate that although similar outcomes can be achieved despite differences in aerobic exercise intensity. Thus moderate exercise should be promoted over high or low intensity programmes given the reduced risks, enhanced compliance, optimal benefits and reduced impact [55].

Exercising at a comfortable intensity for the patient is important in reducing fear avoidance [77], which is important for increasing PA levels [78] as CLBP patients who are more fear avoidant report higher levels of disability [79]. Patients should be encouraged to increase their levels of PA at an intensity that is comfortable for them, and that can be integrated into activities of daily living [53]. Such an approach is more sustainable long term [80]. See Table 1 for a summary of each of the discussed aerobic exercise intervention programmes.

Table 1. Aerobic exercise intervention programmes for NSCLBP patients.

Reference Number	Type of Population	Length of Intervention	Effect on Back Pain	Significance Levels
(Hoffman *et al.*, 2005) [63]	8 individuals with NSCLBP (4 male, 4 female)	25 min of cycle ergometry. 5 min at 50% peak oxygen uptake, then 20 min at 70% peak oxygen uptake	Pressure pain test. Pain significantly decreased by 28% at 2 min and 22% at 32 min post exercise compared to pre-exercise values. No gender/age differences in results	$p < 0.05$
(Shnayderman & Katz-Leurer, 2013) [16]	52 sedentary NSCLBP patients aged 18-65 years	Experimental group (walking on treadmill at 50% heart rate reserve). Control group: specific low back strengthening exercises. Both twice a week for 6 weeks	Low Back Pain Functional Scale: Significantly improved by 20% in experimental group and 15% in control group. No gender/age differences in results	$p < 0.05$
(Chan *et al.*, 2011) [15]	46 NSCLBP patients (10 male, 36 female)	8-week intervention. Both intervention and control groups received conventional physiotherapy. Intervention group only also prescribed aerobic exercise (40%–60% heart rate reserve)	Visual Analogue Scale (VAS): Intervention group: 47% significant reduction post intervention. Control: 42% significant reduction post intervention. No gender/age differences in results	$p < 0.001$
(Chatzitheodorou *et al.*, 2007) [17]	20 NSCLBP patients (11 male, 9 female). Excludes patients with BMI > 30	12-week intervention. Exercise group: high intensity aerobic exercise (running on treadmill at 85% of heart rate reserve). Control group: Passive treatment (ultrasound and did not include any form of PA)	McGill Pain Questionnaire. Exercise group: 41% significant reduction post intervention. Control: no significant change. No gender/age differences in results	$p < 0.001$
(Chatzitheodorou *et al.*, 2008) [18]	64 NSCLBP patients (26 male, 38 female) Excludes patients with BMI > 30	Patients randomly allocated into positive or negative dexamethasone suppression test. Both groups completed 12-week aerobic exercise programme (running on treadmill at 85% heart rate reserve)	McGill Pain Questionnaire. Positive suppression group: 30% significant reduction post intervention. Negative suppression group: 8% significant reduction post intervention. No gender/age differences in results	$p < 0.001$

4.1.2. Summary

Moderate intensity aerobic exercise (40%–60% heart rate reserve) should be promoted for NSCLBP rehabilitation. Aerobic fitness, behavioural treatment and multi-disciplinary treatment programmes are important for reducing CLBP and improving disability [81].

4.2. Muscle Strength and Stabilisation Training

A reduction in core strength can lead to lumbar instability [82], and lumbar instability also reduces the flexibility of the lumbar spine [83]. CLBP patients restrict their trunk movement to reduce the pain in the lumbosacral area, however this only further reduces core strength and increases lumbar instability, resulting in low back pain [84]. Exercises to activate the deep abdominal muscles including the superficial muscles, transversus abdominis muscle and the multifidus are important for CLBP patients [85]. The deep abdominal muscles are essential for supporting the lumbar spine and strengthening these muscles can reduce back pain [86].

A high volume of stress placed on the vertebral column muscles can lead to back pain [87], and poor muscle recruitment of the deep abdominal muscles has been shown in NSCLBP patients [19]. The transversus abdominis is important in muscular stabilisation of the spine which assists in supporting posture [88] and a delayed muscle contraction during movement is often prevalent in patients [89]. Spinal stabilisation exercises aim to increase the strength and endurance of these muscles [90], improving spine stability [91].

Stabilisation exercises have been shown to be effective in reducing NSCLBP [19,21,24], but not acute low back pain [92]. It is important to identify the specific exercises which are most effective for a specific population, as opposed to a generic group [93]. Lumbar stabilisation programmes increase the stability of the spine by training the muscular motor patterns in order to reduce low back pain [94].

Strengthening exercises are considered the most effective treatment for functional gain including walking speed [16]. This is because the deep trunk muscles are active when walking [16], suggesting that strengthening these muscles can help with completing activities of daily living [95].

4.2.1. Muscular Strength and Stabilisation Intervention Programmes

Core stabilisation programmes [19,21,23,24] have been shown to significantly reduce CLBP by 39%–76.8%, and a muscular strength programme significantly reduced CLBP by 61.6% [20].

A 3-month intervention involving 30 NSCLBP patients compared core stabilisation exercises including slow curl ups, bird dog, the plank and sit ups (raising the head and shoulders off the ground with the hands under the head) to conventional spine exercises [19]. The conventional spine exercises included static stretching of muscles found to be tight, however the study does not state which form of assessment was used to identify tight muscles.

Core stabilisation exercises significantly reduced NSCLBP by 76.8% compared to a 62.8% significant reduction following the conventional exercises. These findings suggested both core stabilisation and conventional exercises to be significantly beneficial in reducing CLBP. However the core stabilisation group reported a significantly greater improvement compared to conventional exercises, highlighting the importance of core stability for CLBP patients.

An 8-week core stability intervention programme for 10 NSCLBP patients involved activating core stability responses using unstable standing surfaces and unexpected movements of the upper limbs [21]. CLBP significantly reduced by 39.5%. These results were lower in comparison to the other study [19] which reported a 76.8% significant decrease in CLBP. However this study involved a 3-month intervention [19] compared to the 8-week core stability intervention [21], suggesting the longer a stabilisation intervention programme is, the more positive impact upon CLBP there is.

Another study involved an 8-week stabilisation programme [24] involving 40 NSCLBP patients and investigated the effects of combining ankle dorsiflexion exercises with drawing in the abdominal wall (experimental group), to drawing in the abdominal wall exercises alone (control group). The ankle dorsiflexion exercises were completed at 30% of maximal voluntary isometric contraction of the tibialis anterior muscle, using a resistance band for 10 sets of 20s.

Ankle dorsiflexion exercises were included in the exercise programme because the proprioceptive neuromuscular facilitation irradiation technique, increases core muscular strength by stimulating stronger muscles from the lower body [96], which provides a resistance and stimulus to increase muscle fibres and muscle activity in abdominal muscles [97]. This suggests that to contract the deep target muscle the transversus abdominis, resistance should be applied to the stronger ankle dorsiflexors combined with drawing in the abdominal wall. The transversus abdominis and internal oblique muscles are important for core stability as they are attached to the thoracolumbar fascia, and increase the stiffness of the tissue which improves the core stability [98]. In addition an increase in the stiffness of the tissue in the core, can help to resist the stress placed on the spine and help to reduce back pain [99].

The study reported that the experimental group significantly reduced NSCLBP by 32.5% (according to the VAS), 23.2% (Pain Disability Index) and 21.5% (Pain Rating Scale). The control group significantly reduced CLBP by 16.8% (VAS), 12.4% (Pain Disability Index) and 8% (Pain Rating Scale).

This study [24] also included a follow up measurement after 2 months, in which time patients were instructed to continue the exercises of combining ankle dorsiflexion to drawing in the abdominal wall (experimental group), or only drawing in the abdominal wall (control group). The results identified

CLBP had significantly reduced further to 46.8% (VAS), 39.2% (Pain Disability Index) and 30.7% (Pain Rating Scale) in the experimental group and 38.7% (VAS), 18.8% (Pain Disability Index) and 14.6% (Pain Rating Scale) in the control group. These results provide additional support for the benefits of a longer intervention programme and also for the inclusion of ankle dorsiflexion exercises in rehabilitation of NSCLBP.

Core stability measured by the active straight leg raise was also shown to improve by 56.1% in the experimental group, and 27.4% in the control group after 8 weeks. The results highlighted the importance of core stability in reducing CLBP, especially as core stability had improved by an additional 33.8% at the two month follow up compared to the 8-week measurement in the experimental group, and consequently CLBP had been shown to reduce further. Therefore the results suggested that the addition of ankle dorsiflexion exercises when combined with drawing in the abdominal wall to be an effective exercise in reducing CLBP.

The addition of ankle dorsiflexion exercises to drawing in the abdominal wall is a unique technique for improving core stability for NSCLBP patients, as this technique has only been previously researched in 40 healthy participants [100]. This study [100] reported that the combination of drawing in the abdominal wall and ankle dorsiflexion exercises, resulted in a significantly greater increase in the thickness of the transverse abdominal muscle measured using ultrasonography, compared to drawing in the abdominal wall alone. This is important for improving core strength [101].

The importance of core stability and muscular strength was emphasised by research which had reported that a slumped sitting posture involving lumbar flexion, resulted in a lower activation of the core muscles such as the lumbar multifidus, iliocostalis lumborum pars thoracis and the transverse fibers of internal oblique [102]. Consequently the muscles become weaker which negatively impacts upon the ability to maintain an upright posture [103]. This is because the intervertebral discs are composed of the annulus fibrosus, which connects the spinal vertebrae above and below the disk [104]. The annulus fibrosus requires a highly structured organisation involving aligned collagen fibres within the transverse axis of the spine, which forms an angle-ply laminate structure [105]. However, when the intervertebral disk degenerates the annulus fibrosus becomes unorganised, which can result in low back pain [106]. This is due to mechanical and structural problems such as tears and delamination [107], as the annulus fibrosus distributes force on the intervertebral discs to prevent the gelatinous material in the soft inner core of the intervertebral disc from leaking out [104].

Patients with low back pain adopt a sitting posture with significantly more lumbar flexion than those without low back pain [108,109]. Therefore this suggested a relationship between a poor sitting posture and low back pain, and highlighted the importance of improving core strength and stability [86] to support an upright sitting posture. In contrast no relationship was reported between low back pain and lumbar flexion when sitting in 170 female undergraduate nursing students, with either minor or significant low back pain or without lower back pain [110]. However this study involved only female participants, and males had been shown to be more associated with lumbar flexion when sitting, with an average of 12.2° more flexion than females [103].

A 12-month exercise programme focused on increasing control of the lumbar neutral zone [23] and involved 106 middle aged working men who had a reported episode of non-specific low back pain within the previous 3 months, but did not have severe disability. The participants exercised twice a week undergoing exercises which aimed to improve lumbar stability, such as abdominal curl up with slight rotation and squat exercises. This exercise programme was combined with educating the patients on back pain and providing training on correct techniques for lifting. Low back pain significantly decreased by 39%, suggesting exercises focusing on lumbar stability combined with education to be effective at reducing low back pain. However it was suggested that the participants may have reported a reduced lower back pain as they knew they were involved in the intervention group and therefore expected to experience less back pain [23].

A muscular strength 8-week intervention programme involving 47 women with NSCLBP [20] investigated the effect of different angles of inversion traction on muscular strength and NSCLBP.

The study reported that the inversion −30° group and inversion −60° group was more effective at reducing NSCLBP, and improving core muscular strength than the supine group. NSCLBP significantly reduced by 61.6% in both the inversion −30° group and inversion −60° group, compared to 34.9% in the supine group. In addition extensor back muscle strength was also found to increase by 22.5% (inversion −30° group) and 47% (inversion −60° group), however muscular strength was found to reduce by 6% in the supine group. This suggested that another factor other than muscular strength influenced the decrease in back pain for the supine group.

Trunk extension flexibility was also shown to improve in all three groups. However the biggest increase of 22% was reported in the inversion −60° group compared to an increase of 13.3% in the inversion −30° group, and 4.8% in the supine group. This suggested that a range of factors are responsible for the decrease in NSCLBP, and indicates that a general intervention programme focusing on a range of different areas of fitness is important for NSCLBP rehabilitation.

A 4-week core muscular strength programme (control group) was compared to a core stability programme in addition to core muscular strength exercises (experimental group), in 160 patients with NSCLBP [22]. NSCLBP significantly reduced in the experimental group by 35% compared to 14% in the control group. The results suggested that an intervention programme for NSCLBP which incorporates both core stability and core muscular strength exercises, is more effective at reducing NSCLBP than muscular strength exercises alone.

Four variables exist which may determine the success of a stabilisation exercise programme for CLBP [94]. The four variables include age as participants under the age of 40 have been shown to have higher odds by 3.7 of the stabilisation treatment being a success, an active straight leg raise test higher than 91°, the presence of aberrant movement during lumbar range of motion and a positive prone instability test. Three or more of the four named variables being present is a predictor for the stabilisation exercise programme being successful in reducing CLBP. Therefore it is important to consider the four variables when designing an intervention programme involving stabilisation exercises for CLBP.

Finally, a 15-item questionnaire on clinical instability has been identified [111], which revealed whether patients with NSCLBP respond better to motor control exercises to increase the activation of muscles, including the transversus abdominis, multifidus, and pelvic-floor muscles, or graded activity involving submaximal exercises to increase exercise tolerance. This suggests the questionnaire can help to identify the most effective form of rehabilitation for NSCLBP patients. See Table 2 for a summary of each of the discussed muscular strength and stabilisation intervention programmes.

Table 2. Muscular strength and stabilisation intervention programmes for NSCLBP patients.

Reference Number	Type of Population	Length of Intervention	Effect on Back Pain	Significance Levels
(Inani & Selkar, 2013) [19]	30 NSCLBP patients (20 male, 10 female) aged 20–50 years	3-month intervention. Experimental group: Completed core stabilization exercises including slow curl ups, bird dog, the plank and sit ups (raising head and shoulders off the ground with hands under the head). Control group: Completed conventional spine exercises including static stretching of muscles found to be tight	Visual Analogue Scale. Experimental group: 76.8% significant reduction post intervention. Control group: 62.8% significant reduction post intervention. No gender/age differences in results	$p < 0.001$
(Sarabon, 2011) [21]	10 NSCLBP patients (3 male, 7 female)	8-week core stability intervention programme involving activating core stability responses using unstable standing surfaces and unexpected movements of the upper limbs	Visual Analogue Scale. 39.5% significant reduction post intervention. No gender/age differences in results	$p < 0.01$
(Suni et al., 2006) [23]	106 middle aged working men who had a reported episode of non-specific low back pain within the previous 3 months, but did not have severe disability	12-month programme in which participants exercised twice a week undergoing exercises to improve lumbar stability e.g. abdominal curl up with slight rotation and squat exercises. This exercise programme was combined with educating the patients on back pain and providing training on correct techniques for lifting.	Visual Analogue Scale. Significant 39% reduction	$p < 0.01$
(You et al., 2014) [24]	40 NSCLBP patients (19 male, 21 female)	8-week stabilisation programme and follow up measurement after 2 months. Patients continued exercises throughout 2-month follow up period. Experimental group: Combined ankle dorsiflexion exercises (completed at 30% of maximal voluntary isometric contraction using resistance band for 10 sets of 20 s) with drawing in the abdominal wall. Control group: Drawing in the abdominal wall exercises alone	Experimental group, post intervention: Significant reduction of 32.5% (VAS), 23.2% (Pain Disability Index) and 21.5% (Pain Rating Scale). Control group, post intervention: Significant reduction of 16.8% (VAS), 12.4% (Pain Disability Index) and 8% (Pain Rating Scale). Experimental group, follow up measurement: Significant reduction of 46.8% (VAS), 39.2% (Pain Disability Index) and 30.7% (Pain Rating Scale) compared to pre intervention. Control Group, follow up measurement: Significant reduction of 38.7% (VAS), 18.8% (Pain Disability Index) and 14.6% (Pain Rating Scale) compared to pre intervention. No gender/age differences in results	$p < 0.001$
(Kim et al., 2013) [20]	47 women with NSCLBP	Muscular strength 8-week intervention programme which investigated different angles of inversion traction on NSCLBP. Patients randomly allocated into 3 groups: supine, inversion −30° and inversion −60°. Each group completed a 3 min x 3 set inversion traction protocol at 0°, inverted −30° or inverted −60° for 4 days a week during 8 weeks	Visual Analogue Scale. Significant reduction of 61.6% in both inversion −30° and inversion −60° groups. Significant reduction of 34.9% in the supine group	$p < 0.009$
(Stankovic et al., 2012) [22]	160 NSCLBP patients (63 male, 97 female) 18–75 years	4-week core muscular strength programme (control group) was compared to a core stability programme in addition to core muscular strength exercises (experimental group)	Experimental group: Significantly reduced by 35% post intervention. Control group: Significantly reduced by 14% post intervention. No gender/age differences in results	$p < 0.001$

4.2.2. Summary

Increasing the strength of deep abdominal muscles and improving the stabilisation of the spine is effective at reducing NSCLBP. A core stabilisation programme combined with muscular strength should be considered for NSCLBP patients, as this was shown to be more effective than core muscular strength exercises alone [22]. This suggested a more general programme as opposed to focusing on one particular area of fitness to be more effective at reducing NSCLBP.

4.3. Flexibility Training

Stretching the soft tissues in the back, legs and buttock such as the hamstrings, erector muscles of the spine and hip flexor muscles, ligaments and tendons can help to mobilise the spine, and an increase in the range of motion of the spine can assist back pain [112]. This is because stretching can improve the flexibility of the muscle-tendons and ligaments in the back, which is important to increase the range of motion of the joints [113].Therefore an improved range of motion assists with patients' movement and ability to complete activities of daily living, as most everyday tasks such as lifting and bending require trunk flexion, which involves a complex movement combining lumbar and hip motion [114]. Also stretching exercises decrease the muscle stiffness as a result of changes in viscoelastic properties, due to the decreased actin-myosin cross-bridges and the reflex muscle inhibition [113].

According to the pelvic cross syndrome theory, muscle abnormalities in the postural muscles such as a decreased flexibility and shortening of the hip flexor and back extensor muscles, can result in additional mechanical stress to the joints and soft tissue of the lumbar spine, and can cause lumbar lordosis [87]. Lumbar lordosis is an excessive inward curving of the lumbar spine [115], as a weakening of the abdominal muscles can tilt the pelvis posteriorly, and can result in CLBP [116,117]. In addition the pelvic cross syndrome theory states that hamstring muscle shortening is also important in controlling lumbar lordosis [87]. Hamstring muscle shortening reduces the hip flexion range of motion due to being attached to the posterior leg and the ischial tuberosity, which can affect the lumbopelvic movement during forward bending and can cause low back pain [114].

Flexibility exercises are often used in exercise rehabilitation programmes as they have been shown to be effective at reducing the pain associated with CLBP [25,27]. However CLBP patients must be careful not to perform exercises that result in pain, especially when stretching the flexors and extensors of the trunk and hips [50].

4.3.1. Flexibility Programmes

A 4-week intervention programme involving 40 female NSCLBP patients between 45 and 65 years [27] included 10 exercises for the lumbo-pelvic spine to improve the lumbar flexibility and stability. The exercises were completed in positions which were non-weight bearing such as in a supine position, side lying and prone and were completed twice a week with 10 repetitions of each exercise.

The study reported a 54% significant increase for lumbar flexion and 98% for lumbar extension. Back pain also significantly improved by 58%. The results suggested that completing exercises to improve lumbar flexion and extension is important in reducing NSCLBP in women. This is because during the baseline measurements lumbar flexion was found to be correlated with back pain ($r = -0.581$). However these results cannot be generalised to men.

Lumbar extension exercises can reduce tension in the posterior annular fibers, and alter intradiscal pressure which allows anterior migration of the nucleus pulposus [115] which is important for the vertebral disc to withstand compression [118]. In addition lumbar flexion exercises stretch the hip flexors and lumbar extensors, and decrease the compressive forces on the posterior disc [115].

A further study researched the effect of a 6-week Pilates programme on hamstring and lower back flexibility and CLBP [25]. The study involved 34 NSCLBP patients aged 18–60 years, and were randomly assigned to either the Pilates group or the control group. The Pilates exercises were completed during a one hour class each week taught by a certified Pilates Institute Instructor, and two 30 min sessions each week at home without any supervision. The control group did not participate in the Pilates exercises and continued with their normal PA levels.

The study identified that flexibility significantly increased by 52.9% in the Pilates group, compared to a 7.8% increase in the control group which was not significantly different. Back pain also significantly decreased by 18.5% in the Pilates group, and there was no change in the back pain for the patients in the control group. The results suggested that Pilates exercises can significantly improve back pain and hamstring and lower back flexibility for NSCLBP patients.

The relationship between low back pain, lumbar flexion and hamstring flexibility was researched in a study involving 26 male University rowers who participated in rowing training six times a week [119]. Participants were assigned into groups according to whether they were currently suffering from low back pain (acute, sub-acute or chronic), had suffered from low back pain at some point in their lives or had never suffered from low back pain.

The study reported that the participants with current low back pain (11 participants) had a significantly reduced lumbar flexion compared to the participants without current low back pain (15 participants). However no significant difference was identified in hamstring flexibility between the two groups. In addition no significant difference was identified in lumbar flexion or hamstring flexibility between the participants who had experienced low back pain at some point in their lives (21 participants), or had not experienced low back pain (5 participants).

The results suggested that hamstring flexibility was not associated with low back pain occurrence, and therefore improving hamstring flexibility is not important for preventing low back pain or for an intervention programme for a patient with low back pain. Although, the results did highlight the importance of improving lumbar flexion for patients with current low back pain, and also suggested that a reduced lumbar flexion is an important factor for an occurrence of low back pain.

However the study [119] did not specifically focus on CLBP patients as the participants reported any experiences of low back pain, current or previous, and therefore could have included a range of acute, sub-acute or CLBP. In addition, the results from the study were in contrast to findings previously discussed [25], which suggested that improving hamstring flexibility is important for reducing NSCLBP.

A 3-month intervention programme for 86 NSCLBP patients [26] investigated the effects of progressive therapeutic exercise on spinal and muscle flexibility and back pain by dividing the patients into three groups: intensive training group, home exercise group and the control group. Follow up measurements at 6 and 12 months after baseline tests was also conducted. The intensive training group and home exercise group completed seven exercises for various parts of the body using either gym equipment, such as pulleys and bar bells (intensive training group) or without the use of extra equipment (home exercise group). The control group maintained their normal PA levels throughout the duration of the study and did not participate in an organised exercise programme. However no information was provided on which exercises were completed.

Back pain significantly decreased post intervention by 44% in the intensive training group, 32% in the home exercise group and 39% in the control group. The 6-month follow up identified that back pain had decreased further in the home exercise group to a 47% reduction which was significantly different to baseline. The intensive training group which increased compared to post intervention to a 32% reduction compared to baseline, although this was still significantly different. The control group also increased compared to post intervention to 28% and was not significantly different to baseline.

The flexibility of the hamstrings significantly increased at post intervention from 87°–90° in the intensive training group and 83°–87° in the home exercise group. However at the 12-month follow up hamstring flexibility had reduced to 83° in the intensive training group and 82° in the home exercise group. This suggests the importance of maintaining exercise which is aimed at improving flexibility, as both exercise groups lost the improved degree of hamstring flexibility. Although there was no correlation between back pain and flexibility which suggested the importance of other factors on back pain, such as an increase in core strength and aerobic fitness [16,19,23]. However the study [26] did not measure core strength or aerobic fitness. In addition the study [26] suggested improving flexibility could be important for preventing CLBP from occurring, as opposed to using exercises to improve flexibility as a rehabilitation from CLBP. See Table 3 for a summary of each of the discussed flexibility intervention programmes.

Table 3. Flexibility intervention programmes for NSCLBP patients.

Reference Number	Type of Population	Length of Intervention	Effect on Back Pain	Significance Levels
(Masharawi & Nadaf, 2013) [27]	40 female NSCLBP patients between 45 and 65 years	Study group: Activities of daily living guidance and a 45 min group exercise session aimed at improving lumbar flexibility and stability. Exercise session was completed twice a week for 4 weeks with 10 repetitions of each exercise. Control group: Activities of daily living guidance only	Visual Analogue Scale. Study group: 58% significant improvement following intervention. Control group: no significant change	$p < 0.001$
(Gladwell *et al.*, 2006) [25]	34 NSCLBP patients aged 18–60 years	Pilates group: Completed Pilates exercises during a one hour class each week for 6 weeks, and two 30 min sessions each week at home without any supervision. Control group: Did not participate in the Pilates exercises and continued with their normal PA levels	Visual Analog Scale. Pilates group: 18.5% significant decrease following intervention. Control group: No significant difference. No gender/age differences in results	$p < 0.05$
(Kuukkanen & Malkia, 2006) [26]	86 NSCLBP patients	Intensive training group and home exercise group completed 3-month intervention programme: 7 exercises for various parts of the body using either gym equipment, such as pulleys and bar bells (intensive training group) or without the use of extra equipment (home exercise group). Control group: Maintained their normal PA levels and did not participate in an organised exercise programme	Intensive training: 44% significant reduction post intervention. Control: 39% significant reduction post intervention. Home exercise: 32% significant reduction post intervention. No gender/age differences in results	$p < 0.05$

4.3.2. Summary

Improving the flexibility of the lumbar spine and hamstrings can significantly reduce CLBP by 18.5%–58% [25,27]. This suggests the importance of including flexibility exercises in an intervention programme for CLBP patients. However no association between hamstring flexibility and low back pain was identified in male University rowers [119].

An improvement in lumbar flexibility can increase the range of motion of the spine, which can help to reduce back pain and assist with movement [112]. Hamstring muscle shortening reduces the hip flexion range of motion which impacts upon the lumbopelvic movement [114], and a decrease in the flexibility of the hip flexor and back extensor muscles can lead to lumbar lordosis, which can result in low back pain [87]. Therefore including lumbar flexion exercises in an intervention programme for CLBP is important, as lumbar flexion exercises stretch the hip flexors and lumbar extensors [115].

5. Conclusions

Exercise intervention programmes involving either muscular strength, flexibility or aerobic fitness is beneficial for NSCLBP but not acute low back pain. Non-specific acute low back pain patients recover in 4–6 weeks with or without a treatment [5], and exercising should be avoided to reduce the swelling of the affected area [39].

NSCLBP is multi factorial in nature [110,120], and no single exercise programme is optimal for all NSCLBP patients [50]. In addition, the most appropriate specific intervention for a NSCLBP patient is often unclear [12], and NSCLBP pain should not been considered as a homogenous condition meaning all cases are identical [121]. This suggests that a specific intervention programme focusing on one area of fitness for a group of NSCLBP patients may not be appropriate. This is a limitation of this review as the NSCLBP patients in the included studies may have responded differently to the exercise interventions. Consequently, a general exercise programme which combines muscular strength, flexibility and aerobic fitness would be beneficial for rehabilitation of NSCLBP. Further research is needed into the benefits of a combined exercise intervention programme involving muscular strength, flexibility and aerobic fitness for NSCLBP patients, as the literature has supported the use of each of these fitness areas individually, but more research should be conducted combining all three.

Acknowledgments: Research funded by the University of St Mark & St John.

Author Contributions: Both authors helped to plan the review. The first author conducted the search for intervention programmes, read and reviewed the articles and completed the manuscript. The second author also read and provided improvements to the manuscript. Both authors approved the final manuscript.

Conflicts of Interest: The authors declare no conflict of interest.

References

1. Ricci, J.A.; Stewart, W.F.; Chee, E.; Leotta, C.; Foley, K.; Hochberg, M.C. Back pain exacerbations and lost productive time costs in United States workers. *Spine* **2006**, *31*, 3052–3060. [CrossRef] [PubMed]
2. Van Tulder, M.; Malmivaara, A.; Esmail, R.; Koes, B. Exercise therapy for low back pain: A systematic review within the framework of the cochrane collaboration back review group. *Spine* **2000**, *25*, 2784–2796. [CrossRef] [PubMed]
3. Chen, S.M.; Alexander, R.; Lo, S.K.; Cook, J. Effects of Functional Fascial Taping on pain and function in patients with non-specific low back pain: A pilot randomized controlled trial. *Clin. Rehabil.* **2012**, *26*, 924–933. [CrossRef] [PubMed]
4. Ebadi, S.; Ansari, N.N.; Naghdi, S.; Fallah, E.; Barzi, D.M.; Jalaei, S. A study of therapeutic ultrasound and exercise treatment for muscle fatigue in patients with chronic non specific low back pain: A preliminary report. *J. Back Musculoskelet. Rehabil.* **2013**, *26*, 221–226. [PubMed]
5. Hancock, M.J.; Maher, C.G.; Latimer, J. Spinal manipulative therapy for acute low back pain: A clinical perspective. *J. Man. Manip. Ther.* **2008**, *16*, 198–203. [CrossRef] [PubMed]
6. Kolber, M.J.; Beekhuizen, K. Lumbar stabilization: An evidence-based approach for the athlete with low back pain. *Strength Cond. J.* **2007**, *29*, 26–37. [CrossRef]
7. Lara-Palomo, I.C.; Aguilar-Ferrándiz, M.E.; Matarán-Peñarrocha, G.A.; Saavedra-Hernández, M.; Granero-Molina, J.; Fernández-Sola, C. Short-term effects of interferential current electro-massage in adults with chronic non-specific low back pain: A randomized controlled trial. *Clin. Rehabil.* **2013**, *27*, 439–450. [CrossRef] [PubMed]
8. Waddell, G.; Burton, A.K. Occupational health guidelines for the management of low back pain at work: Evidence review. *Occup. Med.* **2001**, *51*, 124–135. [CrossRef]
9. Thomas, K.J.; MacPherson, H.; Thorpe, L.; Brazier, J.; Fitter, M.; Campbell, M.J. Randomised controlled trial of a short course of traditional acupuncture compared with usual care for persistent non-specific low back pain. *Br. Med. J.* **2006**, *333*, 623–626. [CrossRef] [PubMed]
10. National Health Service (NHS). Backcare Awareness Week. Available online: http://www.nhscareers. nhs.uk/features/2012/october/ (accessed on 16 October 2014).
11. Wynne-Jones, G.; Cowen, J.; Jordan, J.; Uthman, O.; Main, C.J.; Glozier, N.; van der Windt, D. Absence from work and return to work in people with back pain: A systematic review and meta-analysis. *Occup. Environ. Med.* **2014**, *71*, 448–456. [CrossRef] [PubMed]
12. Mayer, J.; Mooney, V.; Dagenais, S. Evidence-informed management of chronic low back pain with lumbar extensor strengthening exercises. *Spine* **2008**, *8*, 96–113. [CrossRef] [PubMed]
13. Bekkering, G.E.; Hendriks, H.J.; Koes, B.W.; Oostendorp, R.A.; Ostelo, R.W.; Thomassen, J.M.; van Tulder, M.W. Dutch physiotherapy guidelines for low back pain. *Physiotherapy* **2003**, *89*, 82–96. [CrossRef]
14. National Health Service (NHS). Back Pain. Available online: http://www.nhs.uk/Conditions/Back-pain/ Pages/Introduction.aspx (accessed on 16 October 2014).
15. Chan, C.W.; Mok, N.W.; Yeung, E.W. Aerobic exercise training in addition to conventional physiotherapy for chronic low back pain: A randomized controlled trial. *Arch. Phys. Med. Rehabil.* **2011**, *92*, 1681–1685. [CrossRef] [PubMed]

16. Shnayderman, I.; Katz-Leurer, M. An aerobic walking programme *versus* muscle strengthening Programme for chronic low back pain: A randomized controlled trial. *Clin. Rehabil.* **2013**, *27*, 207–214. [CrossRef] [PubMed]

17. Chatzitheodorou, D.; Kabitsis, C.; Malliou, P.; Mougios, V. A pilot study of the effects of high-intensity aerobic exercise *versus* passive interventions on pain, disability, psychological strain, and serum cortisol concentrations in people with chronic low back pain. *Phys. Ther.* **2007**, *87*, 304–312. [CrossRef] [PubMed]

18. Chatzitheodorou, D.; Mavromoustakos, S.; Milioti, S. The effect of exercise on adrenocortical responsiveness of patients with chronic low back pain, controlled for psychological strain. *Clin. Rehabil.* **2008**, *22*, 319–328. [CrossRef] [PubMed]

19. Inani, S.B.; Selkar, S.P. Effect of core stabilization exercises *versus* conventional exercises on pain and functional status in patients with non-specific low back pain: A randomized clinical trial. *J. Back Musculoskelet. Rehabil.* **2013**, *26*, 37–43. [PubMed]

20. Kim, J.D.; Oh, H.W.; Lee, J.H.; Cha, J.Y.; Ko, I.G.; Jee, Y.S. The effect of inversion traction on pain sensation, lumbar flexibility and trunk muscles strength in patients with chronic low back pain. *Isokinet. Exerc. Sci.* **2013**, *21*, 237–246.

21. Šarabon, N. Effects of trunk functional stability training in subjects suffering from chronic low back pain: A pilot study. *Kinesiol. Slov.* **2011**, *17*, 25–37.

22. Stankovic, A.; Lazovic, M.; Kocic, M.; Dimitrijevic, L.; Stankovic, I.; Zlatavovic, D. Lumbar stabilization exercises in addition to strengthening and stretching exercises reduce pain and increase function in patients with chronic low back pain: Randomized clinical open-label study. *Turk. J. Phys. Med. Rehabil.* **2012**, *58*, 177–183. [CrossRef]

23. Suni, J.; Rinne, M.; Natri, A.; Statistisian, M.P.; Parkkari, J.; Alaranta, H. Control of the lumbar neutral zone decreases low back pain and improves self-evaluated work ability: A 12-month randomized controlled study. *Spine* **2006**, *31*, 611–620. [CrossRef] [PubMed]

24. You, J.H.; Kim, S.Y.; Oh, D.W.; Chon, S.C. The effect of a novel core stabilization technique on managing patients with chronic low back pain: A randomized, controlled, experimenter-blinded study. *Clin. Rehabil.* **2014**, *28*, 460–469. [CrossRef] [PubMed]

25. Gladwell, V.; Head, S.; Haggar, M.; Beneke, R. Does a program of pilates improve chronic non-specific low Back pain? *J. Sport Rehabil.* **2006**, *15*, 338–350.

26. Kuukkanen, T.; Malkia, E. Effects of a three-month therapeutic exercise programme on flexibility in subjects with low back pain. *Physiother. Res. Int.* **2000**, *5*, 46–61. [CrossRef] [PubMed]

27. Masharawi, Y.; Nadaf, N. The effect of non-weight bearing group-exercising on females with non-specific chronic low back pain: A randomized single blind controlled pilot study. *J. Back Musculoskelet. Rehabil.* **2013**, *26*, 353–359. [PubMed]

28. Hayden, J.A.; van Tulder, M.; Tomlinson, G. Systematic review: Strategies for using exercise therapy to improve outcomes in chronic low back pain. *Ann. Intern. Med.* **2005**, *142*, 776–785. [CrossRef] [PubMed]

29. Smith, J.A.; Osborn, M. Pain as an assault on the self: An interpretative phenomenological analysis of the psychological impact of chronic benign low back pain. *Psychol. Health* **2007**, *22*, 517–534. [CrossRef]

30. Smeets, R.; Severens, J.L.; Beelen, S.; Vlaeyen, J.W.; Knottnerus, J.A. More is not always better: Cost-effectiveness analysis of combined, single behavioral and single physical rehabilitation programs for chronic low back pain. *Eur. J. Pain* **2009**, *13*, 71–81. [CrossRef] [PubMed]

31. Smith, D.; Bissell, G.; Bruce-Low, S.; Wakefield, C. The effect of lumbar extension training with and without pelvic stabilization on lumbar strength and low back pain. *J. Back Musculoskelet. Rehabil.* **2011**, *24*, 241–249. [PubMed]

32. Wai, E.K.; Rodriguez, S.; Dagenais, S.; Hall, H. Evidence informed management of chronic low back pain with physical activity, smoking cessation, and weight loss. *Spine J.* **2008**, *8*, 195–202. [CrossRef] [PubMed]

33. McCarthy, C.J.; Roberts, C.; Gittins, M.; Oldham, J.A. A process of subgroup identification in non-specific low back pain using a standard clinical examination and cluster analysis. *Physiother. Res. Int.* **2012**, *17*, 92–100. [CrossRef] [PubMed]

34. Bupa. Back Pain. Available online: http://www.bupa.co.uk/individuals/health-information/directory/b/backpain#textBlock190676 (accessed on 16 October 2014).

35. McGill, S. Designing Back Exercise: From Rehabilitation to Enhancing Performance. Available online: http://www.backfitpro.com/articles.php (accessed on 11 October 2014).

36. Del Pozo-Cruz, B.; Gusi, N.; Del Pozo-Cruz, J.; Adsuar, J.C.; Hernandez-Mocholí, M.; Parraca, J.A. Clinical effects of a nine-month web-based intervention in subacute non-specific low back pain patients: A randomized controlled trial. *Clin. Rehabil.* **2013**, *27*, 28–39. [CrossRef] [PubMed]

37. Tsauo, J.Y.; Chen, W.H.; Liang, H.W.; Jang, Y. The effectiveness of a functional training programme for patients with chronic low back pain—A pilot study. *Disabil. Rehabil.* **2009**, *31*, 1100–1106. [CrossRef] [PubMed]

38. Wells, C.; Kolt, G.S.; Marshall, P.; Bialocerkowski, A. The definition and application of pilates exercise to treat people with chronic low back pain: A delphi survey of australian physical therapists. *Phys. Ther.* **2014**, *94*, 792–805. [CrossRef] [PubMed]

39. Goertz, M.; Thorson, D.; Bonsell, J.; Bonte, B.; Campbell, R.; Haake, B. *Adult Acute and Subacute Low Back Pain*; Institute for Clinical Systems Improvement: Bloomington, MN, USA, 2012; pp. 1–91.

40. Van Tulder, M.; Becker, A.; Bekkering, T.; Breen, A.; del Real, M.; Hutchinson, A.; Koes, B.; Laerum, E.; Malmivaara, A. Chapter 3 European guidelines for the management of acute nonspecific low back pain in primary care. *Eur. Spine J.* **2006**, *15*, 169–191. [CrossRef] [PubMed]

41. Reme, S.; Shaw, W.; Steenstra, I.; Woiszwillo, M.; Pransky, G.; Linton, S. Distressed, immobilized, or lacking employer support? A sub-classification of acute work-related low back pain. *J. Occup. Rehabil.* **2012**, *22*, 541–552. [CrossRef] [PubMed]

42. Chou, R.; Qaseem, A.; Snow, V.; Casey, D.; Cross, T.; Shekelle, P. Diagnosis and treatment of low back pain: A joint clinical practice guideline from the American College of Physicians and the American Pain Society. *Ann. Intern. Med.* **2007**, *147*, 478–491. [CrossRef] [PubMed]

43. Toye, F.; Barker, K. 'I can't see any reason for stopping doing anything, but I might have to do it differently'—Restoring hope to patients with persistent non-specific low back pain—A qualitative study. *Disabil. Rehabil.* **2012**, *34*, 894–903. [CrossRef] [PubMed]

44. Savigny, P.; Watson, P.; Underwood, M. Early management of persistent non-specific low back pain: Summary of NICE guidance. *Br. Med. J.* **2009**. [CrossRef] [PubMed]

45. Ehrlich, G.E. Low back pain. *Bull. World Health Organ.* **2003**, *81*, 671–676. [PubMed]

46. Nonspecific Lower Back Pain in Adults. Available online: http://www.patient.co.uk/health/nonspecific-lower-back-pain-in-adults (accessed on 16 October 2014).

47. Josephson, I.; Hedberg, B.; Bülow, P. Problem-solving in physiotherapy—Physiotherapists' talk about encounters with patients with non-specific low back pain. *Disabil. Rehabil.* **2013**, *35*, 668–677. [CrossRef] [PubMed]

48. Benjamin, C. Low Back Pain—Acute. Available online: http://www.nlm.nih.gov/medlineplus/ency/article/007425.htm (accessed on 2 December 2014).

49. Koes, B.W.; van Tulder, M.W.; Thomas, S. Diagnosis and treatment of low back pain. *Br. Med. J.* **2006**, *332*, 1430–1434. [CrossRef] [PubMed]

50. Henchoz, Y.; Kai-Lik, S.A. Exercise and nonspecific low back pain: A literature review. *Joint Bone Spine* **2008**, *75*, 533–539. [CrossRef] [PubMed]

51. Winter, E.M.; Fowler, N. Exercise defined and quantified according to the Systeme International d'Unites. *J. Sports Sci.* **2009**, *27*, 447–460. [CrossRef] [PubMed]

52. World Health Organisation. Physical Activity. Available online: http://www.who.int/topics/physical_activity/en/ (accessed on 2 December 2014).

53. Robb, B. Exercise and Physical Activity: What's the Difference? 2009. Available online: http://www.everydayhealth.com/fitness/basics/difference-between-exercise-and-physical-activity.aspx (accessed on 18 November 2014).

54. Hayden, J.A.; van Tulder, M.W.; Malmivaara, A.; Koes, B.W. Exercise therapy for treatment of non-specific low back pain. *Cochrane Database Syst. Rev.* **2005**, *20*, 1–66.

55. Ullrich, P.F. Low Impact Aerobic Exercise. Available online: http://www.spine-health.com/wellness/exercise/low-impact-aerobic-exercise (accessed on 15 November 2014).

56. Kenny, W.L.; Wilmore, J.H.; Costill, D.L. *Physiology of Sport and Exercise*, 5th ed.; Human Kinetics: Champaign, IL, USA, 2012.

57. Stoppler, M.C.; Shiel, W.C. Endorphins: Natural Pain and Stress Fighters. 2014. Available online: http://www.medicinenet.com/script/main/art.asp?articlekey=55001 (accessed on 5 December 2014).

58. Spine-Health. Endorphins Definition. Available online: http://www.spine-health.com/glossary/endorphins (accessed on 5 December 2014).
59. Mayo, T.P.; Weissman, L. The noninvasive path to chronic back pain management. *Rehab Manag. Interdiscip. J. Rehabil.* **2011**, *24*, 18–20.
60. Duque, I.L.; Parra, J.H.; Duvallet, A. Aerobic fitness and limiting factors of maximal performance in chronic low back pain patients. *J. Back Musculoskelet. Rehabil.* **2009**, *22*, 113–119. [PubMed]
61. Lin, C.W.; McAuley, J.H.; Macedo, L.; Barnett, D.C.; Smeets, R.J.; Verbunt, J.A. Relationship between physical activity and disability in low back pain: A systematic review and meta-analysis. *Pain* **2011**, *152*, 607–613. [CrossRef] [PubMed]
62. Smeets, R.; Wittink, H.; Hidding, A.; Knottnerus, J.A. Do patients with chronic low back pain have a lower level of aerobic fitness than healthy controls? Are pain, disability, fear of injury, working status, or level of leisure time activity associated with the difference in aerobic fitness level? *Spine* **2006**, *31*, 90–97. [CrossRef] [PubMed]
63. Hoffman, M.D.; Shepanski, M.A.; Mackenzie, S.P.; Clifford, P.S. Experimentally induced pain perception is acutely reduced by aerobic exercise in people with chronic low back pain. *J. Rehabil. Res. Dev.* **2005**, *42*, 175–181. [CrossRef]
64. Jacob, T.; Baras, M.; Zeev, A.; Epstein, L. Physical activities and low back pain: a community-based study. *Med. Sci. Sports Exerc.* **2004**, *36*, 9–15. [CrossRef] [PubMed]
65. Koho, P.; Orenius, T.; Kautiainen, H.; Haanp, M.; Pohjolainen, T.; Hurri, H. Association of fear of movement and leisure-time physical activity among patients with chronic pain. *J. Rehabil. Med.* **2011**, *43*, 794–799. [CrossRef] [PubMed]
66. Swinkels-Meewisse, I.E.; Roelofs, J.; Oostendorp, R.A.; Verbeek, A.L.; Vlaeyen, J.W. Acute Low Back Pain: Pain-Related Fear and Pain Catastrophizing Influence Physical Performance and Perceived Disability. *Pain* **2006**, *120*, 36–43. [CrossRef] [PubMed]
67. Preuper, H.S.; Reneman, M.F.; Boonstra, A.M.; Dijkstra, P.U.; Versteegen, G.J.; Geertzen, J.H. Relationship between psychological factors and performance-based and self-reported disability in chronic low back pain. *Eur. Spine J.* **2008**, *17*, 1448–1456. [CrossRef] [PubMed]
68. McArthur, D.; Dumas, A.; Woodend, K.; Beach, S.; Stacey, D. Factors influencing adherence to regular exercise in middle-aged women: A qualitative study to inform clinical practice. *BMC* **2014**. [CrossRef] [PubMed]
69. Hanumanthu, V. *Assessment of an Exercise Program on Population with Chronic Medical Conditions*; ProQuest LLC: Ann Arbor, MI, USA, 2008.
70. Balint, T.; Dobrescu, T.; Rata, M.; Cristuta, A. Research regarding the assessment of a body's normal size by using the body mass index. *Gymn. J. Phys. Educ. Sports* **2010**, *11*, 14–17.
71. National Health Service (NHS). What's your BMI? Available online: http://www.nhs.uk/livewell/loseweight/pages/bodymassindex.aspx (accessed on 5 December 2014).
72. Frisco, D.J. Weight Loss for Back Pain Relief. Available online: http://www.spine-health.com/wellness/nutrition-diet-weight-loss/weight-loss-back-pain-relief (accessed on 1 December 2014).
73. Hurley, D.; O'Donoghue, G.; Tully, M.; Klaber Moffett, J.; van Mechelen, W.; Daly, L. A walking programme and a supervised exercise class *versus* usual physiotherapy for chronic low back pain: A single-blinded randomised controlled trial. *BMC Musculoskelet. Disord.* **2009**. [CrossRef] [PubMed]
74. National Institute of Arthritis and Musculoskeletal and Skin Diseases (NIAMS). Handout on Health: Back Pain. Available online: http://www.niams.nih.gov/Health_Info/Back_Pain/ (accessed on 8 December 2014).
75. Hill, E.E.; Zack, E.; Battaglini, C.; Viru, M.; Viru, A.; Hackney, A.C. Exercise and circulating cortisol levels: The intensity threshold effect. *J. Endocrinol. Investig.* **2008**, *31*, 587–591. [CrossRef] [PubMed]
76. Muhtz, C.; Rodriguez-Raecke, R.; Hinkelmann, K.; Moeller-Bertram, T.; Kiefer, F.; Wiedemann, K. Cortisol response to experimental pain in patients with chronic low back pain and patients with major depression. *Pain Med.* **2013**, *14*, 498–503. [CrossRef] [PubMed]
77. Nagarajan, M.; Nair, M.R. Importance of fear-avoidance behavior in chronic non-specific low back pain. *J. Back Musculoskelet. Rehabil.* **2010**, *23*, 87–95. [PubMed]
78. Hanney, W.J.; Kolber, M.J.; Beekhuizen, K.S. Implications for physical activity in the population with low back pain. *Am. J. Lifestyle Med.* **2009**, *3*, 63–70. [CrossRef]

79. Basler, H.D.; Luckmann, J.; Wolf, U.; Quint, S. Fear-avoidance beliefs, physical activity, and disability in elderly individuals with chronic low back pain and healthy controls. *Clin. J. Pain* **2008**, *24*, 604–610. [CrossRef] [PubMed]
80. Lante, K.; Stancliffe, R.J.; Bauman, A.; van der Ploeg, H.P.; Jan, S.; Davis, G.M. Embedding sustainable physical activities into the everyday lives of adults with intellectual disabilities: A randomised controlled trial. *BMC Public Health* **2014**. [CrossRef] [PubMed]
81. Krismer, M.; van Tulder, M. Low back pain (non-specific). *Best Pract. Res. Clin. Rheumatol.* **2007**, *21*, 77–91. [CrossRef] [PubMed]
82. Willson, J.D.; Dougherty, C.P.; Ireland, M.L.; Davis, I.M. Core stability and its relationship to lower extremity function and injury. *J. Am Acad Orthop. Surg.* **2005**, *13*, 316–325. [CrossRef] [PubMed]
83. Cho, H.Y.; Kim, E.H.; Kim, J. Effects of the CORE exercise program on pain and active range of motion in patients with chronic low back pain. *J. Phys. Ther. Sci.* **2014**, *26*, 1237–1240. [CrossRef] [PubMed]
84. Danneels, L.A.; Vanderstraeten, G.G.; Cambier, D.C.; Witvrouw, E.E.; de Cuyper, H.J. CT imaging of trunk muscles in chronic low back pain patients and healthy control subjects. *Eur. Spine J.* **2000**, *9*, 266–272. [CrossRef] [PubMed]
85. Franca, F.R.; Burke, T.N.; Hanada, E.S.; Marques, A.P. Segmental stabilisation and muscular strengthening in chronic low back pain—A comparative study. *Clinics* **2010**, *65*, 1013–1017. [CrossRef] [PubMed]
86. Amit, K.; Manish, G.; Taruna, K. Effect of trunk muscles stabilization exercises and general exercises on pain in recurrent non specific low back ache. *Int. Res. J. Med. Sci.* **2013**, *1*, 23–26.
87. Nourbakhsh, M.R.; Arabloo, A.M.; Salavati, M. The relationship between pelvic cross syndrome and chronic low back pain. *J. Back Musculoskelet. Rehabil.* **2006**, *19*, 119–128.
88. Standaert, C.J.; Weinstein, S.M.; Rumpeltes, J. Evidence-informed management of chronic low back pain with lumbar stabilisation exercises. *Spine J.* **2008**, *8*, 114–120. [CrossRef] [PubMed]
89. Hodges, P.W.; Richardson, C.A. Inefficient muscular stabilization of the lumbar spine associated with low back pain: a motor control evaluation of transversus abdominis. *Spine* **1996**, *21*, 2640–2650. [CrossRef] [PubMed]
90. Arokoski, J.P.; Valta, T.; Airaksinen, O.; Kankaanpää, M. Back and abdominal muscle function during stabilization exercises. *Arch. Phys. Med. Rehabil.* **2001**, *82*, 1089–1098. [CrossRef] [PubMed]
91. Kavcic, N.; Grenier, S.; McGill, S. Determining the stabilizing role of individual torso muscles during rehabilitation exercises. *Spine* **2004**, *29*, 1254–1265. [CrossRef] [PubMed]
92. Ferreira, P.H.; Ferreira, M.L.; Maher, C.G.; Herbert, R.D.; Refshauge, K. Specific stabilisation exercise for spinal and pelvic pain: A systematic review. *Aust. J. Physiother.* **2006**, *52*, 79–88. [CrossRef]
93. Hodges, P. Transversus abdominis: A different view of the elephant. *Br. J. Sports Med.* **2008**, *42*, 941–944. [CrossRef] [PubMed]
94. Hicks, G.E.; Fritz, J.M.; Delitto, A.; McGill, S.M. Preliminary development of a clinical prediction rule for determining which patients with low back pain will respond to a stabilization exercise program. *Arch. Phys. Med. Rehabil.* **2005**, *86*, 1753–1762. [CrossRef] [PubMed]
95. Maeo, S.; Takahashi, T.; Takai, Y.; Kanehisa, H. Trunk muscle activities during abdominal bracing: comparison among muscles and exercises. *J. Sports Sci. Med.* **2013**, *12*, 467–474. [PubMed]
96. Adler, S.; Beckers, D.; Buck, M. *PNF in Practice: An Illustrated Guide*, 3rd ed.; Springer: Berlin, Germany, 2008.
97. Shimura, K.; Kasai, T. Effects of proprioceptive neuromuscular facilitation on the initiation of voluntary movement and motor evoked potentials in upper limb muscles. *Hum. Mov. Sci.* **2002**, *21*, 101–113. [CrossRef]
98. Richardson, C.; Hodges, P.W.; Hides, J. *Therapeutic Exercise for Lumbopelvic Stabilization: A Motor Control Approach for the Treatment and Prevention of Low Back Pain*, 2nd ed.; Churchill Livingstone: Edinburgh, UK, 2004.
99. Stanton, T.; Kawchuk, G. The effect of abdominal stabilization contractions on posteroanterior spinal stiffness. *Spine* **2008**, *33*, 694–701. [CrossRef] [PubMed]
100. Chon, S.C.; Chang, K.Y.; You, J.H. Effect of the abdominal draw-in manoeuvre in combination with ankle dorsiflexion in strengthening the transverse abdominal muscle in healthy young adults: a preliminary, randomised, controlled study. *Physiotherapy* **2010**, *96*, 130–136. [CrossRef] [PubMed]
101. Katsura, Y.; Ueda, S.Y.; Yoshikawa, T.; Usui, T.; Orita, K.; Sakamoto, H.; Sotobayashi, D.; Fujimoto, S. Effects of aquatic exercise training using new water-resistance equipment on trunk muscles, abdominal circumference, and activities of daily living in elderly women. *Int. J. Sport Health Sci.* **2011**, *9*, 113–121. [CrossRef]

102. Dankaerts, W.; O'Sullivan, P.; Burnett, A.; Straker, L. Altered patterns of superficial trunk muscle activation during sitting in nonspecific chronic low back pain patients: importance of subclassification. *Spine* **2006**, *31*, 2017–2023. [CrossRef] [PubMed]

103. O'Sullivan, P.B.; Smith, A.; Beales, D.J.; Straker, L.M. Association of biopsychosocial factors with degree of slump in sitting posture and self-report of back pain in adolescents: A cross-sectional study. *Phys. Ther.* **2011**, *91*, 470–484. [CrossRef] [PubMed]

104. Spine-Health. Annulus Fibrosus Definition. Available online: http://www.spine-health.com/glossary/annulus-fibrosus (accessed on 15 December 2014).

105. Nerurkar, N.L.; Sen, S.; Huang, A.H.; Elliott, D.M.; Mauck, R.L. Engineered disk-like angle-ply structures for intervertebral disk replacement. *Spine* **2012**, *35*, 867–873. [CrossRef] [PubMed]

106. Reitmaier, S.; Shirazi-Adl, A.; Bashkuev, M.; Wilke, H.J.; Gloria, A.; Schmidt, H. *In vitro* and in silico investigations of disc nucleus replacement. *J. R. Soc.* **2012**, *9*, 1869–1879. [CrossRef] [PubMed]

107. Guerin, H.L.; Elliott, D.M. Quantifying the contributions of structure to annulus fibrosus mechanical function using a nonlinear, anisotropic, hyperelastic model. *J. Orthop. Res.* **2007**, *25*, 508–516. [CrossRef] [PubMed]

108. O'Sullivan, P.B.; Mitchell, T.; Bulich, P.; Waller, R.; Holte, J. The relationship between posture and back muscle endurance in industrial workers with flexion-related low back pain. *Man. Ther.* **2006**, *11*, 264–271. [CrossRef] [PubMed]

109. Womersley, L.; May, S. Sitting posture of subjects with postural backache. *J. Manip. Physiol. Ther.* **2006**, *29*, 213–218. [CrossRef] [PubMed]

110. Mitchell, T.; O'Sullivan, P.B.; Burnett, A.F.; Straker, L.; Smith, A. Regional differences in lumbar spinal posture and the influence of low back pain. *BMC Musculoskelet. Disord.* **2008**. [CrossRef] [PubMed]

111. Gazzi, M.L.; Maher, C.G.; Hancock, M.J.; Kamper, S.J.; McAuley, J.H.; Stanton, T.R. Predicting response to motor control exercises and graded activity for patients with low back pain: preplanned secondary analysis of a randomized controlled trial. *Phys. Ther.* **2014**, *94*, 1543–1554.

112. Ullrich, P.F. Stretching for Back Pain Relief. Available online: http://www.spine-health.com/wellness/exercise/stretching-back-pain-relief (accessed on 17 December 2014).

113. MacAuley, D.; Best, T. *Evidence-Based Sports Medicine*, 2nd ed.; Blackwell Publishing: Oxford, UK, 2007.

114. Li, Y.; McClure, P.W.; Pratt, N. The effect of hamstring muscle stretching on standing posture and on lumbar and hip motions during forward bending. *Phys. Ther.* **1996**, *76*, 836–845. [PubMed]

115. DeLisa, J.A.; Gans, B.M.; Walsh, N.E. *Physical Medicine and Rehabilitation: Principles and Practice*, 4th ed.; Lippincott Williams and Wilkins: Philadelphia, PA, USA, 2005.

116. Youdas, J.W. Lumbar lordosis and pelvic inclination in adults with chronic low back pain. *Phys. Ther.* **2000**, *80*, 261–275. [PubMed]

117. Kim, H.; Chung, S.; Kim, S.; Shin, H.; Lee, J.; Kim, S. Influences of trunk muscles on lumbar lordosis and sacral angle. *Eur. Spine J.* **2006**, *15*, 409–414. [CrossRef] [PubMed]

118. Spine-Health. Nucleus Pulposus Definition. Available online: http://www.spine-health.com/glossary/nucleus-pulposus (accessed on 19 December 2014).

119. Stutchfield, B.M.; Coleman, S. The relationships between hamstring flexibility, lumbar flexion, and low back pain in rowers. *Eur. J. Sport Sci.* **2006**, *6*, 255–260. [CrossRef]

120. O'Sullivan, P. Diagnosis and classification of chronic low back pain disorders: maladaptive movement and motor control impairments as underlying mechanism. *Man. Ther.* **2005**, *10*, 242–255. [CrossRef] [PubMed]

121. Brennan, G.P.; Fritz, J.; Hunter, S.J.; Thackeray, A.; Delitto, A.; Erhard, R. Identifying subgroups of patients with acute/subacute "nonspecific" low back pain: results of a randomized clinical trial. *Spine* **2006**, *31*, 623–631. [CrossRef] [PubMed]

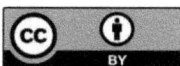

Article

A Controlled and Retrospective Study of 144 Chronic Low Back Pain Patients to Evaluate the Effectiveness of an Intensive Functional Restoration Program in France

Isabelle Caby [1,2,*], **Nicolas Olivier** [1,3], **Frédérick Janik** [1,2], **Jacques Vanvelcenaher** [4] and **Patrick Pelayo** [1,3]

[1] Univ. Lille, Univ. Artois, Univ. Littoral Cote d'Opale, EA 7369, Unité de Recherche Pluridisciplinaire Sport Santé Société (URePSSS), F-59000 Lille, France; oliviern@neuf.fr (N.O.); frederick.janik@free.fr (F.J.); patrick.pelayo@univ-lille2.fr (P.P.)
[2] Department of Sports Sciences, University Artois, 62800 Liévin, France
[3] Department of Sports Sciences, University Lille, 59790 Ronchin, France
[4] Department of Physical Medicine and Readaptation, Functional Re-Education and Rehabilitation Center, "L'Espoir", 59260 Hellemmes, France; jacques.vanvelcenaher@centre-espoir.com
* Correspondence: i.caby@wanadoo.fr or Isabelle.caby@univ-artois.fr; Tel.: +33-321-45-85-06

Academic Editor: Robert J. Gatchel
Received: 29 February 2016; Accepted: 19 April 2016; Published: 27 April 2016

Abstract: *Study Design*: A controlled and retrospective study of 144 chronic low back pain patients to evaluate the effectiveness of an intensive functional restoration program in France. *Objective*: Evaluating the efficiency of an intensive, dynamic and multidisciplinary functional restoration program in patients with chronic low back pain (LBP), during 6 and 12 months follow up. *Summary of background data*: Chronic low back pain disease has a multifactor nature, involving physical, psychological professional and social factors. A functional restoration program (FRP) has been included in a multidisciplinary training program which provides an efficient therapeutic solution. However, the effectiveness of an FRP has not been yet established. *Methods*: 144 subjects (71 males, 73 females) with chronic low back pain were included in a functional restoration program. The FRP includes physiotherapy and occupational therapy interventions together with psychological counselling. Patients participated as in- or outpatients 6 h per day, 5 days a week over 5 weeks. Pain intensity, trunk flexibility, trunk strength, lifting ability, quality of life and return to work were recorded before, immediately after, and at 6 months and 12 months after the treatment period. *Results*: All outcome measures were significantly higher just after the FRP (144 patients) and at 6 and 12 months (from available data in 31 subjects) compared to pre-treatment values. This FRP for chronic low back pain maintained its benefits whatever the patient's activities. *Conclusions*: The effects reflected on all outcome measures, both on short and long term follow-up. The multidisciplinary FRP for chronic low back pain patients durably stopped the de-conditioning syndrome and involved new life-style habits for the patient, daily pain management and a return to work.

Keywords: chronic low back pain; functional restoration program; de-conditioning syndrome; short term and long term follow-up

1. Introduction

In many countries, industrialisation has been instrumental in the development of musculoskeletal disorders, of which low back pain (LBP) is the most common and expensive [1,2]. Thus, today, LBP remains a public health issue. About 60% to 80% of the population in the western world will experience low back pain at some stage in life. The main low back pain subjects (90%) will recover in 6 weeks without any intervention, while some of the sufferers will report pain at 3 months (5% to 10%) [3]. There appears to be a trend toward chronic low back pain [4,5]. The multi-factorial nature of chronic low back pain, including physical, functional, psychological, professional and social factors, is now acknowledged [6].

Chronic low back pain (CLBP) programs have been developed during the past two decades [7–12], based on the concept developed by Tom Mayer and Robert J. Gatchel: the deconditoning syndrome [13, 14]. These programs have had significant results [15–21], so the exercise therapy program included daily global reconditioning activities, and the objective was to improve some aspects of health-related quality of life in addition to reducing pain and improving function. Include multidisciplinary interventions with the objective of resuming activities and returning to work. A functional restoration program (FRP) was first introduced in France by Vanvelcenaher *et al.* at the end of the 20th century [22,23]. The evaluation of such programs includes the cost-effectiveness factor and requires long-term follow-up. Thus, several cohorts of CLBP patients with a functional restoration program treatment have been surveyed in a re-education and rehabilitation structure since 2000.

Hence, the aim of this present paper was to assess the short and long term effectiveness of a French-specific RFP. More precisely, the objective of this follow up was to evaluate the efficiency of a 6 and 12 month intensive, dynamic and multidisciplinary functional restoration program in patients with chronic low back pain (CLBP).

2. Materials and Methods

2.1. Study Design

The study was designed as a controlled, retrospective and non-randomized study in chronic low back pain patients to evaluate the effectiveness of an intensive functional restoration program.

2.2. Study Population

A total of 144 CLBP subjects (71 females, 73 males) of the eligible patients referred by their general practitioner or medical specialist were included in the FRP of a re-education and rehabilitation centre. All 144 subjects participated in the 5 coverage weeks. A total of 31 subjects correspond to the patients who have participated in all the evaluations. Low back pain patients fit for following a reconditioning program have been included in this protocol. Employees, the intermediate professions and the working class are the socioprofessional classes dominant in low back pain populations. 61% of the 31 patients do not practice any physical activity. Of the others, half practice regular activity (twice or more/week), and half practice occasional activity. Among the 31 patients taking part in the study, 38% have an IMC > 25, among those, only two subject have an ĪMC > 30.

The inclusion criteria were: aged between 18 and 65 years, presence of CLBP or lumbo radiculalgy existing for at least 3 months according to the criteria of the French health evaluation agency [24], suffering from the deconditioning syndrome (loss of flexibility, muscular strength or daily capability). Exclusion criteria were: secondary LBP; osteoarthritis or neurological disease precluding physical exercise; cardiac and/or pulmonary conditions (diagnosed after cyclo ergometer stress tests); psychiatric disorders incompatible with the participation in a group program; secondary profits (financial interest); severe addiction to drugs, narcotics, or alcohol, and finally pregnancy. In our protocol, 15 subjects were excluded.

2.3. Interventions

The intervention included participation in a FRP. The FRP, imported from the American rehabilitation institute of Dallas for Ergonomics (PRIDE), was standardised and proposed by a rehabilitation centre. This program included a multidisciplinary team of physicians, physiotherapists, occupational therapists, psychotherapists, sports therapists and social workers. The FRP involves the treatment of low back pain with a primary focus on return of function [25], rather than simply suppressing pain. Patients in RFP have to tolerate some temporary discomfort while participating in sports medicine, and detoxifying from habit-forming narcotic medication. The patients' active role and motivation is essential to make a success of this rehabilitation program. The patients trained 6 h a day over 5 weeks, 5 days a week with complete or outpatient hospitalization.

The physical program consisted of muscle-strengthening (for the trunk, lower and upper limbs), cardiovascular exercises, stretching and proprioceptive practice.

A physiotherapist supervised the performed exercises and adjusted the exercise intensity to each CLBP patient. During the first week, patients learned muscular warm-up and stretching techniques, improved their flexibility and performed cardio-respiratory exercises. During the second week, patients began muscular-strengthening exercises. During the third week, muscular-strengthening increased with endurance exercises. Patients performed weightlifting as well as proprioception and coordination exercises. During the fourth and the fifth weeks, the intensity of strengthening exercises increased progressively.

The endurance training (cycling) was adapted to each patient's heart rate and to the exercise stress test performed before the program. The training program (cycling) was individualized according to heart rate and was intermittent in nature. It consisted of several series of low- or moderate-intensity exercises alternated with active recovery periods. In order to adapt the protocol to the exercise therapy program constraints, the subjects were trained for 21 min, by alternating 3 min at 70% and 3 min at 85% of peak heart rate (peak heart rate = 220-age).

The CLBP patients also received ergonomic care and performed work simulations during occupational therapy sessions.

Patients were referred to the psychologist at least once in the first week and for further treatment if necessary.

In order to prepare the patients' return to work, the social workers made contact with appropriate authorities. In this way, they could envisage the conditions for resumption of work (a full-time or part-time job, part-time work on medical grounds, an adapted workstation, disabled worker redeployment).

Each week, the patients attended a clinic with the specialist in physical medicine rehabilitation, who was the medical supervisor of the program.

2.4. Outcome Measures

The FRP was based on five evaluations: before the program (T1), at the beginning (T0), immediately after the 5 weeks of the RFP (T5 weeks), and at 6 and 12 month (T6mo, T12mo) follow-up visits.

Demographic Data and Clinical Characteristics: For each patient, the age, weight, height, gender, duration of complaints and disability, history of back surgery, sick leave duration, practice of physical and sports activities and tobacco consumption were recorded (Table 1).

Table 1. Demographic data and clinical characteristics before rehabilitation.

	Male (n = 73)	Female (n = 71)	*p*	Total
Age (yrs)	41.3 ± 8.5	42.4 ± 9,2	0.415	41.9 ± 8.8
Mass (kg)	84.4 ± 13	63.8 ± 11,1	*p* < 0.001	74 ± 15.9
Height (cm)	1.78 ± 6.8	1.64 ± 6.2	*p* < 0.001	1.71 ± 0.1
BMI (Kg/m^2)	26.4 ± 3.8	23.6 ± 4	*p* < 0.001	25 ± 4.1
Sick leave prior to inclusion (weeks)	38.7 ± 38.9	29.6 ± 39.3	0.069	33.1 ± 39.1
Length of ongoing back pain (mo)	79 ± 61	70 ± 61	0.352	74 ± 63
History of spinal surgery	16	21	0.481	37
Smokers (cigarettes/day)	9 ± 13	4 ± 7	0.055	6 ± 11
Leisure time Sport and physical Activity: twice or more a week	14	14	0.059	21
Average time of inclusion in FRP (mo)	5 ± 3	5 ± 4	0.857	5 ± 3
Pain (VAS, mm)	49 ± 18	48 ± 22	0.546	49 ± 20
FTF distance (cm)	18 ± 14	10 ± 12	*p* < 0.001	14 ± 14

Values are mean ± SD (range) or percentage. BMI = Body Mass Index; VAS = visual analogue scale; FTF = finger to floor.

Pain Intensity: A 100-mm long visual analogue scale (VAS) with "no pain" on the left side and "unbearable pain"on the right side was used. Relevance, validity, and reliability have been sufficiently tested for patients with CLPB [26–28].

Trunk Flexibility: Finger-to-floor distance (FTF) was used to evaluate flexibility [29].

Trunk Strength: The strength of the trunk flexors and extensors was evaluated by using standardized iso-kinetic and iso-inertial lifting performance measurements on the Cybex Norm. Reciprocal concentric trunk flexion and extension peak torque values at different angular velocities using the Cybex NORM Trunk Modular Component^{TM} isokinetic dynamometer were assessed at 30 degrees/s 60 degrees/s and 90 degrees/s angular velocities [30,31]. The iso-kinetic measurements used were peak torque (PT), work, power-in the best repetition and total work (TW).

Muscle strength assessment by isokinetic dynamometer was carried out with a Cybex Norm. The spinal flexors and extensors are concentrically explored at speeds of 60 degrees/s and 90 degrees/s. The parameters studied were peak torque (PT), work, power in the best repetition and total work (TW).

Lifting Ability: The Progressive Iso-Inertial Lifting Evaluation (PILE) test evaluates the lifting ability of the CLBP patients [32].

Quality of life: The self-administrated Dallas Pain Questionnaire (DPQ) assesses the impact of the chronic low back pain in four aspects of the patients' life: daily activities, work and leisure activities, perceived anxiety-depression, and sociability [33].

Working ability: Working ability was analysed by the social workers' questionnaire to inform the duration to return to work, work status.

2.5. Statistical Analyses

The statistical analysis was performed with sigma Stat version 2.03. The evolution of FTF, VAS, PILE, DPQ and trunk strength scores between men and women at T0 and T5 weeks were analysed by using a "*t*" test or a two way ANOVA. The results from post-treatment (T5 weeks) and follow-up sessions (T6mo, T12mo) were compared to the pre-treatment results (T0). Paired "*t*" test and repeated measure ANOVA were used to test differences over time for each variable.

3. Results

3.1. Pre-Treatment Characteristics

One hundred and forty-four patients (71 women, 73 men) were included in the trial. The mean age was 41.9 years. 31 patients (22%) performed all the tests. 144 patients performed only the pre- and post-tests.

Regarding the demographic data and to the clinical characteristics (Table 1), no statistically significant difference was found between men and women concerning age, sick leave prior to inclusion, length of ongoing back pain, sporting and physical activities, average time of inclusion in the FRP and pain. Although the men were taller, heavier and had a higher BMI ($p < 0.001$) and higher lifting results, their flexibility was less than women's. Men were also heavier smokers in comparison with women.

Regarding the percentages of the clinical characteristics before the FRP (Table 2), nearly half of the population (46%) of the CLBP patients was overweight (BMI > 25), a third smokers, 19.4% practiced a sport or a physical activity twice a week, or more and a third had a history of spinal surgery (32%).

Table 2. Male and female percentages of clinical characteristics before rehabilitation.

	Male (n = 73)	Female (n = 71)	Mean
BMI > 25 (%)	55	37	46
History of spinal surgery (%)	34	30	32
Smokers (%)	33	28	31
Leisure time Sport and physical Activity: twice or more a week (%)	19	20	19.4

The percentages above refer to the percentage of men and women that answered the questions.

3.2. Evolution after Treatment

Significant improvements were found in physical performances (trunk strength, FFD, PILE), and working ability after the treatment, compared to before ($p < 0.001$). This improvement was maintained at the 6 and 12 month follow-ups. The FRP considerably increased trunk strength, but principally the strength of the trunk extensors: maximal force, endurance force and speed force (Table 3).

Table 3. Short term (n = 144) and long term (n = 31) effects of the FRP on physical, psychological and occupational measures in CLBP patients.

Variable	Short Term Effects of FRP (n = 144)			Long Term Effects of FRP (n = 31)			
	T0	T5 weeks	p value for time effect	T5 weeks	T6mo	T12mo	p value for time effect
Pain (VAS, mm)	50 ± 22	27 ± 21	$p < 0.001$	23 ± 13	26 ± 22	25 ± 22	0.585
FTF distance (cm)	13 ± 15	-6 ± 8	$p < 0.001$	-6 ± 9	-3 ± 10	-2 ± 10	0.252
PILE (% of mass)	25 ± 12	44 ± 15	$p < 0.001$	45 ± 16	41 ± 14	39 ± 13	0.254
DPQ daily activities (%)	75 ± 11	47 ± 26	$p < 0.001$	51 ± 28	59 ± 30	56 ± 32	0.874
DPQ work and leisure (%)	68 ± 16	43 ± 27	$p < 0.001$	49 ± 29	59 ± 32	58 ± 35	0.798
DPQ anxiety and depression (%)	46 ± 20	29 ± 26	$p < 0.05$	30 ± 22	49 ± 27	50 ± 26	0.265
DPQ sociability (%)	27 ± 18	28 ± 24	0.958	35 ± 25	39 ± 25	38 ± 32	0.968
Trunk strength 30° sec (ratios F/E, % of body weight)	1.09 ± 0.28	0.86 ± 0.18	$p < 0.001$	0.83 ± 0.18	0.83 ± 0.19	0.89 ± 0.26	0.503
Trunk strength 120° sec (ratios F/E, % of body weight)	1.56 ± 1.19	1.07 ± 0.43	$p < 0.001$	1.25 ± 0.62	1.10 ± 0.27	1.06 ± 0.36	0.926
Extensors Trunk strength, maximal force 30° sec (peak torque, % of body weight)	222 ± 81	307 ± 89	$p < 0.001$	318 ± 98	306 ± 94	301 ± 103	0.831
Extensors Trunk strength, endurance force 120° sec (total work, % of body weight)	104 ± 63	211 ± 70	$p < 0.001$	209 ± 89	186 ± 72	184 ± 69	0.182
Extensors Trunk strength, speed force 90° sec (power, % of mass)	128 ± 69	236 ± 80	$p < 0.001$	230 ± 87	219 ± 91	224 ± 91	0.898

VAS = Visual Analogue Scale; FTF = Finger To Floor; PILE = Progressive Iso-inertial Lifting Evaluation; DPQ = Dallas Pain Questionnaire; ratios F/E = ratio Flexors/ Extensors.

Pain severity on VAS and every score on the DPQ except for the social interest score were significantly lower at T5 weeks than at T0. The results remained stable at the 6 and 12 month follow-up periods.

The majority of the CLBP patients considered their physical fitness to be improved. Indeed, after the FRP, 81% of the CLBP patients return to work (57% without special facilities and 24% with special facilities). Two-thirds of the patients returned to work after an average of one month.

4. Discussion

Our study was as a controlled, retrospective and non-randomized study in chronic low back pain patients. Our main objective was to assess the effectiveness of an intensive functional restoration program and show the medium- and long-term efficiency. We studied a homogeneous population of 144 CLBP patients living in the same area of France comprising a majority of employees. A total of 81% of the CLPB patients in our study returned to work, 57% without special facilities and 24% with such facilities (a part-time job, part-time work on medical grounds, adapted workstation, *etc.*). Similar results were found in a systematic review by Guzman *et al.* [7]. These authors found strong evidence that intensive interdisciplinary rehabilitation with functional restoration reduces pain and improves function in patients with CLBP significantly more than less intensive programs or usual care. The cost-comparison savings data in a study by Mayer *et al.* [13] were quite impressive: a less intensive program cost twice as much as the FRP over a 1-year period because the treatment-as-usual group had five times as many patient visits to health-care professionals and higher rates of recurrence or injury.

In the last few years, the outcome and cost effectiveness of intensive functional restoration programs have been studied because of their high costs for the health care system [34,35]. For example, the average overall cost per patient in France is 15,000 €, the largest part being indirect costs because of sick leave payments [36]. Most studies consider the main outcome to be return to work and/or the numbers of days of sick leave taken [37–40].

57% of the study patients were working full time in their former jobs after the end of the FRP (Table 4). This is consistent with the results found by Keel *et al* [21] after a reconditioning program similar to ours. At the end of the program, 60% of the patients returned to work. Waldburger *et al.* [41] found that 66% of 50 patients returned to work after a reconditioning program. In the United States, with a reconditioning program similar to ours, full time return-to-work rates ranged from 70% to 80% [37]. These better results could be linked to the more limited unemployment benefits available in the United States than in Europe, so that reconditioning is often the patient's only chance to maintain an income [40].

Table 4. Return to work after 5 weeks of FRP.

	Mean
Return to work without facilitation (%)	57
Return to work with facilitations (%)	24
No return to work (%)	19
Average time to return to work (days)	30 ± 59

In this study, the direct effectiveness of the FRP was assessed by clinical, physical, functional and psychosocial data [42]. The FRP was effective both for males and females in reducing back pain intensity, functional disability and in improving their quality of life, flexibility and trunk strength between T0 and T5 weeks (Table 5). Moreover, these results were maintained at T6mo and T12mo. Nevertheless, some significant differences in values at T5 weeks may be noticed between male and female subjects. These differences could be linked to muscular force assessed in the PILE and isokinetic tests. Thus, the present results could be analysed without differentiation between genders, according to Gagnon *et al.* [12].

Physical parameter values were significantly higher at T5 weeks (Table 3). Before the FRP, all the CLBP patients suffered from a lack of endurance force, speed force and maximal force of back extensors. The decreased endurance of back extensors is considered to be a risk factor for CLPB [43]. After the five-week intensive functional program, all the types of back extensor strength were significantly higher than in T0 (Table 3). Thus, at the end of the program, regarding the flexor–extensor ratios, trunk extensors became stronger than the flexors, as shown in the literature [44]. Isokinetic training could explain the back strength recovery in providing feedback to patients on their performance level and in quantifying their progress. Table 5 outlines the descriptive values for strength and identifies a significant gender effect in all relative strength values ($p < 0.001$), in accordance with other results [45]. Although differences between males and females were noticed, the same functional restoration program may be proposed as it will not disturb individual improvement, which represents the main objective of the FRP. Moreover, it could also improve personal, motivation and sociability.

Table 5. Male and female data at T0 and T5 weeks.

Variable	Male n = 73			Female n = 71			p value for Gender effect T0	p value for Gender effect T5
	T0	T5 weeks	p value for time effect	T0	T5 weeks	p value for time effect		
Pain (VAS, mm)	50 ± 19	25 ± 20	$p < 0.001$	50 ± 22	29 ± 22	$p < 0.001$	0.944	0.449
FTF distance (cm)	17 ± 15	-5 ± 8	$p < 0.001$	9 ± 12	-8 ± 7	$p < 0.001$	$p < 0.001$	0.140
PILE (% of mass)	30 ± 13	52 ± 14	$p < 0.001$	20 ± 7	35 ± 9	$p < 0.001$	$p < 0.001$	$p < 0.001$
DPQ daily activities (%)	75 ± 11	49 ± 28	$p < 0.05$	45 ± 23	76 ± 12	$p < 0.001$	0.860	0.520
DPQ work and leisure (%)	66 ± 18	49 ± 29	$p < 0.05$	70 ± 13	37 ± 24	$p < 0.001$	0.526	0.126
DPQ anxiety and depression (%)	49 ± 22	37 ± 31	0.130	43 ± 18	20 ± 18	$p < 0.001$	0.529	0.056
DPQ sociability (%)	24 ± 15	31 ± 29	0.368	31 ± 21	25 ± 18	0.511	0.484	0.389
Trunk strength 30° sec (ratios F/E, % of body weight)	1.10 ± 0.30	0.85 ± 0.19	$p < 0.001$	1.08 ± 0.25	0.88 ± 0.18	$p < 0.001$	0.564	0.541
Trunk strength 120° sec (ratios F/E, % of body weight)	1.77 ± 1.64	1.08 ± 0.45	$p < 0.001$	1.40 ± 0.48	1.03 ± 0.3	$p < 0.05$	$p < 0.05$	0.709
Extensors Trunk strength, maximal force 30° sec (peak torque, % of body weight)	251 ± 87	348 ± 96	$p < 0.001$	195 ± 52	262 ± 58	$p < 0.001$	$p < 0.001$	$p < 0.001$
Extensors Trunk strength, endurance force 120° sec (total work, % of body weight)	119 ± 70	243 ± 75	$p < 0.001$	91 ± 47	176 ± 47	$p < 0.001$	0.053	$p < 0.001$
Extensors Trunk strength, speed force 90° sec (power, % of mass)	148 ± 75	277 ± 83	$p < 0.001$	109 ± 43	190 ± 45	$p < 0.001$	$p < 0.05$	$p < 0.001$

VAS = Visual Analogue Scale; FTF = Finger to Floor; PILE = Progressive Iso-inertial Lifting Evaluation; DPQ = Dallas Pain Questionnaire; ratios F/E = ratio Flexors/ Extensors.

At the end of the FRP, the CLBP patients in the present study recovered 75% of the isokinetic values at 30 °/s (peak torque, % of body weight), 55% at 120 °/s (power, % of body weight) at T5 weeks and 73% and 47% respectively at T6mo of the standard values reported by Vanvelcenaher *et al.* [23] in a previous study. In the latter, strength of the back extensors was measured in a healthy population aged between 25 and 30. These results could partly be explained both by the young age of the healthy population, while the mean age of our population was nearly 42 years old, and furthermore by their leisure time and physical activities. Stevenson *et al.* [6] also advanced the hypothesis of an association between muscle fiber type at the lumbar sites (reduced slow twitch fibers, type I) and LBP.

The FTF distance was significantly reduced after the FRP program. The improvement in flexibility could be the result of the frequency and the duration of stretching exercises performed every day in various forms: passive training with the physiotherapist, active training on an isokinetic machine, collective and active training during stretching sessions, and collective and active training in balneotherapy. Sessions of relaxation therapy and occupational therapy are also efficient in improving flexibility, alleviating distress and managing pain [46]. Recently, Mc Geary *et al.* highlighted the role of pain intensity and reported that high pain intensities before the program are often associated with bad outcomes both in LBP and other musculoskeletal diseases [47]. In our study, 75% of the CLBP patients evaluated their pain between 25 and 75 at T0 when 52% of the patients were painless (VAS < 25) at T5 weeks. Furthermore, pain regression was similar both in male and female subjects. Nevertheless, the findings of previous studies suggest analysing men and women separately in trials concerning pain treatment, because of different responses to pain treatments between genders [48]. Moreover, pain regression is not dependent on the endorphinic or opioïde effect but is due to repetitive rhythmic movements involving antagonist muscles used in the same manner, with increased local cellular metabolism.

In the present study, psychosocial measures were significantly improved (Tables 3 and 5). The reduction of subjective feelings of disability and of general emotional distress is decisive in enabling a successful return to work. DPQ scores improved significantly after the FRP and the benefits were maintained over the medium and long term. The improvement in DPQ daily activities, together with work and leisure activities could be related to the self-reported ability to resume work and leisure activities and to the decline of fears concerning physical and work activities.

In this study, it would have been interesting to learn about good and bad prognostic factors; however, this was not possible. In a future investigation, we plan to compare our results with those of a control group and to calculate correlation to the modalities included and the dose of therapy applied in order to increase our understanding of the physical therapy benefits for chronic low back pain patients.

5. Conclusions

An intensive and multidisciplinary functional restoration program seems to stop the deconditioning syndrome (medium and long term effects) in CLBP and to improve functional, physical and psychosocial values. The stabilization of these values would depend on the active way of life of the subjects after the treatment. FRP would teach the CLBP patient new lifestyle habits, daily management of pain and a return to work.

The reluctance of third–party payers to authorize the use of intensive interdisciplinary rehabilitation with functional restoration is due to its perceived high cost. This study confirms that such perceptions are misguided and incorrect in terms of the potential long-term cost savings of such programs.

Author Contributions: Isabelle Caby and Patrick Pelayo wrote the first draft of the manuscript, Nicolas Olivier contributed to revisions of the manuscript. Jacques Vanvelcenaher supervised the study and contributed to data aquisition, procedural protocols. All authors contributed to the study design, procedural protocols, data acquisition, and the drafting of this paper. All authors read and approved the final manuscript.

Conflicts of Interest: The authors declare no conflict of interest.

References

1. Van Tulder, M.; Malmivaara, A.; Esmail, R.; Koes, B. Exercise therapy for low back pain: A systematic review within the framework of the cochrane collaboration back. *Spine* **2000**, *25*, 2784–2796. [CrossRef] [PubMed]
2. Anderson, G.B.J. Epidemiological features of chronic low-back pain. *Lancet* **1999**, *354*, 581–585. [CrossRef]
3. Waddell, G. A new clinical model for the treatment of low back. *Spine* **1987**, *12*, 165–175.
4. Lewis, J.S.; Hewitt, J.S.; Billington, L.; Cole, S.; Byng, J.; Karayiannis, S. A randomized clinical trial comparing two physiotherapy interventions for chronic low back pain. *Spine* **2005**, *30*, 711–721. [CrossRef] [PubMed]
5. Olivier, N.; Lepretre, A.; Caby, I.; Dupuis, M.A.; Prieur, F. Does exercise therapy for chronic lower-back pain require daily isokinetic reinforcement of the trunk muscles? *Ann. Readapt. Med. Phys.* **2008**, *51*, 284–291. [CrossRef] [PubMed]
6. Stevenson, J.M.; Weber, C.L.; Smith, J.T.; Dumas, G.A.; Albert, W.J. A longitudinal study of the development of low back pain in an industrial population. *Spine* **2001**, *26*, 1370–1377. [CrossRef] [PubMed]
7. Guzmán, J.; Esmail, R.; Karjalainen, K.; Malmivaara, A.; Irvin, E.; Bombardier, C. Multidisciplinary rehabilitation for chronic low back pain: Systematic review. *BMJ* **2001**, *322*, 1511–1516. [CrossRef] [PubMed]
8. Maul, I.; Läubli, T.; Oliveri, M.; Krueger, H. Long-term effects of supervised physical training in secondary prevention of low back pain. *Eur. Spine* **2005**, *14*, 599–611. [CrossRef] [PubMed]
9. Smeets, R.J.; Vlaeyen, J.W.; Hidding, A.; Kester, A.D.; van der Heijden, G.J.; van Geel, A.C.; Knottnerus, J.A. Active rehabilitation for chronic low back pain: Cognitive-behavioral, physical, or both? First direct post-treatment results from a randomized controlled trial. *BMC Musculoskelet. Disord.* **2006**. [CrossRef] [PubMed]
10. Verfaille, S.; Delarue, Y.; Demangeon, S.; Beuret-Blanquart, F. Evaluation after four years of exercise therapy for chronic low back pain. *Ann. Readapt. Med. Phys.* **2005**, *48*, 53–60. [CrossRef] [PubMed]
11. Bontoux, L.; Roquelaure, Y.; Billabert, C.; Dubus, V.; Sancho, P.O.; Colin, D.; Brami, L.; Moisan, S.; Fanello, S.; Penneau-Fontbonne, D.; *et al.* Prospective study of the outcome at one year of patients with chronic low back pain in a program of intensive functional restoration and ergonomic intervention. Factors predicting their return to work. *Ann. Readapt. Med. Phys.* **2004**, *47*, 563–572. [CrossRef]
12. Gagnon, S.; Lensel-Corbeil, G.; Duquesnoy, B. Multicenter multidisciplinary training program for chronic low back pain: French experience of the Renodos back pain network (Réseau Nord-Pas-de-Calais du DOS). *Ann. Phys. Rehabil. Med.* **2009**, *52*, 3–16. [CrossRef] [PubMed]
13. Mayer, T.G.; Gatchel, R.J.; Kishino, N.; Keeley, J.A.; Capra, P.A.; Mayer, H.O.; Barnett, J.; Mooney, V.E. Objective assessment of spine function following industrial injury. A prospective study with comparison group and one-year follow-up. *Spine* **1985**, *10*, 482–493. [CrossRef] [PubMed]
14. Mayer, T.G.; Smith, S.S.; Kondraske, G.; Gatchel, R.J.; Carmichael, T.W.; Mooney, V. Quantification of lumbar function. Part 3: Preliminary data on isokinetic torso rotation testing with myoelectric spectral analysis in normal and low-back pain subjects. *Spine* **1985**, *10*, 912–920. [CrossRef] [PubMed]
15. Bendix, T.; Bendix, A.; Labriola, M.; Hæstrup, C.; Ebbehøj, N. Functional restoration *versus* outpatient physical training in chronic low back pain: A randomized comparative study. *Spine* **2000**, *25*, 2494–2500. [CrossRef] [PubMed]
16. Frost, H.; Klaber Moffett, J.A.; Moser, J.S.; Fairbank, J.C.T. Randomised controlled trial for evaluation of fitness programme for patients with chronic low back pain. *BMJ* **1995**, *310*, 151–154. [CrossRef] [PubMed]
17. Hansen, F.R.; Bendix, T.; Skov, P.; Jensen, C.V.; Kristensen, J.H.; Krohn, L.; Schioeler, H. Intensive, dynamic back-muscle exercises, conventional physiotherapy, or placebo-control treatment of low-back pain. A randomized, observer-blind trial. *Spine* **1993**, *18*, 98–108. [CrossRef] [PubMed]
18. Hlobil, H.; Staal, J.B.; Twisk, J.; Köke, A.; Ariëns, G.; Smid, T.; Van Mechelen, W. The effects of a graded activity intervention for low back pain in occupational health on sick leave, functional status and pain: 12-Month results of a randomized controlled trial. *J. Occup. Rehabil.* **2005**, *15*, 569–580. [CrossRef] [PubMed]
19. Hlobil, H.; Uegaki, K.; Staal, J.B.; de Bruyne, M.C.; Smid, T.; van Mechelen, W. Substantial sick-leave costs savings due to a graded activity intervention for workers with non-specific sub-acute low back pain. *Eur. Spine J.* **2007**, *16*, 919–924. [CrossRef] [PubMed]
20. Jousset, N.; Fanello, S.; Bontoux, L.; Dubus, V.; Billabert, C.; Vielle, B.; Roquelaure, Y.; Penneau-Fontbonne, D.; Richard, I. Effects of functional restoration *versus* 3 hours per week physical therapy: A randomized controlled study. *Spine* **2004**, *29*, 487–493. [CrossRef] [PubMed]

21. Keel, P.J.; Wittig, R.; Deutschmann, R.; Diethelm, U.; Knüsel, O.; Löschmann, C.; Matathia, R.; Rudolf, T.; Spring, H. Effectiveness of in-patient rehabilitation for sub-chronic and chronic low back pain by an integrative group treatment program (Swiss Multicentre Study). *Scand. J. Rehabil. Med.* **1998**, *30*, 211–219. [PubMed]

22. Vanvelcenaher, J.; Voisin, P.; Struk, P.; Weissland, T.; Goethals, M.; Masse, P.; Bibré, P.; Aernoudts, E.; Raevel, D.; O'Miel, G.; *et al.* La restauration fonctionnelle du rachis® (RFR®) chez les lombalgiques chroniques: Bilan 1997. *Ann. Phys. Rehabil. Med.* **1997**, *40*, 444–453. [CrossRef]

23. Vanvelcenaher. *Restauration Fonctionnelle du Rachis Dans les Lombalgies Chroniques*; Frison-Roche: Paris, France, 2003.

24. Agence Nationale d'Accréditation et d'Evaluation en Santé (ANAES). Diagnostic, prise en charge et suivi des malades atteints de lombalgie chronique: Décembre 2000. *Douleurs* **2001**, *2*, 283–289. (In French)

25. Van Geen, J.W.; Edelaar, M.J.; Janssen, M.; van Eijk, J.T.M. The long-term effect of multidisciplinary back training: A systematic review. *Spine* **2007**, *32*, 249–255. [CrossRef] [PubMed]

26. Huskisson, E.C. Measurement of pain. *Lancet* **1974**, *2*, 1127–1131. [CrossRef]

27. Price, D.D.; McGrath, P.A.; Rafii, A.; Buckingham, B. The validation of visual analogue scales as ratio scale measures for chronic and experimental pain. *Pain* **1983**, *7*, 45–56. [CrossRef]

28. Carlsson, A.M. Assessment of chronic pain. I. Aspects of the reliability and validity of the visual analogue scale. *Pain* **1983**, *16*, 87–101. [CrossRef]

29. Perret, C.; Poiraudeau, S.; Fermanian, J.; Colau, M.; Benhamou, M.; Revel, M. Validity, reliability, and responsiveness of the fingertip-to-floor test. *Arch. Phys. Med. Rehabil.* **2001**, *82*, 1566–1570. [CrossRef] [PubMed]

30. Byl, N.N.; Sadowsky, H.S. Intersite reliability of repeated isokinetic measurments: Cybex backsystems including trunk rotation, trunkextension-flexion, and liftask. *Iso. Exerc. Sci.* **1993**, *3*, 139–147.

31. Delto, A.; Rose, S.J.; Crandell, C.E.; Strube, M.J. Reliability of isokinetic measurments of trunk muscle performance. *Spine* **1991**, *16*, 800–803. [CrossRef]

32. Mayer, T.G.; Barnes, D.; Kishino, N.D.; Nichols, G.; Gatchel, R.J.; Mayer, H.; Mooney, V. Progressive isoinertial lifting evaluation. I. A standardized protocol and normative database. *Spine* **1988**, *13*, 993–997. [CrossRef] [PubMed]

33. Marty, M.; Blotman, F.; Avouac, B.; Rozenberg, S.; Valat, J.P. Validation of the French version of the Dallas Pain Questionnaire in chronic low back pain patients. *Rev. Rhum. Engl.* **1998**, *65*, 126–134.

34. Roche, G.; Ponthieux, A.; Parot-Shinkel, E.; Jousset, N.; Bontoux, L.; Dubus, V.; Penneau-Fontbonne, D.; Roquelaure, Y.; Legrand, E.; Colin, D.; *et al.* Comparison of a functional restoration program with active individual physical therapy for patients with chronic low back pain: A randomized controlled trial. *Arch. Phys. Med. Rehabil.* **2000**, *88*, 1229–1235. [CrossRef] [PubMed]

35. Gatchel, R.J.; Mayer, T.G. Evidence-informed management of chronic low back pain with functional restoration. *Spine* **2008**, *8*, 65–69. [CrossRef] [PubMed]

36. Haumesser, D.; Becker, P.; Grosso-Lebon, B.; Weill, G. Medical, social and economics aspects of the management of chronic low-back pain. *Rev. Méd. l'Assur. Mal.* **2004**, *35*, 27–36.

37. Hazard, R.G.; Fenwick, J.W.; Kalisch, S.M.; Redmond, J.; Reeves, V.; Reid, S.; Frymoyer, J.W. Functional restoration with behavioral support. A one-year prospective study of patients with chronic low-back pain. *Spine* **1989**, *14*, 157–161. [CrossRef] [PubMed]

38. Bendix, A.E.; Bendix, T.; Haestrup, C.; Busch, E. A prospective, randomized 5-year follow-up study of functional restoration in chronic low back pain patients. *Eur. Spine J.* **1998**, *7*, 111–119. [CrossRef] [PubMed]

39. Bendix, A.F.; Bendix, T.; Labriola, M.; Bœkgaard, P. Functional restoration for chronic low back pain. Two-year follow-up of two randomized clinical trials. *Spine* **1998**, *23*, 717–725. [CrossRef] [PubMed]

40. Casso, G.; Cachin, C.; van Melle, G.; Gerster, J.C. Return-to-work status 1 year after muscle reconditioning in chronic low back pain patients. *Jt. Bone Spine* **2004**, *71*, 136–139. [CrossRef]

41. Waldburger, M.; Stucki, R.F.; Balagué, F.; Wittig, R. Early multidisciplinary approach in lumbar pain to prevent development of chronicity. *Rev. Med. Suisse Romande* **2001**, *121*, 581–584. [PubMed]

42. Gatchel, R.J. The Continuing and Growing Epidemic of Chronic Low Back Pain. *Healthcare* **2015**, *3*, 838–845. [CrossRef]

43. Biering-Sørensen, F. Physical measurements as risk indicators for low-back trouble over a one-year period. *Spine* **1984**, *9*, 106–119. [CrossRef] [PubMed]

44. Langrana, N.A.; Lee, C.K.; Alexander, H.; Mayott, C.W. Quantitative assessment of back strength using isokinetic testing. *Spine* **1984**, *9*, 287–290. [CrossRef] [PubMed]
45. Marshall, P.W.; Mannion, J.; Murphy, B.A. The eccentric, concentric strength relationship of the hamstring muscles in chronic low back pain. *J. Electromyogr. Kinesiol.* **2010**, *20*, 39–45. [CrossRef] [PubMed]
46. VanDalfsen, P.J.; Syrjala, K.L. Psychological strategies in acute pain management. *Crit. Care Clin.* **1990**, *6*, 421–431. [PubMed]
47. McGeary, D.D.; Mayer, T.G.; Gatchel, R.J. High pain ratings predict treatment failure in chronic occupational musculoskeletal disorders. *J. Bone Jt. Surg. Am.* **2006**, *88*, 317–325. [CrossRef] [PubMed]
48. Kääpä, E.H.; Frantsi, K.; Sarna, S.; Malmivaara, A. Multidisciplinary group rehabilitation *versus* individual physiotherapy for chronic nonspecific low back pain: A randomized trial. *Spine* **2006**, *31*, 371–376. [CrossRef] [PubMed]

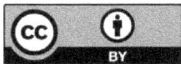

healthcare

Article

Getting "Unstuck": A Multi-Site Evaluation of the Efficacy of an Interdisciplinary Pain Intervention Program for Chronic Low Back Pain

Timothy Clark [1,*], Jean Claude Wakim [1,†] and Carl Noe [2,†]

1   Baylor Center for Pain Management, 3600 Gaston Ave, Wadley Tower, Suite 360, Dallas, TX 75246, USA;
    Jean.Wakim@BSWHealth.org
2   Eugene McDermott Center for Pain Management—University of Texas Southwestern Medical Center,
    1801 Inwood Avenue, Suite WA 7.5, Dallas, TX 75390, USA; Carl.Noe@utsouthwestern.edu
*   Correspondence: Timothy.Clark@BSWHealth.org; Tel.: +1-214-820-7526; Fax: +1-214-820-8080
†   These authors contributed equally to this work.

Academic Editors: Robert J. Gatchel and Sampath Parthasarathy
Received: 16 December 2015; Accepted: 3 June 2016; Published: 14 June 2016

Abstract: Chronic low back pain is one of the major health problems in the U.S., resulting in a large number of years of disability. To address the biopsychosocial nature of pain, interdisciplinary pain programs provide integrated interventions by an interdisciplinary team in a unified setting with unified goals. This study examined outcomes of an interdisciplinary program located at two sites with different staff, yet with a unified model of treatment and documentation. Efficacy at the combined sites was examined by comparing standard measures obtained upon admission to the program with measures at completion of a 3–4 week long program for 393 patients with chronic low back pain (CLBP). Repeated measures included pain severity, pain interference, efficacy of self-management strategies, hours of activity, depression, ability to do ADLs, and physical endurance. All repeated measures differed at the $p < 0.001$ level, with large effect sizes (0.66–0.85). Eighty-two percent of graduates reported being "very much improved" or "much improved". A second analyses provided evidence that treatment effects were robust across sites with no differences (<0.001) found on five of seven selected outcome measures. A third analysis found that number of days of treatment was correlated on three of seven measures at the <0.01 level. However, the amount of variance explained by days of treatment was under 5% on even the most highly correlated measure. These finding are consistent with previous research and explore short-term effectiveness of treatment across treatment sites and with variable duration of treatment.

Keywords: low back pain; interdisciplinary treatment; effectiveness; biopsychosocial; outcome measures

---

1. Introduction

"Whenever I see my doctor for another visit; he seems to do the Michael Jackson moonwalk—I can feel him backing out of the room at the same time he is walking in". Patient with chronic pain.

This patient's (probably accurate) perception captures the frustration of both healthcare providers and patients facing chronic low back pain (CLBP). This subjective impression of being "stuck" is reflected in the continued suffering and disability despite the high cost of ongoing healthcare. As evidenced by recent reports by the Institute of Medicine [1,2], between $560 and $630 billion is spent annually on direct and indirect costs of chronic pain. These costs continue, or may in fact increase, despite advancements in pain medicine, in new pain medication, assessment of genotypes predicting medication response [3], and new surgical and interventional procedures and devices, among others.

As the most common type of musculoskeletal pain, low back pain continues to be a primary source of disability, as evidenced in both emergency department and inpatient medical stays [4].

In an effort to better understand the problem of CLBP, some have suggested that the problem is more accurately understood and more effectively treated by use of a biopsychosocial model [5]. The biopsychosocial understanding of pain suggests that perceived pain and ensuing disability result from a complex array of factors interacting over time. This model suggests that success in the treatment of chronic pain is diminished by a simplistic focus on medical intervention for nociception. In fact, some recent literature indicates that CLBP is processed differently than acute back pain [6]. The present article will review basic biopsychosocial issues impacting chronic low back pain, the use of interdisciplinary programs as an appropriate treatment, and the results of a large prospective series of patients treated with this type of program.

1.1. Psychosocial Factors

The role of psychosocial factors has been well documented in both the development of CLBP and the resulting disability. These factors have been found to increase risk for acute low back pain developing into chronic pain, and for increased risk of disability associated with low back pain [7–9]. In addition, these factors adversely impact outcomes of both surgical intervention as well as success of interventional technologies such as spinal cord stimulation or intrathecal pumps for pain control [10–13].

A variety of psychosocial factors have been found to be of relevance [8,14]. Clinical assessment often examines an array of factors [11]: contextual factors such as work related factors, co-occurring life stressors, financial and social reinforcement for pain behavior and disability, and patterns of medical practice, all of which impact outcomes. Other factors evaluated include psychosocial factors such as depression and anxiety, as well as patient expectations, fear of movement (kinesiophobia), reactivity to pain such as pain catastrophizing, and external locus of control. Information is often obtained through both interview and psychometric testing.

In light of data indicating the impact of a biopsychosocial model, interventions based on these factors are used with varying degrees of frequency and have become commonly recommended [15,16]. The most common nonsurgical or non-medication intervention has been physical therapy with most patients being prescribed therapy at some point in their treatment. A second well-established approach has been cognitive behavioral therapy (CBT) to address the psychosocial factors. [17,18].

1.2. Interdisciplinary Pain Management Programs

In light of the interactive nature of many factors using the biopsychosocial model, one response has been the development of the interdisciplinary pain management program [19]. To address this complex array of factors, interdisciplinary pain programs began to appear in the United States initially led by John Bonica. Over the last 40 years, such pain programs have been created throughout the United States. These programs have been described by a primary accreditation organization, CARF International. They define a program in this way: "An interdisciplinary pain rehabilitation program provides outcomes-focused, coordinated, goal-oriented interdisciplinary team services". p.12 [20]. They include goals such as a reduction of impairment and activity limitations, while maximizing quality of life.

These programs include multiple types of providers (physicians, psychologists, nurses, occupational therapists, physical therapists) offering coordinated services "under one roof", with frequent communication through team meetings around a unified vision and goals. They utilize standardized measurement of functioning of physical ability, pain and suffering, emotional distress, utilization of medical resources, and functional activities of living. The model emphasizes the use of structured supervised physical activation with treatment to change behavioral and social patterns which have evolved from, and have changed, the patients' experience of pain as well as their life functioning. Treatment is designed to address the array of factors impacting patients' pain, distress, and subsequent disability. It is interesting that some of these factors are ones found by Pincus [8], which predict chronicity/disability in prospective cohorts with low back pain.

Over the last 30 years, the effectiveness of these programs has been extensively examined for both treatment efficacy and cost-effectiveness [19,21–26]. Fullen *et al.* [27] documented effectiveness of treatment of 553 patients with pain over an 8-year period of time. Chou and colleagues in 2009 [28], in the American Pain Society's Guidelines for Low Back Pain, gave a "strong" recommendation for the use of interdisciplinary treatment and rated evidence as "high" quality. More recently, a Cochrane System Review and meta-analysis found moderate-quality evidence of programs reducing pain and disability [29]. When clinical efficacy and cost efficacy of interdisciplinary pain programs were compared to conventional treatment [23,30], the programs resulted in greater pain reduction, medication reduction, reduction of emotional distress, decreased health care utilization, reduction of iatrogenic consequences, increased activity/return to work, and closure of disability claims. These same reviews compared cost of interdisciplinary programs to surgical intervention, and conventional care including the cost of initial treatment, subsequent surgery, medical treatment in the year following, and lifetime disability. Interdisciplinary treatment was found to be nine times more cost-effective than conservative treatment. Some studies have documented the economic cost of patients being placed on waitlists for interdisciplinary pain facilities [24]. In addition to these group changes, Federoff *et al.* [31] documented the efficacy of programs at the level of individuals, rather just on a group basis. Significant variability was found in response to treatment, but no clear predictors of response were found. In an extension of work by Morley [32], Smith *et al.* [33] repeated an analysis of both group and individual response. They also found that outcomes changed when outcomes from two different time sequences were compared.

Several issues warrant further exploration. First, few studies have examined the impact of providing similar programs at multiple sites to see if effectiveness is similar in various treatment settings. Second, the role of the duration of treatment has been explored in a limited fashion [34–36] without evidence of strong effect of duration of treatment. Oslund *et al.* [36] in an unpublished dissertation compared outcomes for patients with three levels of treatment: 120 h, 72 h, and 24 h. It was found that patients with higher dysfunction pretreatment (*i.e.*, greater number of hours resting a day and high levels of pain) profited more with high intensity treatment, whereas persons with lower dysfunction did not respond differentially to levels of intensity of treatment.

In order to further evaluate these issues, the present study utilized a large data set collected over 14 years from two programs with similar models but different locations to address three questions. First, prior to analyzing site and duration, did the program as a whole produce clinically significant change at the completion of treatment across a broad range of outcomes in a large sample of persons with low back pain? Second, were outcomes at the two sites of the program similar or significantly different? Third, did a range of intensity (days of treatment) create differences in outcomes?

2. Experimental Section

Data were collected from a larger data set accumulated for quality control purposes of patients attending the comprehensive interdisciplinary program (Baylor Center for Pain Management) from 2000 to 2014. Four hundred eighty five patients (40%) had a primary diagnosis of back pain according to the Pain Region, as defined by the International Association for the Study of Pain [37]. Of these, 393 (81%) completed treatment. Patients provided written consent to have data included for outcomes analysis. This retrospective study was approved by the IRB at the Baylor Research Institute.

2.1. Program Description

The comprehensive outpatient program at the Baylor Center for Pain Management in Dallas, Texas, has provided interdisciplinary treatment since 1995. This program was carried at two sites—in Dallas and Richardson—with the same treatment protocol, staffing patterns, program direction, and standard outcomes measures and procedures. Each site utilized a psychologist, a licensed professional counselor providing biofeedback, an occupational therapist, a physical therapist, and a case manager. Both sites were under the direction of the same program director over the 15 years providing broad stability in treatment and data collection. Program size would range from 2–12 patients at a time. Patients were included if pain was chronic (over 6 months), it interfered with functional activities and/or demonstrated elevated emotional distress, and patients reported desire for improvement and functional goals. Patients were excluded if their level of psychiatric problems or cognitive functions would interfere with participation and understanding in a group-oriented program. As an outpatient program, patients were required to be safe and independent for all self-care, ambulation, and transfers. Patients were also required to set goals and to commit to regular participation in the programs.

Initially, the program consisted of 20 days of treatment (approximately 100 h) but, over time, has been reduced to 12 days of treatment (approximately 60 h) to adapt to scheduling needs of patients and insurance carriers. Daily patients participated in one hour of physical therapy, one hour of aquatics therapy, one hour of counseling or biofeedback, one hour CBT group, one hour occupational therapy group, one mind/body technique for pain control, and one hour occupational therapy with focus on lifestyle management for adaptive living including return to work. Training in meditative practice, biofeedback, as well as consultation with chaplain services and nutrition services were included.

2.2. Measurement

Data were gathered upon admission to the program (Day 1) and at the final day of treatment. Outcomes included changes in pain, emotional distress, activity levels, medical utilization, physical abilities, instrumental activities of living, and patients' perception of change. These data are used to measure primary outcomes indicated by the IMPACCT group [16,38].

2.2.1. Descriptive Statistics

Upon admission, patients completed a questionnaire which included demographic data, duration of pain (in months), and estimate of utilization of medical resources in the year prior.

2.2.2. Outcome Measures

Abbreviations are as follows: the Multidimensional Pain Inventory (MPI) [39]; Beck Depression Inventory (BDI); Canadian Occupational Performance Measure (COPM) [40]. Daily Life Questionnaire measured patient rating of hours active, efficacy of non-medication pain management techniques, and physical therapy including distance walked in 5 min (measured in laps).

2.2.3. Patients' Rating of Change

In addition, at graduation, patients completed the Patients' Global Impression of Change (PGIC) scale [41] and a rating of changes in use of medication.

2.3. Data Analysis

Initial analysis was made by combining data from graduates from the two sites. Descriptive analysis was conducted for the program's primary descriptors of the participants, including frequency of categorical variables and means and standard deviations for continuous variables with the exception of duration for which median and range were chosen due to the extreme variability. Shapiro-Wilk tests for normality of distribution were carried out on variables. Because distributions did not meet assumptions of normality, a series of Wilcoxon signed rank tests were used to measure the effects of treatment. Effect size was measured using the value of r, which is appropriate for Wilcoxon tests.

Second, outcome variables from the two sites were carried out using repeated-measures ANOVAs, with treatment site as one variable and individual patient's change in scores from pre to post as the second variable. It should be noted that, although some measures were not normally distributed, ANOVAs are robust to minor deviations from normality. Chi-square tests were used for categorical variables, such as the Patient's Global Impression of Change.

Third, the relationship between the numbers of days of treatment and the amount of change was calculated using a series of correlation coefficients.

3. Results and Discussion

3.1. Descriptive Data from Both Sites

Analysis of descriptive statistics (see Tables 1 and 2) found significant differences on almost all variables except gender distribution, suggesting that populations were somewhat different. Patients at Site 1 were significantly ($t(392)= -2.78$, $p = 0.004$) younger (mean = 51.8, SD = 12.4) than those at Site 2 (mean = 56.6, SD = 12.0). The duration of pain in months was also significantly shorter ($t(354)= 3.0$, $p = 0.002$) in Site 1 (mean = 95.6, SD = 117.1) than in Site 2 (mean = 146, SD = 138.9), although the distribution was so broad as to undermine meaningfulness of central tendency. Gender distribution was not different (chi square = 0.38, $p = 0.53$). Payer source was also significantly different (chi square = 11.09, $p = 0.01$).

Table 1. Descriptive statistics of each sample site. (Group 1 = Dallas; Group 2 = Richardson).

Variable	Group	N	Mean	SD	SEM
Age	1	326	51.877	12.377	0.686
	2	68	56.603	12.019	1.457
Duration of pain (months)	1	291	95.680	117.109	6.865
	2	65	146.400	138.923	17.231
Pain Treatment in Last Year (Mean/SD)					
# of MD Office visits due to pain	1	317	0.934	0.775	0.044
	2	67	0.955	0.475	0.058
# of mental health visits for pain	1	300	3.063	7.091	0.409
	2	67	3.836	7.168	0.876
# of ED visits for pain	1	298	0.977	1.704	0.099
	2	68	0.500	1.029	0.125
# of diagnostic procedures for pain	1	306	2.278	1.867	0.107
	2	65	1.815	1.776	0220
# of treatment procedures for pain	1	311	2.103	2.194	0.124
	2	67	2.836	5.918	0.723
# of surgeries for pain	1	308	0.786	1.377	0.078
	2	67	0.433	0.857	0.105

Note: SEM: Standard error, SD = standard deviation, MD = Visits to a physician, ED = Visits to the emergency department.

Table 2. Additional descriptive statistics (categorical) of each sample site. (Group 1 = Dallas; Group 2 = Richardson).

Payer Source	Group	N	Percent
Worker's Comp	1	44	15.1
	2	1	1.5
Commercial	1	142	48.8
	2	36	53.7
Medicare	1	100	34.4
	2	30	44.8
Others	1	5	1.7
	2	0	0.0

3.2. Outcomes from Combined Sites

Seven standard measures (see Table 3) were used to determine outcome by comparing scores from the start of the program (pre) to the completion of the program (post). None of the seven measures met assumptions for the normality of distribution as measured by the Shapiro–Wilk test. Paired sample t-tests found that changes for all variables were significant at the 0.001 level using Wilcoxon signed rank t-tests.

These changes were found for both self-report repeated measures—self-reported perception of clinical progress and objective measures obtained by a physical therapist (laps walked in 5 min). Changes were large as evidenced by effect sizes (ES's), ranging from 0.66–0.85. All changes were at $p = 0.001$.

Table 3. Comparison of pre- and post- program treatment outcomes using Wilcoxon signed rank tests.

Variable	Pretreatment Mean + SEM	Posttreatment Mean + SEM	Statistic (df)	*p* Value	Effect Size *
Pain severity (n = 375)	8.61 ± 0.10	6.74 ± 0.11	45,498 (374)	<0.001	0.66
Pain interference (n = 375)	10.18 + 0.10	7.21 + 0.15	48,217 (374)	<0.001	0.77
Depression (n = 376)	21.52 + 0.54	10.18 + 0.44	63,676 (375)	<0.001	0.82
Hours active (n = 360)	4.88 ± 0.15	8.26 ± 0.15	2725 (357)	<0.001	0.78
Helpfulness (n = 341)	3.28 + 0.11	7.53 + 0.10	509 (340)	<0.001	0.85
Ability to do ADLs (n = 259)	3.35 + 0.12	7.50 + 0.32	252 (258)	<0.001	0.85
Distance walked (n = 377)	14.17 + 0.28	20.49 + 0.33	701.97	<0.001	0.85

Pain severity, Pain Interference, (Modified Multidimensional Pain Inventory—Pain Severity, Pain Interference, Range = 0–12), Depression (Beck Depression Inventory-II), Helpfulness (How helpful are your techniques to manage your pain? Range 0–10), Ability to do ADLs (Canadian Occupational Performance Measure), Distance walked (laps walked in 5 min). * The r statistic (the z score divided by the square root of the number of observations) was used for determining Effect Size: Small ES = 0.10, Medium = −0.30, Large = 0.50.

3.2.1. Pain

Although only 36% of patients (see Table 4) achieved a pain severity reduction of 30% as a recommended target, [42], change was significant as demonstrated by a a large ES (0.6), and the helpfulness of nonmedical techniques used to manage pain had improved by 129% (ES = 0.85). In addition, it has been noted that pain reduction alone may not be an appropriate primary goal for chronic back pain [43].

Table 4. Percent of patient's achieving 30% or greater change.

Variable	# Achieving 30%/Total N	Percent Achieving 30%
Pain severity	136/375	36%
Pain interference	177/375	47%
Depression	296/376	78%
Hours active	251/360	70%
Helpfulness	278/341	82%
Ability to do ADLs	236/259	91%
Distance walked	231/377	61%

Note: # = Number.

3.2.2. Functional Activities

Prominent changes in function were also found. Interference by pain was reduced by at least 30% for 47% of patients (ES = 0.77), 70% of patients increased hours of activity by 30% (ES = 0.78), and 91% of patients increased by at least 30% in their ability to carry out primary desired activities of living as measured by the COPM (ES = 0.85).

3.2.3. Physical Measures

These self-reported changes in activity and functional ADLs were mirrored by changes in physical functioning. Distance walked in a 5-min timed task improved by at least 30% in 61% of patients (ES = 0.85).

3.2.4. Psychological Functioning

Ratings of emotional distress markedly improved. Using standard interpretation of scores, depression decreased by at least 30% in 78% of patients (ES = 0.82) with mean scores changing from moderate (pre-treatment mean = 21.5) to minimal (post-treatment mean = 10.2) range of depression using standard interpretation of the scores.

3.2.5. Medication Use

Due to the challenges in quantifying medication usage in this clinical setting, data were not collected on specific types or dosages of medication used by each patient. However, patients were asked at graduation to report any change in the use of pain medication. Of the 344 patients in this group: 13 (9%) reported taking no medications; 162 (47%) reported taking fewer; 138 (40%) were unchanged in the use of medication; and 31 (9%) reported taking more medication.

3.2.6. Patient Rating of Change

Patients reported positive changes on global impression of change. Eighty-two percent of 281 patients reporting met the *a priori* goal of either "much improved" (n = 103, 36%) or "very much improved (n = 131, 46%)". Forty-four (15%) reported "minimal improvement", and only 3 (1%) reported "no change". No patients reported being "minimally worse", "much worse", or "very much worse".

3.3. Comparison of Outcomes from the Two Sites

It should be noted that, although some measures were not normally distributed, it was decided that parametric tests would be conducted because of the clarity of presentation, as well as the fact that ANOVAs are quite robust to minor deviations from normality. Therefore, repeated-measures ANOVAs (see Table 5) were conducted for a subset of outcomes chosen from various domains using the site as one variable and the change in repeated measures as another. Three analyses were conducted. Site outcomes were similar in most variables. Overall scores, combining pre- and post-scores at the two sites were similar with differences in only 2 of 7 measures: interference by pain ($F = 9.46$, $p = 0.002$) and distance walked in five minutes ($F = 24.56$, $p = 0.001$). Second, as reviewed above in Table 4, when sites were combined, the comparison of individuals pre/post measures were different at the $p < 0.05$ level and, in fact, were at the $p = 0.001$ level.

Table 5. Changes in outcome variables with 95% confidence intervals for both groups (program sites), within subjects (pre/post differences for combined sites), and interaction of group (program site by within subjects).

Variable	Site 1	Site 2	Between Group	Within Subjects	Within Sub Group
Pain severity			$F = 2.07, p = 0.15$	$F = 103.5, p = 0.001$	$F = 1.90, p = 0.16$
Pre-program	8.7 (2.0)	8.1 (1.9)			
Post-program	6.8 (2.2)	6.7 (2.6)			
Pain interference			$F = 9.46, p = 0.02$	$F = 219.80, p = 0.001$	$F = 3.68, p = 0.06$
Pre-program	10.3 (2.0)	9.8 (2.3)			
Post-program	7.4 (2.9)	6.1 (3.4)			
Helpfulness of Pain Techniques			$F = 1.49, p = 0.22$	$F = 863.1, p = 0.000$	$F = 2.78, p = 0.09$
Pre-program	3.3 (2.1)	3.7 (2.4)			
Post-program	7.5 (2.0)	7.5 (1.8)			
Hours active			$F = 0.00, p = 0.98$	$F = 406.8, p = 0.000$	$F = 6.84, p = 0.009$
Pre-program	4.7 (2.8)	5.4 (7.8)			
Post-program	8.3 (2.9)	7.8 (2.8)			
Depression			$F = 2.03, p = 0.15$	$F = 306.8, p = 0.001$	$F = 0.210, p = 0.65$
Pre-program	21.7 (10.4)	20.4 (11.5)			
Post-program	10.5 (8.8)	8.6 (7.9)			
Distance Walked			$F = 24.56, p = 0.001$	$F = 323.4, p = 0.001$	$F = 7.62, p = 0.006$
Pre-program	14.7 (5.7)	11.9 (4.0)			
Post-program	21.3 (6.5)	16.8 (4.5)			
Performance of ADLS			$F = 0.69, p = 0.79$	$F = 147.9, p = 0.000$	$F = 1.10, p = 0.315$
Pre-program	3.3 (2.2)	3.6 (1.5)			
Post-program	7.6 (5.9)	7.1 (1.6)			

Pain severity, Pain Interference (Modified Multidimensional Pain Inventory—Pain Severity and Pain Interference scales, Range = 0–12), Depression (Beck Depression Inventory-II), Helpfulness (How helpful are your techniques to manage your pain? Range 0–10), Performance of ADLs (Canadian Occupational Performance Measure), Distance walked (laps walked in 5 min)).

Some variability was found between measures in the interaction of the site and outcome measures. For four of the seven measures (pain intensity, pain interference, helpfulness of pain techniques, depression, satisfaction with ADL), the interaction of Site $\times$ Change was not significant at the $p = 0.05$ level. Hours of activity and distance walked each demonstrate an interaction effect of Site $\times$ Change and an amount of change (F = 406.8, $p = 0.009$; F = 7.62, $p = 0.006$). Chi-square tests of patient ratings of five ratings of improvement by pain site revealed no significant difference between sites (chi square = 4.620, $p = 0.33$).

3.4. Impact of Intensity of Treatment with Outcomes

Finally, the amount of change for selected variables was evaluated to determine correlation with the number of days of treatment completed. Although several change scores were correlated at the $p = 0.01$ level (*i.e.*, helpfulness of techniques) and at the $p = 0.001$ level (*i.e.*, hours active, distance walked), these correlations were quite low. For example, although significant, the number of days of treatment completed only accounted for 4% of the variance ($r^2 = 0.41$) in the change in hours active per day.

4. Conclusions

This study explored three aspects of interdisciplinary programs for treatment of chronic pain. In the first analysis, results were consistent with previous literature indicating that interdisciplinary pain management programs can provide broad-based change, even for patients with entrenched CLBP associated with high pain, emotional distress, functional disability, and excessive use of medications and medical resources. Consistent with recommendations by the Initiative on Methods, Measurement, and Pain Assessment in Clinical Trials (IMMPACT) group and others for research with chronic low back pain [38,44], it included repeated measures of pain, physical functioning, emotional functioning, and participants ratings of improvement. These changes were both highly significant statistically, as well as having large effect sizes. These findings are consistent with the previous studies of the effectiveness of interdisciplinary pain programs for patients with low back pain [22,23]. Of note, the types of change and size of change are comparable to those obtained with more invasive or intensive medical measures, which are more costly or have higher iatrogenic risks. Interdisciplinary pain programs have produced an analgesic effect comparable to opioids for CLBP or back pain with chronic radiculitis, but without the risk of overdose, addiction, and diversion [45,46]. The functional benefits noted are also important because they are not associated with the risks and complications associated either with spine surgery or even spinal cord stimulation [19].

Although this study was confirmatory of previous studies, a number of potential limitations should be noted. First, this was not a randomized controlled trial, but data were collected on a prospective basis as part of a quality assurance assessment. As such, there was no control group, so a potential placebo effect could not be measured or ruled out. Second, 20% of patients discontinued treatment for a variety of reasons, and, due to the focus of this study, no analysis was made of factors predicting non-completion or the degree of change during the program. A previous study of these programs, however, with all diagnostic groups included, found predictors for non-completion and identified factors predicting a response to treatment [36].

In addition, these changes reflect immediate effects of treatment at program completion. Additional literature [31–33] suggests that the psychological effects of intervention tend to lessen over time. This was found in an earlier study with this same program [47]. Continued change from pre-treatment was found on all measures at the $p > 0.001$ level, both six months and one year following treatment. However, six months later, some measures had regressed towards the pre-treatment scores, yet others had remained stable, and some had even continued to improve. All measures had regressed somewhat one year following treatment.

In the second analysis, this study also documented that interdisciplinary programs were effective across treatment sites. Patient populations were somewhat different based on descriptive data, such as age and duration of pain. Despite this, groups did not differ globally on a variety of measures selected to represent an array of domains. In addition, there were no differences in change at the two sites on six of seven measures, although difference in response was noted on one measure: change in distance walked in five minutes. This study suggests that, even with somewhat different populations, interdisciplinary programs were robust in the change they produced.

In the third analysis, this study also provided evidence that change was only minimally correlated with the number of days of treatment. Despite statistically significant correlations between the numbers of days of treatment, days of treatment only accounted for 4% of variance at most. This finding is consistent with the results of a previous review [35].

As Gatchel *et al.* [19] noted in their recent review, it is troubling that interdisciplinary pain programs have often been allowed to fail. It continues to be puzzling that a treatment protocol with well-documented improvements in patient quality of life and patient satisfaction is so often unavailable or not offered to patients (and healthcare providers) who are "stuck". The benefit to healthcare systems would likely be even greater if treatment programs were provided to patients much sooner following the onset of pain. This study provides additional confirmation that these programs may robustly provide effective treatment, even with variation between program staff and settings and with variable duration of treatment.

Acknowledgments: The authors wish to acknowledge the contributions of the members of the interdisciplinary team at the Baylor Center for Pain Management in Dallas and Richardson.

Author Contributions: Primary collection of data was carried out under the supervision of Timothy Clark, analysis of data was carried out by Jean-Claude Wakim, and writing was carried out by Timothy Clark, Jean-Claude Wakim, and Carl Noe.

Conflicts of Interest: The authors declare no conflicts of interest.

References

1. Mackey, S. National Pain Strategy Task Force: The strategic plan for the IOM Pain Report. *Pain Med.* **2014**, *15*, 1070–1071. [CrossRef] [PubMed]
2. Institute of Medicine (US) Committee on Advancing Pain Research, Care, and Education. *Relieving Pain in America: A Blueprint for Transforming Prevention, Care, Education, and Research*; National Academies Press (US): Washington, DC, USA, 2011.
3. Brennan, M.J. The clinical implications of cytochrome p450 interactions with opioids and strategies for pain management. *J. Pain Symptom Manag.* **2012**, *44*, S15–S22. [CrossRef] [PubMed]
4. Murray, C.J.; Abraham, J.; Ali, M.K.; Alvarado, M.; Atkinson, C.; Baddour, L.M.; Bartels, D.H.; Benjamin, E.J.; Bhalla, K.; Birbeck, G.; *et al.* The state of US health, 1990–2010: Burden of diseases, injuries, and risk factors. *JAMA* **2013**, *310*, 591–608. [CrossRef] [PubMed]
5. Gatchel, R.J.; Peng, Y.B.; Peters, M.L.; Fuchs, P.N.; Turk, D.C. The biopsychosocial approach to chronic pain: Scientific advances and future directions. *Psychol. Bull.* **2007**, *133*, 581–624. [CrossRef] [PubMed]
6. Hashmi, J.A.; Baliki, M.N.; Huang, L.; Baria, A.T.; Torbey, S.; Hermann, K.M.; Schnitzer, T.J.; Apkarian, A.V. Shape shifting pain: Chronification of back pain shifts brain representation from nociceptive to emotional circuits. *Brain* **2013**, *136*, 2751–2768. [CrossRef] [PubMed]
7. Hill, J.C.; Whitehurst, D.G.; Lewis, M.; Bryan, S.; Dunn, K.M.; Foster, N.E.; Konstantinou, K.; Main, C.J.; Mason, E.; Somerville, S.; *et al.* Comparison of stratified primary care management for low back pain with current best practice (STarT Back): A randomised controlled trial. *Lancet* **2011**, *378*, 1560–1571. [CrossRef]
8. Pincus, T.; Burton, A.K.; Vogel, S.; Field, A.P. A systematic review of psychological factors as predictors of chronicity/disability in prospective cohorts of low back pain. *Spine* **2002**, *27*, E109–E120. [CrossRef] [PubMed]
9. Mehling, W.E.; Ebell, M.H.; Avins, A.L.; Hecht, F.M. Clinical decision rule for primary care patient with acute low back pain at risk of developing chronic pain. *Spine J.* **2015**, *15*, 1577–1586. [CrossRef] [PubMed]
10. Block, A.R.; Marek, R.J.; Ben-Porath, Y.S.; Kukal, D. Associations between pre-implant psychosocial factors and spinal cord stimulation outcome: Evaluation using the MMPI-2-RF. *Assessment* **2015**. [CrossRef] [PubMed]
11. Block, A.R.; Ohnmeiss, D.D.; Guyer, R.D.; Rashbaum, R.F.; Hochschuler, S.H. The use of presurgical psychological screening to predict the outcome of spine surgery. *Spine J.* **2001**, *1*, 274–282. [CrossRef]

12. Davis, C.E.; Kyle, B.N.; Thorp, J.; Wu, Q.; Firnhaber, J. Comparison of pain, functioning, coping, and psychological distress in patients with chronic low back pain evaluated for spinal cord stimulator implant or behavioral pain management. *Pain Med.* **2015**, *16*, 753–760. [CrossRef] [PubMed]

13. Marek, R.J.; Block, A.R.; Ben-Porath, Y.S. The Minnesota Multiphasic Personality Inventory-2-Restructured Form (MMPI-2-RF): Incremental validity in predicting early postoperative outcomes in spine surgery candidates. *Psychol. Assess.* **2015**, *27*, 114–124. [CrossRef] [PubMed]

14. Campbell, P.; Bishop, A.; Dunn, K.M.; Main, C.J.; Thomas, E.; Foster, N.E. Conceptual overlap of psychological constructs in low back pain. *Pain* **2013**, *154*, 1783–1791. [CrossRef] [PubMed]

15. Chou, R.; Qaseem, A.; Snow, V.; Casey, D.; Cross, J.T., Jr.; Shekelle, P.; Owens, D.K. Diagnosis and treatment of low back pain: A joint clinical practice guideline from the American College of Physicians and the American Pain Society. *Ann. Intern. Med.* **2007**, *147*, 478–491. [CrossRef] [PubMed]

16. Deyo, R.A.; Dworkin, S.F.; Amtmann, D.; Andersson, G.; Borenstein, D.; Carragee, E.; Carrino, J.; Chou, R.; Cook, K.; DeLitto, A.; *et al.* Report of the NIH Task Force on research standards for chronic low back pain. *J. Pain.* **2014**, *15*, 569–585. [CrossRef] [PubMed]

17. Williams, A.C.C.; Eccleston, C.; Morley, S. Psychological Therapies for the Management of Chronic Pain (Excluding Headache) in Adults. In *Cochrane Database of Systematic Reviews*; John Wiley & Sons, Ltd.: New York, NY, USA, 2012.

18. Ehde, D.M.; Dillworth, T.M.; Turner, J.A. Cognitive-Behavioral therapy for individuals with chronic pain: Efficacy, innovations, and directions for research. *Am. Psychol.* **2014**, *69*, 153–166. [CrossRef] [PubMed]

19. Gatchel, R.J.; McGeary, D.D.; McGeary, C.A.; Lippe, B. Interdisciplinary chronic pain management: Past, present, and future. *Am. Psychol.* **2014**, *69*, 119–130. [CrossRef] [PubMed]

20. Committee on the Accreditation of Rehabiliation Facilities (CARF). 2015 Medical Rehabilitation Program Descriptions. Available online: www.carf.org/ProgramDescriptions/MED-InterdisciplinaryPain-Outpatient/ (accessed on 16 December 2015).

21. Flor, H.; Fydrich, T.; Turk, D.C. Efficacy of multidisciplinary pain treatment centers: A meta-analytic review. *Pain* **1992**, *49*, 221–230. [CrossRef]

22. Rainville, J.; Nguyen, R.; Suri, P. Effective Conservative Treatment for Chronic Low Back Pain. *Semin. Spine Surg.* **2009**, *21*, 257–263. [CrossRef] [PubMed]

23. Gatchel, R.J.; Okifuji, A. Evidence-based scientific data documenting the treatment and cost-effectiveness of comprehensive pain programs for chronic nonmalignant pain. *J. Pain* **2006**, *7*, 779–793. [CrossRef] [PubMed]

24. Guerriere, D.N.; Choinière, M.; Dion, D.; Peng, P.; Stafford-Coyte, E.; Zagorski, B.; Banner, R.; Barton, P.M.; Boulanger, A.; Clark, A.J.; *et al.* The Canadian STOP-PAIN project - Part 2: What is the cost of pain for patients on waitlists of multidisciplinary pain treatment facilities? *Can. J. Anaesth.* **2010**, *57*, 549–558. [CrossRef] [PubMed]

25. Stanos, S. Focused review of interdisciplinary pain rehabilitation programs for chronic pain management. *Curr. Pain Headache Rep.* **2012**, *16*, 147–152. [CrossRef] [PubMed]

26. Morley, S.; Williams, A.; Hussain, S. Estimating the clinical effectiveness of cognitive behavioural therapy in the clinic: Evaluation of a CBT informed pain management programme. *Pain* **2008**, *137*, 670–680. [CrossRef] [PubMed]

27. Fullen, B.M.; Blake, C.; Horan, S.; Kelley, V.; Spencer, O.; Power, C.K. Ulysses: The effectiveness of a multidisciplinary cognitive behavioural pain management programme-an 8-year review. *Ir. J. Med. Sci.* **2014**, *183*, 265–275. [CrossRef] [PubMed]

28. Chou, R.; Loeser, J.D.; Owens, D.K.; Rosenquist, R.W.; Atlas, S.J.; Baisden, J.; Carragee, E.J.; Grabois, M.; Murphy, D.R.; Resnick, D.K.; *et al.* Interventional therapies, surgery, and interdisciplinary rehabilitation for low back pain: An evidence-based clinical practice guideline from the American Pain Society. *Spine* **2009**, *34*, 1066–1077. [CrossRef] [PubMed]

29. Kamper, S.J.; Apeldoorn, A.T.; Chiarotto, A.; Smeets, R.J.; Ostelo, R.W.; Guzman, J.; van Tulder, M.W. Multidisciplinary biopsychosocial rehabilitation for chronic low back pain: Cochrane systematic review and meta-analysis. *BMJ* **2015**. [CrossRef] [PubMed]

30. Sveinsdottir, V.; Eriksen, H.R.; Reme, S.E. Assessing the role of cognitive behavioral therapy in the management of chronic nonspecific back pain. *J. Pain Res.* **2012**, *5*, 371–380. [PubMed]

31. Fedoroff, I.C.; Blackwell, E.; Speed, B. Evaluation of group and individual change in a multidisciplinary pain management program. *Clin. J. Pain* **2014**, *30*, 399–408. [CrossRef] [PubMed]

32. Morley, S. Efficacy and effectiveness of cognitive behaviour therapy for chronic pain: Progress and some challenges. *Pain* **2011**, *152*, S99–S106. [CrossRef] [PubMed]

33. Smith, J.G.; Knight, L.; Stewart, A.; Smith, E.L.; McCracken, L.M. Clinical effectiveness of a residential pain management programme—Comparing a large recent sample with previously published outcome data. *Br. J. Pain* **2016**, *10*, 46–58. [CrossRef]

34. Rose, M.J.; Reilly, J.P.; Pennie, B.; Bowen-Jones, K.; Stanley, I.M.; Slade, P.D. Chronic low back pain rehabilitation programs: A study of the optimum duration of treatment and a comparison of group and individual therapy. *Spine* **1997**, *22*, 2246–2251. [CrossRef] [PubMed]

35. Scascighini, L.; Toma, V.; Dober-Spielmann, S.; Sprott, H. Multidisciplinary treatment for chronic pain: A systematic review of interventions and outcomes. *Rheumatology* **2008**, *47*, 670–678. [CrossRef] [PubMed]

36. Oslund, S.R. Predictors of Success Across Differing Interdisciliary Pain Programs: Who Benefits from Which Treatment? Available online: https://repositories.tdl.org/utswmed-ir/handle/2152.5/301 (accessed on 10 November 2015).

37. Task Force on the Taxonomy of the International Association for the Study of Pain. *Classification of Chronic Pain: Descriptions of Chronic Pain Syndromes and Definitions of Pain Terms*, 2nd ed.; Merskey, H., Bogduk, N., Eds.; Intl Assn for the Study of Pain: Seattle, DC, USA, 1994.

38. Dworkin, R.H.; Turk, D.C.; Farrar, J.T.; Haythornthwaite, J.A.; Jensen, M.P.; Katz, N.P.; Kerns, R.D.; Stucki, G.; Allen, R.R.; Bellamy, N.; *et al.* Core outcome measures for chronic pain clinical trials: IMMPACT recommendations. *Pain* **2005**, *113*, 9–19. [CrossRef] [PubMed]

39. Walker, K.E. Correlates of the Scales of a Modified Screening Version of the Multidimensional Pain Inventory with Depression and Anxiety on a Chronic Pain Sample. Available online: http://gradworks.umi.com/33/77/3377470.html (accessed on 10 November 2015).

40. Canadian Occupational Performance Measure (COPM). Available online: http://www.thecopm.ca/ (accessed on 24 November 2015).

41. Kamper, S.J.; Maher, C.G.; Mackay, G. Global Rating of Change Scales: A Review of Strengths and Weaknesses and Considerations for Design. *J. Man Manip. Ther.* **2009**, *17*, 163–170. [CrossRef] [PubMed]

42. Ostelo, R.W.J.G.; Deyo, R.A.; Stratford, P.; Waddell, G.; Croft, P.; Von Korff, M.; Bouter, L.M.; de Vet, H.C. Interpreting change scores for pain and functional status in low back pain: Towards international consensus regarding minimal important change. *Spine* **2008**, *33*, 90–94. [CrossRef] [PubMed]

43. Ballantyne, J.C.; Sullivan, M.D. Intensity of chronic pain—The wrong metric? *N. Engl. J. Med.* **2015**, *373*, 2098–2099. [CrossRef] [PubMed]

44. Younger, J.; McCue, R.; Mackey, S. Pain outcomes: A brief review of instruments and techniques. *Curr. Pain Headache Rep.* **2009**, *13*, 39–43. [CrossRef] [PubMed]

45. Khoromi, S.; Cui, L.; Nackers, L.; Max, M.B. Morphine, nortriptyline and their combination *vs.* placebo in patients with chronic lumbar root pain. *Pain* **2007**, *130*, 66–75. [CrossRef] [PubMed]

46. Jamison, R.N.; Raymond, S.A.; Slawsby, E.A.; Nedeljkovic, S.S.; Katz, N.P. Opioid therapy for chronic noncancer back pain. A randomized prospective study. *Spine* **1998**, *23*, 2591–2600. [CrossRef] [PubMed]

47. Oslund, S.; Robinson, R.C.; Clark, T.C.; Garofalo, J.P.; Behnk, P.; Walker, B.; Walker, K.E.; Gatchel, R.J.; Mahaney, M.; Noe, C.E. Long-Term effectiveness of a comprehensive pain management program: Strengthening the case for interdisciplinary care. *Bayl. Univ. Med. Cent. Proc.* **2009**, *22*, 211–214.

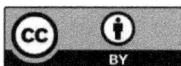

healthcare

MDPI

Article

Enhanced Brain Responses to Pain-Related Words in Chronic Back Pain Patients and Their Modulation by Current Pain

Alexander Ritter [1,2,†], Marcel Franz [1,†], Christian Puta [3], Caroline Dietrich [1], Wolfgang H. R. Miltner [1] and Thomas Weiss [1,*]

[1] Department of Biological and Clinical Psychology, Friedrich Schiller University of Jena, Am Steiger 3, Haus 1, Jena D-07743, Germany; alexander.ritter@uni-jena.de (A.R.); marcel.franz@uni-jena.de (M.F.); caroline.dietrich@uni-jena.de (C.D.); wolfgang.miltner@uni-jena.de (W.H.R.M.)
[2] Section of Neurological Rehabilitation, Hans–Berger Department of Neurology at Jena University Hospital, Erlanger Allee 101, Jena D-07747, Germany
[3] Department of Sports Medicine and Health Promotion, Friedrich Schiller University of Jena, Wöllnitzer Str. 42, Jena D-07749, Germany; christian.puta@uni-jena.de
*   Correspondence: Thomas.Weiss@uni-jena.de; Tel.: +49-3641-945143; Fax: +49-3641-945142
†   These authors contributed equally to this work.

Academic Editor: Robert J. Gatchel
Received: 14 April 2016; Accepted: 1 August 2016; Published: 10 August 2016

Abstract: Previous functional magnetic resonance imaging (fMRI) studies in healthy controls (HC) and pain-free migraine patients found activations to pain-related words in brain regions known to be activated while subjects experience pain. The aim of the present study was to identify neural activations induced by pain-related words in a sample of chronic back pain (CBP) patients experiencing current chronic pain compared to HC. In particular, we were interested in how current pain influences brain activations induced by pain-related adjectives. Subjects viewed pain-related, negative, positive, and neutral words; subjects were asked to generate mental images related to these words during fMRI scanning. Brain activation was compared between CBP patients and HC in response to the different word categories and examined in relation to current pain in CBP patients. Pain-related words vs. neutral words activated a network of brain regions including cingulate cortex and insula in subjects and patients. There was stronger activation in medial and dorsolateral prefrontal cortex (DLPFC) and anterior midcingulate cortex in CPB patients than in HC. The magnitude of activation for pain-related vs. negative words showed a negative linear relationship to CBP patients' current pain. Our findings confirm earlier observations showing that pain-related words activate brain networks similar to noxious stimulation. Importantly, CBP patients show even stronger activation of these structures while merely processing pain-related words. Current pain directly influences on this activation.

Keywords: chronic back pain; semantic processing; current pain; fMRI

1. Introduction

Processing and perceptual evaluation of noxious events and their underlying neural substrates are strongly modulated by psychological variables such as attention [1–4], emotion [5–10], expectation [11,12], and learning [13,14]. Furthermore, several studies indicate that environmental semantic and visual pain-related cues can induce activity in structures of the brain that process, among others, nociceptive information [15–17] even when no noxious stimulus is applied [18,19]. Based on Hebb's concept of cell assemblies, it can be assumed that whenever we experience pain, its semantic and emotional representations are activated simultaneously with neural structures that process noxious events and constitute the experience of pain [20,21]. Consequently, words that are used to describe pain-related experiences were found to alter pain itself [22,23], and to activate brain structures engaged in the processing of noxious stimuli, e.g., anterior cingulate cortex, insula, secondary somatosensory cortex (SII), prefrontal cortex, and parietal cortex [24,25].

It has been shown that chronic back pain (CBP) patients differ from healthy controls (HC) in structural [26], functional [27,28], and neurochemical brain parameters [29,30]. In CBP patients, pain is a common everyday experience and pain has been expressed hundreds of times throughout the course of chronic pain development. It was suggested that CBP patients as chronic pain sufferers should have developed a strong pain network and a strong link of this network to their lexicon of pain terms. Accordingly, chronic pain patients exhibit larger event-related potentials (ERPs) to painful stimuli [31], larger late ERP amplitudes when noxious stimuli were primed by pain-related words [14], and stronger blood oxygenation level dependent (BOLD) responses even when pain was not attended [32–34]. Furthermore, chronic pain patients showed larger late ERP magnitudes in response to pain-related words and rated such words more negatively than neutral words, indicating that pain-related words draw similar attention and information processing as if an actually painful stimulus would have been processed [35]. In summary, the processing of pain-related words leads to enhanced behavioral and neuronal responses even when semantic processing is precluded from conscious access.

The present study aimed to extend previous findings by investigating the processing of pain-related words in CBP patients with actually ongoing (current) back pain. It was expected that the presence of current pain would activate the brain regions important for the analysis of pain and, thereby, enhance the processing of pain-related words. These assumptions lead to the following hypotheses: H1—CBP patients exhibit different valence, arousal, and pain relevance to pain-related words compared to HC; H2—CBP patients vs. HC show a stronger activation during the processing of pain-related than non-pain-related word categories and to negative words; and H3—There is a linear relationship between the strength of current pain and the measured BOLD response during the processing of pain-related words in CBP patients.

2. Materials and Methods

2.1. Patients and Controls

Participants of this study were recruited by advertisement at the university or by personal contact. Thirteen patients with CBP (2 men; 23–56 years old, mean age = 44.3 years) and thirteen pain-free HC (2 men; 24–58 years old, mean age = 46.5 years), matched for gender, age, and education, participated in this study as paid volunteers. Sociodemographic and clinical characteristics of participants are summarized in Table 1. The CBP patients have been examined by physicians and met the following criteria: (1) minimum duration of low back pain: for 6 months; (2) pain classified as 'non-specific low back pain' (no indication for nerve root problems and radiation to foot or toes, numbness and/or paraesthesia; straight leg raising test caused no leg pain); (3) magnetic resonance imaging (MRI) of the spine only indicated age-related wear and tear but no spinal disorders or disc pathology; (4) no psychiatric disorders, no disease associated to small fiber pathology (e.g., diabetes mellitus), no other chronic disorder; (5) no use of medication (except contraceptive) for at least 48 h prior to the experiment (requested before scanning). All participants were native German speakers and right-handed as assessed by the Edinburgh Handedness Inventory (EHI) [36]. None of the healthy controls reported former subacute or chronic pain episodes (longer than one month), any neurological, psychiatric or other chronic disorder. Because depression may alter the processing of pain-related words [37], depressive symptoms were assessed with a German version of the Beck Depression Inventory-II (BDI-II) [38]. For the assessment of catastrophizing thoughts and persuasions, all subjects completed the Pain Catastrophizing Scale (PCS, [39]; German version: [40]). In accordance with the

Declaration of Helsinki, written informed consent was obtained from each participant before the study, and the Ethics Committee of the Friedrich Schiller University approved the experiment.

Table 1. Demographic and clinical characteristics as well as behavioral data of chronic back pain patients (CBP) and healthy controls (HC).

	CBP	HC			
Sex					
Male/Female	2/11	2/11			
Age (in years)	44.31 ± 12.15	46.46 ± 10.19			
Range	23–56	24–58			
Pain history					
6–12 months	$N = 2$	$N = 0$			
2–5 years	$N = 4$	$N = 0$			
>5 years	$N = 7$	$N = 0$			
Pain intensity			*t*	*df*	*p*
Mean pain intensity (VAS [a] recent 4 weeks)	3.31 ± 1.83	0.09 ± 0.30	5.72	10.53	<0.001
Strongest pain (VAS recent 4 weeks)	5.14 ± 1.85	0.27 ± 0.90	6.27	12.76	<0.001
Current pain (VAS post scanning)	1.72 ± 1.34	0.05 ± 0.15	4.15	10.25	0.002
BDI [b] *score*	7.77 ± 5.13	2.62 ± 1.76	3.50	12.12	0.004
Pain Catastrophizing Scale (PCS)	14.08 ± 6.11	11.82 ± 7.04	0.61	24	0.550
Rumination	5.46 ± 3.46	5.09 ± 3.27	0.12	24	0.905
Helplessness	4.85 ± 3.11	4.00 ± 2.61	0.49	24	0.632
Magnification	3.77 ± 2.32	2.73 ± 2.19	0.98	24	0.351
Task difficulty [c]	1.38 ± 1.50	1.38 ± 1.50	0	24	1
			χ^2		
Correct word categorization [d]	15.66 ± 0.79	15.45 ± 1.65	0.04	1	0.865

Note: Values are mean ± SD; [a] Visual Analogue Scale (VAS): 0 = "no pain", 10 = "strongest pain imaginable"; [b] BDI = Beck Depression Inventory; [c] Visual Analogue Scale (VAS): 0 = "very easy", 10 = "very difficult"; [d] correct categorizations out of 16 judgments.

2.2. Verbal Stimuli

Verbal stimuli included pain-related and non-pain-related negative, neutral, and positive adjectives. In a pilot study, 40 words were selected, and rated for valence, arousal, and pain relevance. Pain-related adjectives, affectively negative adjectives, and positive adjectives were matched for arousal. In addition, pain-related and negative adjectives were also matched for valence. Furthermore, word categories were matched according to the number of syllables and frequency in German language (COSMAS II database, http://www.ids-mannheim.de/cosmas2/). For a more detailed description of stimulus selection and the stimulus set, see Richter, Eck, Straube, Miltner and Weiss [32].

2.3. Experimental Procedure

Examples of each word category were presented while participants were familiarized with the experimental procedure prior to the experiment. A video beamer projected the stimuli onto a screen mounted on the head coil of the MRI scanner. The experimental design is displayed in Figure 1. Subjects were instructed to focus on the semantics of the words by generating a mental image of a situation associated with the word. To increase compliance, subjects were told that they would be asked for examples of their imaginations after the experiment. All subjects were able to associate appropriate mental images to the words. For example, neutral word "traubenförmig" ("aciniform") was frequently associated with wine grapes and positive word "wärmend" ("warming") was commonly associated with an oven. Word stimuli were presented in 16 blocks (4 blocks of each word category). Each block consisted of five words (belonging to one word category); each word was displayed for 4.1 s and was followed by a blank screen for 0.1 s. Each block was followed by a delay phase in which a fixation cross was presented for 11 s and a subsequent interval of 7 s. During this interval, subjects were requested to choose the correct word category from two categories presented (e.g., A = pain-related, B = negative). Subjects responded by a MRI-compatible button response box fixed below their right hand. After the selection, a fixation cross was presented for 13 s. Each word was presented twice throughout the experiment. The order of the words within each block and the order of blocks were pseudo-randomized with the restriction that the same word category was not presented twice in succession. The whole fMRI run lasted 14 min.

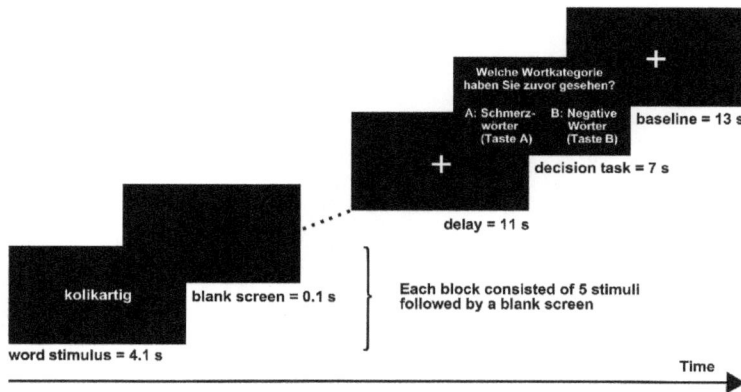

Figure 1. Stimulus protocol.

After the scanning session, participants rated the mean valence, arousal, and pain relevance of each word category on a 10-point numerical rating scale (NRS), with 0 = "negative/no arousal/not relevant", and 10 = "positive/maximum arousal/highly relevant". Following the scanning procedure, all subjects also rated their current back pain on a VAS (visual analogue scale, = "no pain", 10 = "worst pain imaginable"). The pain ratings were obtained at the end of the experiment to avoid any mutual influence between the rating of words and the pain rating. Furthermore, a rating of task difficulty was requested using a VAS (0 = "very easy", 10 = "very difficult"). During the study, we introduced the vividness of imagination scale [41] measuring emotional imagination, i.e., the ability to create emotional scenarios in mind. Higher ratings are associated with enhanced vividness of imagination.

2.4. Analysis of Behavioral Data

All statistical calculations were carried out using IBM SPSS Statistics 19 (IBM, Armonk, NY, USA). Normal distribution of behavioral data was determined by Kolmogorov-Smirnov Test. Levene's test was applied to assess the equality of variances across the two groups. Variables were statistically analyzed using Student's *t*- test if they were distributed normally; otherwise, χ^2-tests were applied. Welch's *t*-test was used for variables with unequal variances across groups. Differences between CBP patients and HC were evaluated for the ratings of arousal, valence, pain relevance, and vividness of imagination of word material [41].

To test differences of word category between patients and HC, separate two-way repeated measurements ANOVAs for mixed experimental design (between-subject factor Group and within-subject factor Word Category) were conducted. We considered values of $p < 0.05$ to be statistically significant.

2.5. fMRI-Data Acquisition and Analysis

MRI was obtained by a 3-Tesla magnetic resonance scanner (Tim Trio, Siemens, Medical Systems, Erlangen, Germany). For fMRI, 305 volumes were recorded using a T2* weighted echo-planar sequence (time to echo (TE) = 30 ms, flip angle = 90°, matrix = 64 × 64, field of view (FOV) = 192 mm, scan repeat time (TR) = 2.8 s). Each volume was comprised of 40 axial slices (thickness = 3 mm, no gap, in-plane resolution = 3 × 3 mm) parallel to the intercommissural plane (AC–PC-plane). Additionally, a high-resolution T1-weighted anatomical volume was obtained based on 192 slices with TE = 5 ms, matrix = 256 × 256 mm and resolution = 1 × 1 × 1 mm. Imaging data were pre-processed and analyzed using BrainVoyagerQX, Version 2.8 (Brain Innovation, Maastricht, The Netherlands) and NeuroElf V0.9 (Jochen Weber, SCAN Unit, Columbia University, New York City, NY, USA, http://www.neuroelf.net).

All volumes were realigned to the first volume in order to minimize the effects of head movements on data analysis. Further data pre-processing comprised spatial (6 mm full-width half-maximum isotropic Gaussian kernel) as well as temporal smoothing (high pass filter: 3 cycles per run). Anatomical and functional images were co-registered and normalized to the Talairach space [42]. Statistical analysis of fMRI-data was performed by multiple linear regression of the signal time course at each voxel. The expected blood oxygen level-dependent (BOLD) signal change for each event type (predictor) was modeled by a canonical hemodynamic response function (modified gamma function). A random-effects General Linear Model was used to identify associated brain activity in all acquired slices. To balance between type I and type II errors, we tested whether the detected clusters survived a correction for multiple comparisons. We used the approach as implemented in Brain Voyager which is based on a 3D extension of the randomization procedure described by Forman and colleagues [43,44]. First, voxel-level threshold was set at $p < 0.05$ (uncorrected). Threshold maps were then submitted to a correction for multiple comparisons for each contrast. The correction criterion was based on the estimate of the map's spatial smoothness and on a Monte Carlo simulation (1000 iterations) for estimating cluster-level false-positive rates. The minimum cluster size threshold yielding a cluster level false-positive rate of 1% was applied to the statistical maps of each contrast [45]. All clusters reported in this article survived this control of multiple comparisons. Main effects were analyzed for the contrast between pain-related words vs. baseline (hypothesis 1; H1). Separate interaction analyses including the factor Group were performed for the relevant contrasts between word categories according to H2: pain-related (weighted 3 times according to the other word categories) vs. all other word categories (negative, neutral, and positive words) and pain-related vs. negative words. For the comparison between CBP patients and HC, the variance of depression (BDI-II) served as covariate in the General Linear Model.

In the next step, we analyzed correlations between VAS pain ratings after the scanning procedure with the relevant differences of parameter estimates (difference: pain vs. negative) for the group of the CBP patients only (HC were excluded because they had no pain, so there is no variance in these parameters allowing a correlative analysis) according to H3. Voxel-level threshold was set at $p < 0.01$ (uncorrected). The map was submitted to a correction for multiple comparisons (see above). After 1000 iterations, the minimum cluster size threshold yielding a cluster level false-positive rate of 1% was applied to the statistical maps.

3. Results

3.1. Questionnaire and Behavioral Data

Questionnaire data. On average, CBP patients reported significantly higher current pain ratings ($M = 1.69$, $SD = 1.36$) than healthy controls (HC) ($M = 0.04$, $SD = 0.14$), Welch's t (12.25) = 4.34, $p < 0.001$ (Table 1). In addition, total BDI-2 scores of CBP patients ($M = 7.77$, $SD = 5.13$) were significantly higher than those of HC ($M = 2.62$, $SD = 1.76$), Welch's $t(14.78) = 3.424$, $p = .004$ (Table 1). According to BDI-scores, only one patient expressed a clinically meaningful depression (score of 20; [38]). Since results remained essentially unchanged after exclusion of this subject, we kept this subject in all further analyses. BDI showed no linear relationship to VAS ratings for current pain ($r(26) = 0.353$, $p = 0.77$). fMRI group differences were calculated with BDI II values as a covariate. There was no significant difference between groups in pain catastrophizing according to the Pain Catastrophizing Scale (PCS; Table 1).

H1: Behavioral Effects of Group and Word Category

During the experiment, all participants categorized the words properly (M_{CBP} = 15.66 and M_{HC} = 15.45 correct out of 16 judgments, see Table 1). ANOVA results of the differences between CBP patients' and HC subjects' ratings (regarding post-scanning arousal, valence, and pain relevance) of the word categories are depicted in Figure 2.

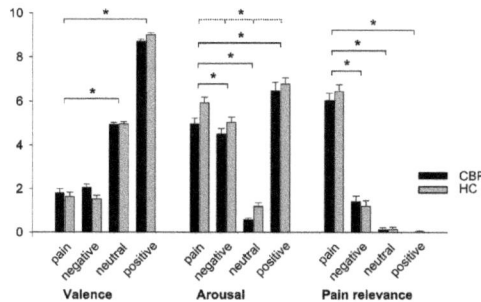

Figure 2. Mean ratings (standard errors) of valence, arousal, and pain relevance of each word category for CBP patients and HC. Valence (0 = "negative"; 10 = "positive"), arousal (0 = "no arousal"; 10 = "maximal arousal"), and pain relevance (0 = "not relevant"; 10 = "highly relevant"). Asterisks (*) indicate significant contrasts of Word Category (black line) and significant main effects of Group (dotted line).

Valence: Valence of word categories was rated differently as indicated by a significant main effect of Word Category ($F_{3, 54}$ = 940.31, $p < 0.001$, η^2 = 0.981). Contrasts were performed by comparing the pain-related word category to the remaining categories: This analysis revealed significant contrasts for neutral vs. pain-related words ($F_{1, 18}$ = 315.49, $p < 0.001$, η^2 = 0.946) and positive vs. pain-related words ($F_{1, 18}$ = 1803.89, $p < 0.001$, η^2 = 0.990). The contrast negative vs. pain-related words were not significant ($F_{1, 18}$ = 0.139, p = 0.714, η^2 = 0.008) indicating similar valence of these word categories. No significant main effect of Group ($F_{1, 18}$ = 494, p = 0.491, η^2 = 0.027) and no significant interaction of Word Category*Group ($F_{3, 54}$ = 2.41, p = 0.077, η^2 = 0.118) was observed on any valence rating.

Arousal: Mauchly's test indicated that the assumption of sphericity was violated for the main effect of Word Category, ($\chi^2(5)$ = 11.66, p = 0.040). Therefore, degrees of freedom were corrected using the Greenhouse–Geisser estimate of sphericity (ε = 0.67). As expected, there was a significant main effect of the factor Word Category on arousal ratings ($F_{2.02, 36.35}$ = 181.14, $p < 0.001$, η^2 = 0.910), with pain-related words being rated as more arousing than neutral words ($F_{1, 18}$ = 505.98, $p < 0.001$, η^2 = 0.966). A significant contrast was observed for the comparison between pain-related and positive words ($F_{1, 18}$ = 13.32, p = 0.002, η^2 = 0.425) as well as between pain-related and negative words ($F_{1, 18}$ = 11.87, p = 0.003). Likewise, there was a significant main effect of Group on arousal ratings ($F_{1, 18}$ = 13.26, p = 0.002, η^2 = 0.424) with CBP patients showing lower arousal ratings than HC. No significant interaction Word Category × Group was observed ($F_{2.02, 36.35}$ = 0.53, p = 0.597, η^2 = 0.028).

Pain Relevance: Mauchly's test indicated that the assumption of sphericity was violated for the main effect of Word Category, ($\chi^2(5)$ = 25.57, $p < 0.001$). Therefore, degrees of freedom were corrected using Greenhouse–Geisser estimate of sphericity (ε = 0.65). A repeated measure ANOVA confirmed the effect of Word Category on the rating scores of pain relevance ($F_{1.94, 34.85}$ = 413.15, $p < 0.001$, η^2 = 0.958). Contrasts of the factor Word Category confirmed that pain-related words were rated as more pain relevant than negative ($F_{1, 18}$ = 487.09, $p < 0.001$, η^2 = 0.947), neutral ($F_{1, 18}$ = 763.58, $p < 0.001$, η^2 = 0.977), and positive words ($F_{1, 18}$ = 714.04, $p < 0.001$, η^2 = 0.975). There was no significant main effect of Group ($F_{1, 18}$ = 0.13, p = 0.722, η^2 = 0.007) and no significant interaction between Word Category × Group ($F_{1.94, 34.85}$ = 0.83, p = 0.440, η^2 = 0.044).

There was also no significant main effect of Vividness of Imagination ($F_{3, 36} = 1.626$, $p = 0.2$, $\eta^2 = 0.119$) between word categories and no significant interaction Word Category × Group ($F_{3, 36} = 0.463$, $p = 0.71$, $\eta^2 = 0.037$). Average vividness ratings for both groups were 5.58 for neutral words, 5.85 for positive words, 5.65 for negative words and 5.19 for pain-related words. Higher ratings are associated with enhanced vividness of imagination. These data show that both groups were similarly able to generate the requested emotive images associated with the presented words.

3.2. Imaging

CBP patients and HC showed activations in a similar network of brain regions in response to viewing pain-related words vs. a fixation cross (baseline). This network includes—among others—the striate and extrastriate cortex of the occipital lobe extending into the fusiform gyrus, widely distributed activations in the frontal lobe bilaterally, bilateral activations of the supplementary motor area (SMA) and pre-SMA, the primary motor cortex (MI) and the anterior cingulate cortex (ACC) (Supplementary Materials Table S1). These activations are in line with previous research [32,34].

3.2.1. H2: Effects of Group and Word Category

The interaction between Group and Word category (pain-related vs. negative words) revealed increased activations in CBP patients in the medial prefrontal cortex (mPFC), the anterior midcingulate cortex (aMCC), and in the dorsolateral prefrontal cortex (DLPFC; Figure 3A and Table 2). These results are in line with H2. For separate main effects of word category (pain-related words versus negative words), see Supplementary Materials Tables S3 and S4.

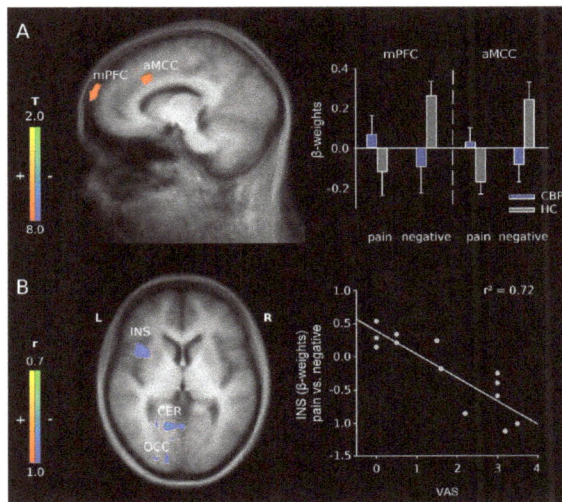

Figure 3. (**A**) activation maps illustrating the interaction between group (CBP patients vs. HC) and word category (pain-related vs. negative adjectives) with activations in the medial prefrontal cortex (mPFC) and anterior midcingular cortex (aMCC) including the dorsolateral prefrontal cortex (DLPFC); x = −10. Right: schematic overview of the β-weights for the aforementioned structures; mean + Standard Error; and (**B**) correlation of current pain (VAS) with the differences in parameter estimates for the contrast pain-related vs. negative adjectives in CBP patients in insula (INS), cerebellum (CER) and occipital cortex (OCC); z = 4. Activations are superimposed on a Talairach template (average of all subjects). Right: correlation plot for the relation of current pain (VAS) and differences in parameter estimates for the contrast pain-related vs. negative adjectives for the anterior insula.

Table 2. Activations to pain-related versus negative words in the comparison between CBP patients and HC.

x	y	z	Cluster Size	*t*-Value	Brain Region	Laterality	Brodmann Area
−20	13	35	76	4.92	anterior cingulate cortex/ dorsolateral prefrontal cortex	R/L	32
−10	−76	64	54	3.97	medial prefrontal cortex	L	10

Listed are clusters of activation with an uncorrected cluster threshold of $p < 0.05$. Talairach coordinates are provided for the maxima of the respective cluster. The corresponding neuroanatomical regions, the Brodmann areas, and the laterality (L, left; R, right) are described.

We also tested the interaction between Group and Word category for pain-related words and all other word categories [32,34]. This comparison revealed activations in the subgenual anterior cingulate cortex (sACC), the MCC, the posterior cingulate cortex (PCC), bilaterally in the posterior insula, the primary somatosensory cortex (SI) and MI, the fusiform gyrus, the posterior parietal cortex, the mPFC, and in the limbic parahippocampal gyrus (Supplementary Materials Table S2). These results confirm H2.

3.2.2. H3: Correlation Analyses of Word Category in CBP Patients

To test whether the current pain affects the processing of adjectives (H3), a correlation analysis between ratings (VAS) of current pain and the differences in activation between pain-related vs. negative words was performed for the group of CBP patients. We found clusters of negatively correlated activity in several regions including MI and the anterior insula (Figure 3B and Table 3).

Table 3. Correlations between current pain ratings (VAS) and the differences in activation between pain-related vs. negative words in CBP patients.

x	y	z	Cluster Size	*r*-Value	Brain Region	Laterality	Brodmann Area
39	13	2	48	−0.83	insula	R	13/44
45	−65	21	56	−0.84	medial temporal cortex	R	39
−16	−62	−11	108	−0.84	cerebellum	L	
5	−87	18	193	−0.88	occipital cortex	R	17/18/23
−43	−15	41	40	−0.90	precentral cortex (MI)	L	4
−4	−77	39	106	−0.91	parietal cortex/occipital cortex	L	19/7
14	−55	−8	211	−0.96	cerebellum	R	19

Listed are clusters of activation with an uncorrected cluster threshold of $p < 0.01$. Talairach coordinates are provided for the maxima of the respective cluster. The corresponding neuroanatomical regions, the Brodmann areas, and the laterality (L, left; R, right) are described.

4. Discussion

The present fMRI study revealed several important results. Firstly, our results support previous findings [32,34] that showed an increase of activation during the processing of pain-related words in several regions of the brain including parts of brain areas that also become activated when exposed to painful stimuli. Secondly, patients suffering from CBP showed stronger activations than HC for pain-related vs. other word categories in several brain structures including the insula and parts of the cingulate cortex. Thirdly, data revealed linear relationships between patients' current pain and brain activations in CBP patients in a variety of brain structures that are known to be involved in the processing of pain. Behavioral data showed only one effect including factor Group, i.e., a main effect of Group on arousal.

4.1. H1: Behavioral Effects of Group and Word Category

Behavioral data show the only effect including factor Group as main effect or interaction for arousal evoked by the different word categories. This effect results from lower arousal ratings in CBP patients compared to HC. There are several reasons that might account for this effect as well as for the absence of significant differences with respect to valence and pain relevance. First, in our sample, CBP patients had relatively low chronic back pain. We discuss this point extensively in Section 4.4 (Study Limitations). Second, ratings of CBP were especially low when the experiment took place. This has previously been reported and might result from distraction and excitement along with the scanning procedure [2,46]. Third, these partly unexpected behavioral results might be due to the permanent exposure to CBP and CBP-related stimuli that the patients suffer from. As a result, habituation to pain-related stimuli may have taken place. Fifth, we also have to take into account that pain-related words were well matched with the other word categories, but they were not specific for CBP; instead, they were referred to pain in general. This might have lowered the impact on our patients specifically suffering from CBP. Nevertheless, there were clear main effects of factor Word Category demonstrating that the expected valence and arousal were specific for each of the word categories. This might serve as a manipulation check of the stimulus material. Moreover, as there were no interaction effects of Word Category × Group on valence, arousal, or pain relevance, these effects could not account for the fMRI results.

4.2. H2: Effects of Group and Word Category

CBP patients showed stronger activations than HC during the processing of pain-related words vs. negative words in the medial prefrontal cortex and in a cluster including the aMCC and the DLPFC. In comparison, HC showed stronger brain activation during the processing of negative words and lower brain activation to pain-related words in these structures. Thus, a general difference in processing of pain-related verbal material was observed in CBP patients. Frontal lobe activity during the experience of pain was regularly observed and is generally linked to attention and cognitive processes [47,48]. The mPFC was found to be activated whenever contextual information was used to guide behavior [49]. This structure additionally exerts top-down pain modulation when cognitively demanding tasks interfere with the pain sensation [12,50–52]. Thus, activity in the mPFC seems to be strongly modulated during expectation of painful events [12]. In the sense of a priming mechanism, the pain-associated adjectives might have pre-activated a network of structures that were associated with the neuromatrix of pain in the past as a larger neural network. Thus, the cluster including the face area of M1 might be pre-activated due to painful facial expressions [53,54] according to current pain. In a broader sense, similar priming effects have also been shown for action verbs and activation of the sensorimotor cortex [55–57]. In the sense of such a priming mechanism and as the mPFC is involved in the recall of recent and remote memory traces [58], we suggest that the processing of painful words is associated with pain-related memories in CBP patients. The DLPFC is known to mediate the cognitive dimension of pain [18,59–62]. In previous studies, a stronger activation of the DLPFC was found in response to pain-related words as well [32,34]. In the present study, the activation in DLPFC is stronger in CBP patients than in HC, presumably, because these patients are prone to perceive pain more frequently and more seriously than HC. Activity of the aMCC has repeatedly been found for the subjective experience of pain [63]. More specifically, the aMCC seems to integrate pain processing and motor function [64,65]. Thus, structures that are commonly activated when CBP patients are exposed to current painful stimuli seem to be equally activated by words that indicate or connote pain.

In line with previous findings [32], the interaction between pain-related and other word categories revealed enhanced activation in several brain regions including sACC, the aMCC, the ventral posterior cingulate gyrus, the fusiform gyrus, the parahippocampal gyrus, and the posterior insula. Most of these brain areas are implicated in the experience of pain. For example, sACC is involved in the processing of emotional aspects of pain [66], but also in the processing of anxiety and stress [67]. The stronger activation of this structure in CBP patients suggests that pain-related words bear an elevated level of emotional salience and increased stress relatively to non-pain-related words of negative valence for CBP sufferers. It thus might be that their attention is more frequently focused on potential painful threats in the environment.

4.3. H3: Relationship to Current Pain

The correlation between current pain (VAS) and differences in activation between pain-related vs. negative words revealed negative correlations in MI and the anterior insula. This is in contrast to our hypothesis H3, i.e., we only found structures where the difference in activation between pain-related and negative words correlated negatively with VAS, but no structure with a positive linear correlation. This result might be due to several reasons. One possible explanation might be that current pain results in a constant activation of these structures. With fMRI, it is not possible to demonstrate this activation as the statistics belong to differences. However, if a pre-activation exists, then the activation of these structures by pain-related words might become less efficient due to pre-activation. Thus, the anterior insula might be pre-activated as a result of current pain due to its significance for the processing of salience information [17,68], which is a core feature of pain [15]. An alternative interpretation might result from the pain-inhibiting pain effect [69,70]. It is well known that two pain stimuli interact by different mechanisms influencing each other [52]. In this sense, chronic pain might result in a lower activation to a pain-related stimulus, even when this stimulus is a pain-related word.

4.4. Study Limitations

One limitation of the present study is its relative small number of participants. Strict inclusion criteria and exact matching of participants' gender and age in both groups made recruitment difficult. However, even in this rather small sample of 13 subjects per group, we revealed significant differences in fMRI activations. Another important limitation of our study is that the CBP patients showed a comparatively low CBP intensity and a relatively low tendency to pain catastrophizing. These characteristics of our CBP patients might result from our inclusion criteria that were already at the advertisement, namely the request not to use any medication (beside contraceptive) 48 h prior to the experiment. This might have deterred more seriously affected CBP patients from participating in our experiment. This limitation is not only important with respect to explaining part of the behavioral results, but it should also be taken into account for the generalizability of the fMRI results. Nevertheless, the magnitudes of pain intensity ratings differed highly significantly from HC. In addition, CBP patients were significantly more depressed than HC, indicating an impairment of everyday life due to chronic pain states. Therefore, in the sense of generalizability, we would expect that our results rather underestimate the effect of CBP. Another limitation is that fMRI group differences were calculated using depression (BDI values) as covariates. Furthermore, our subjects were requested to attend to the presented words and to produce images in their mind with respect to these words. However, we were not able to control whether subjects fulfilled the requests. Future research might investigate whether the present results will remain stable when subjects do not attend or are not requested to imagine related scenes, as well as when CBP patients are more affected than those patients of our sample.

5. Conclusions

In summary, the present results revealed that CBP patients compared to HC show enhanced activations to pain-related words in brain structures commonly activated while processing painful events and while processing words with strong associations to pain. Thus, processing of verbal pain-related information is emphasized and particularly meaningful for chronic pain sufferers. However, as differences in brain activations to verbal expressions of pain vs. negative words became smaller, the stronger the current pain was in the CBP patients. These results are in accordance with the associative network theory [56], indicating a significant and systematic interplay between word and pain processing that is enhanced during chronic pain states.

Supplementary Materials: The following are available online at www.mdpi.com/2227-9032/4/3/54/s1, Table S1: Activations to pain-related words versus baseline for CBP patients and HC, Table S2: Activations to pain-related versus all other word categories in the comparison between CBP patients and HC, Table S3: Activations to pain-related words versus negative words for HC, Table S4: Activations to pain-related words versus negative words for CBP patients.

Acknowledgments: This study was supported by the German Federal Ministry of Education and Research BMBF (01EC1003).

Author Contributions: Thomas Weiss designed the experiment, Alexander Ritter, Thomas Weiss, Marcel Franz, Caroline Dietrich, Christian Puta and Wolfgang H. R. Miltner wrote the manuscript. Alexander Ritter and Marcel Franz analyzed the data.

Conflicts of Interest: The authors declare no conflict of interest.

Abbreviations

The following abbreviations are used in this manuscript:

CBP	chronic back pain
HC	healthy control
fMRI	functional magnetic resonance imaging
BOLD	blood oxygen level-dependent
DLPFC	dorsolateral prefrontal cortex
ERP	event-related potential
VAS	visual analogue scale
NRS	numerical rating scale
mPFC	medial prefrontal cortex
INS	insula
CER	cerebellum
OCC	occipital cortex
SMA	supplementary motor area
MI	primary motor cortex
ACC	anterior cingulate cortex
PCC	posterior cingulate cortex
MCC	midcingular cortex
sACC	subgenual anterior cingulate cortex
aMCC	anterior midcingulate cortex

References

1. Kenntner-Mabiala, R.; Weyers, P.; Pauli, P. Independent effects of emotion and attention on sensory and affective pain perception. *Cogn. Emot.* **2007**, *21*, 1615–1629. [CrossRef]
2. Villemure, C.; Slotnick, B.M.; Bushnell, M.C. Effects of odors on pain perception: Deciphering the roles of emotion and attention. *Pain* **2003**, *106*, 101–108. [CrossRef]
3. Seminowicz, D.A.; Davis, K.D. Interactions of pain intensity and cognitive load: The brain stays on task. *Cereb. Cortex* **2007**, *17*, 1412–1422. [CrossRef] [PubMed]
4. Valet, M.; Sprenger, T.; Boecker, H.; Willoch, F.; Rummeny, E.; Conrad, B.; Erhard, P.; Tolle, T.R. Distraction modulates connectivity of the cingulo-frontal cortex and the midbrain during pain—An FMR1 analysis. *Pain* **2004**, *109*, 399–408. [CrossRef] [PubMed]
5. Loggia, M.L.; Mogil, J.S.; Bushnell, M.C. Empathy hurts: Compassion for another increases both sensory and affective components of pain perception. *Pain* **2008**, *136*, 168–176. [CrossRef] [PubMed]
6. Rainville, P.; Bao, Q.V.H.; Chretien, P. Pain-related emotions modulate experimental pain perception and autonomic responses. *Pain* **2005**, *118*, 306–318. [CrossRef] [PubMed]
7. Godinho, F.; Magnin, M.; Frot, M.; Perchet, C.; Garcia-Larrea, L. Emotional modulation of pain: Is it the sensation or what we recall? *J. Neurosci.* **2006**, *26*, 11454–11461. [CrossRef] [PubMed]
8. Decety, J.; Jackson, P.L.; Brunet, E.; Meltzoff, A.N. Empathy examined through the neural mechanisms involved in imagining how I feel versus how you feel pain. *Neuropsychologia* **2006**, *44*, 752–761.
9. Kenntner-Mabiala, R.; Pauli, P. Affective modulation of brain potentials to painful and nonpainful stimuli. *Psychophysiology* **2005**, *42*, 559–567. [CrossRef] [PubMed]
10. Singer, T.; Seymour, B.; O'Doherty, J.; Kaube, H.; Dolan, R.J.; Frith, C.D. Empathy for pain involves the affective but not sensory components of pain. *Science* **2004**, *303*, 1157–1162. [CrossRef] [PubMed]

11. Coghill, R.C.; Koyama, T.; McHaffie, J.G.; Laurienti, P.J. The subjective experience of pain: Where expectations become reality. *Proc. Natl. Acad. Sci. USA* **2005**, *102*, 12950–12955.

12. Wager, T.D.; Rilling, J.K.; Smith, E.E.; Sokolik, A.; Casey, K.L.; Davidson, R.J.; Kosslyn, S.M.; Rose, R.M.; Cohen, J.D. Placebo-induced changes in fMRI in the anticipation and experience of pain. *Science* **2004**, *303*, 1162–1167. [CrossRef] [PubMed]

13. Miltner, W.H.R.; Braun, C.; Arnold, M.; Witte, H.; Taub, E. Coherence of gamma-band eeg activity as a basis for associative learning. *Nature* **1999**, *397*, 434–436. [CrossRef] [PubMed]

14. Weiss, T.; Miltner, W.H.R.; Dillmann, J. The influence of semantic priming on event-related potentials to painful laser-heat stimuli in migraine patients. *Neurosci. Lett.* **2003**, *340*, 135–138. [CrossRef]

15. Iannetti, G.D.; Hughes, N.P.; Lee, M.C.; Mouraux, A. Determinants of laser-evoked EEG responses: Pain perception or stimulus saliency? *J. Neurophysiol.* **2008**, *100*, 815–828. [CrossRef] [PubMed]

16. Iannetti, G.D.; Mouraux, A. From the neuromatrix to the pain matrix (and back). *Exp. Brain Res.* **2010**, *205*, 1–12. [CrossRef] [PubMed]

17. Legrain, V.; Iannetti, G.D.; Plaghki, L.; Mouraux, A. The pain matrix reloaded: A salience detection system for the body. *Prog. Neurobiol.* **2011**, *93*, 111–124. [CrossRef] [PubMed]

18. Apkarian, A.V.; Bushnell, M.C.; Treede, R.D.; Zubieta, J.K. Human brain mechanisms of pain perception and regulation in health and disease. *Eur. J. Pain* **2005**, *9*, 463–484. [CrossRef] [PubMed]

19. Melzack, R. From the gate to the neuromatrix. *Pain* **1999**, S121–S126. [CrossRef]

20. Bower, G.H. Mood and memory. *Am. Psychol.* **1981**, *36*, 129–148. [CrossRef] [PubMed]

21. Hebb, D.O. *The Organization of Behavior: A Neuropsychological Theory*; Wiley: New York, NY, USA, 1949; p. 335.

22. Dutt-Gupta, J.; Bown, T.; Cyna, A.M. Effect of communication on pain during intravenous cannulation: A randomized controlled trial. *Br. J. Anaesth.* **2007**, *99*, 871–875. [CrossRef] [PubMed]

23. Ott, J.; Aust, S.; Nouri, K.; Promberger, R. An everyday phrase may harm your patients the influence of negative words on pain during venous blood sampling. *Clin. J. Pain* **2012**, *28*, 324–328. [CrossRef] [PubMed]

24. Gu, X.; Han, S. Neural substrates underlying evaluation of pain in actions depicted in words. *Behav. Brain Res.* **2007**, *181*, 218–223. [CrossRef] [PubMed]

25. Osaka, N.; Osaka, M.; Morishita, M.; Kondo, H.; Fukuyama, H. A word expressing affective pain activates the anterior cingulate cortex in the human brain: An fMRI study. *Behav. Brain Res.* **2004**, *153*, 123–127. [CrossRef] [PubMed]

26. Apkarian, A.V.; Sosa, Y.; Sonty, S.; Levy, R.M.; Harden, R.N.; Parrish, T.B.; Gitelman, D.R. Chronic back pain is associated with decreased prefrontal and thalamic gray matter density. *J. Neurosci.* **2004**, *24*, 10410–10415. [CrossRef] [PubMed]

27. Flor, H.; Braun, C.; Elbert, T.; Birbaumer, N. Extensive reorganization of primary somatosensory cortex in chronic back pain patients. *Neurosci. Lett.* **1997**, *224*, 5–8. [CrossRef]

28. Baliki, M.N.; Chialvo, D.R.; Geha, P.Y.; Levy, R.M.; Harden, R.N.; Parrish, T.B.; Apkarian, A.V. Chronic pain and the emotional brain: Specific brain activity associated with spontaneous fluctuations of intensity of chronic back pain. *J. Neurosci.* **2006**, *26*, 12165–12173. [CrossRef] [PubMed]

29. Wand, B.M.; Parkitny, L.; O'Connell, N.E.; Luomajoki, H.; McAuley, J.H.; Thacker, M.; Moseley, G.L. Cortical changes in chronic low back pain: Current state of the art and implications for clinical practice. *Man. Ther.* **2011**, *16*, 15–20. [CrossRef] [PubMed]

30. Siddall, P.J.; Stanwell, P.; Woodhouse, A.; Somorjai, R.L.; Dolenko, B.; Nikulin, A.; Bourne, R.; Himmelreich, U.; Lean, C.; Cousins, M.J.; et al. Magnetic resonance spectroscopy detects biochemical changes in the brain associated with chronic low back pain: A preliminary report. *Anesth. Analg.* **2006**, *102*, 1164–1168. [CrossRef] [PubMed]

31. Lutzenberger, W.; Flor, H.; Birbaumer, N. Enhanced dimensional complexity of the eeg during memory for personal pain in chronic pain patients. *Neurosci. Lett.* **1997**, *226*, 167–170. [CrossRef]

32. Richter, M.; Eck, J.; Straube, T.; Miltner, W.H.R.; Weiss, T. Do words hurt? Brain activation during the processing of pain-related words. *Pain* **2010**, *148*, 198–205. [CrossRef] [PubMed]

33. Simon, D.; Craig, K.D.; Miltner, W.H.R.; Rainville, P. Brain responses to dynamic facial expressions of pain. *Pain* **2006**, *126*, 309–318. [CrossRef] [PubMed]

34. Eck, J.; Richter, M.; Straube, T.; Miltner, W.H.R.; Weiss, T. Affective brain regions are activated during the processing of pain-related words in migraine patients. *Pain* **2011**, *152*, 1104–1113. [CrossRef] [PubMed]

35. Flor, H.; Knost, B.; Birbaumer, N. Processing of pain- and body-related verbal material in chronic pain patients: Central and peripheral correlates. *Pain* **1997**, *73*, 413–421. [CrossRef]

36. Oldfield, R.C. Assessment and analysis of handedness - edinburgh inventory. *Neuropsychologia* **1971**, *9*, 97–113. [CrossRef]

37. Nikendei, C.; Dengler, W.; Wiedemann, G.; Pauli, P. Selective processing of pain-related word stimuli in subclinical depression as indicated by event-related brain potentials. *Biol. Psychol.* **2005**, *70*, 52–60. [CrossRef] [PubMed]

38. Hautzinger, M.; Kühner, C.; Keller, F. *Bdi-ii Beck-Depressions-Inventar*; Harcourt Test Services: Frankfurt, Germany, 2006.

39. Sullivan, M.J.L.; Bishop, S.R.; Pivik, J. The pain catastrophizing scale: Development and validation. *Psychol. Assess.* **1995**, *7*, 524–532. [CrossRef]

40. Meyer, K.; Sprott, H.; Mannion, A.F. Cross-cultural adaptation, reliability, and validity of the german version of the pain catastrophizing scale. *J. Psychosom. Res.* **2008**, *64*, 469–478. [CrossRef] [PubMed]

41. Guy, M.E.; Mccarter, R.E. Scale to measure emotive imagery. *Percept. Mot. Skill* **1978**, *46*, 1267–1274. [CrossRef]

42. Talairach, J.; Tournoux, P. *Coplanar Stereotaxic atlas of the Human Brain*; Thieme: Stuttgart, Germany, 1988.

43. Forman, S.D.; Cohen, J.D.; Fitzgerald, M.; Eddy, W.F.; Mintun, M.A.; Noll, D.C. Improved assessment of significant activation in functional magnetic-resonance-imaging (fmri)—Use of a cluster-size threshold. *Magn. Reson. Med.* **1995**, *33*, 636–647. [CrossRef] [PubMed]

44. Goebel, R.; Esposito, F.; Formisano, E. Analysis of functional image analysis contest (FIAC) data with brainvoyager QX: From single-subject to cortically aligned group general linear model analysis and self-organizing group independent component analysis. *Hum. Brain Mapp.* **2006**, *27*, 392–401. [CrossRef] [PubMed]

45. Straube, T.; Schmidt, S.; Weiss, T.; Mentzel, H.J.; Miltner, W.H.R. Sex differences in brain activation to anticipated and experienced pain in the medial prefrontal cortex. *Hum. Brain Mapp.* **2009**, *30*, 689–698. [CrossRef] [PubMed]

46. Bantick, S.J.; Wise, R.G.; Ploghaus, A.; Clare, S.; Smith, S.M.; Tracey, I. Imaging how attention modulates pain in humans using functional MRI. *Brain* **2002**, *125*, 310–319. [CrossRef] [PubMed]

47. Bornhovd, K.; Quante, M.; Glauche, V.; Bromm, B.; Weiller, C.; Buchel, C. Painful stimuli evoke different stimulus-response functions in the amygdala, prefrontal, insula and somatosensory cortex: A single-trial fMRI study. *Brain* **2002**, *125*, 1326–1336. [CrossRef] [PubMed]

48. Tolle, T.R.; Kaufmann, T.; Siessmeier, T.; Lautenbacher, S.; Berthele, A.; Munz, F.; Zieglgansberger, W.; Willoch, F.; Schwaiger, M.; Conrad, B.; et al. Region-specific encoding of sensory and affective components of pain in the human brain: A positron emission tomography correlation analysis. *Ann. Neurol.* **1999**, *45*, 40–47. [CrossRef]

49. Euston, D.R.; Gruber, A.J.; McNaughton, B.L. The role of medial prefrontal cortex in memory and decision making. *Neuron* **2012**, *76*, 1057–1070. [CrossRef] [PubMed]

50. Bingel, U.; Schoell, E.; Buchel, C. Imaging pain modulation in health and disease. *Curr. Opin. Neurol.* **2007**, *20*, 424–431. [CrossRef] [PubMed]

51. Petrovic, P.; Ingvar, M. Imaging cognitive modulation of pain processing. *Pain* **2002**, *95*, 1–5. [CrossRef]

52. Tracey, I.; Mantyh, P.W. The cerebral signature and its modulation for pain perception. *Neuron* **2007**, *55*, 377–391. [CrossRef] [PubMed]

53. Kunz, M.; Chen, J.I.; Lautenbacher, S.; Vachon-Presseau, E.; Rainville, P. Cerebral regulation of facial expressions of pain. *J. Neurosci.* **2011**, *31*, 8730–8738. [CrossRef] [PubMed]

54. Kunz, M.; Lautenbacher, S.; LeBlanc, N.; Rainville, P. Are both the sensory and the affective dimensions of pain encoded in the face? *Pain* **2012**, *153*, 350–358. [CrossRef] [PubMed]

55. Pulvermuller, F. Brain embodiment of syntax and grammar: Discrete combinatorial mechanisms spelt out in neuronal circuits. *Brain Lang.* **2010**, *112*, 167–179. [CrossRef] [PubMed]

56. Pulvermuller, F.; Fadiga, L. Active perception: Sensorimotor circuits as a cortical basis for language. *Nat. Rev. Neurosci.* **2010**, *11*, 351–360. [CrossRef] [PubMed]

57. Pulvermuller, F. Brain reflections of words and their meaning. *Trends Cogn. Sci.* **2001**, *5*, 517–524. [CrossRef]

58. Hugues, S.; Garcia, R. Reorganization of learning-associated prefrontal synaptic plasticity between the recall of recent and remote fear extinction memory. *Learn. Mem.* **2007**, *14*, 520–524. [CrossRef] [PubMed]

59. Brighina, F.; De Tommaso, M.; Giglia, F.; Scalia, S.; Cosentino, G.; Puma, A.; Panetta, M.; Giglia, G.; Fierro, B. Modulation of pain perception by transcranial magnetic stimulation of left prefrontal cortex. *J. Headache Pain* **2011**, *12*, 185–191. [CrossRef] [PubMed]

60. Lorenz, J.; Minoshima, S.; Casey, K.L. Keeping pain out of mind: The role of the dorsolateral prefrontal cortex in pain modulation. *Brain* **2003**, *126*, 1079–1091. [CrossRef] [PubMed]

61. Ung, H.; Brown, J.E.; Johnson, K.A.; Younger, J.; Hush, J.; Mackey, S. Multivariate classification of structural MRI data detects chronic low back pain. *Cereb. Cortex* **2014**, *24*, 1037–1044. [CrossRef] [PubMed]

62. Bushnell, M.C.; Ceko, M.; Low, L.A. Cognitive and emotional control of pain and its disruption in chronic pain. *Nat. Rev. Neurosci.* **2013**, *14*, 502–511. [CrossRef] [PubMed]

63. Shackman, A.J.; Salomons, T.V.; Slagter, H.A.; Fox, A.S.; Winter, J.J.; Davidson, R.J. The integration of negative affect, pain and cognitive control in the cingulate cortex. *Nat. Rev. Neurosci.* **2011**, *12*, 154–167. [CrossRef] [PubMed]

64. Misra, G.; Coombes, S.A. Neuroimaging evidence of motor control and pain processing in the human midcingulate cortex. *Cereb. Cortex* **2015**, *25*, 1906–1919. [CrossRef] [PubMed]

65. Peyron, R.; Faillenot, I.; Mertens, P.; Laurent, B.; Garcia-Larrea, L. Motor cortex stimulation in neuropathic pain. Correlations between analgesic effect and hemodynamic changes in the brain. A pet study. *Neuroimage* **2007**, *34*, 310–321. [CrossRef] [PubMed]

66. Vogt, B.A. Pain and emotion interactions in subregions of the cingulate gyrus. *Nat. Rev. Neurosci.* **2005**, *6*, 533–544. [CrossRef] [PubMed]

67. Peyron, R.; Laurent, B.; Garcia-Larrea, L. Functional imaging of brain responses to pain. A review and meta-analysis (2000). *Neurophysiol. Clin.* **2000**, *30*, 263–288. [CrossRef]

68. Wiech, K.; Lin, C.S.; Brodersen, K.H.; Bingel, U.; Ploner, M.; Tracey, I. Anterior insula integrates information about salience into perceptual decisions about pain. *J. Neurosci.* **2010**, *30*, 16324–16331. [CrossRef] [PubMed]

69. Diers, M.; Koeppe, C.; Diesch, E.; Stolle, A.M.; Holzl, R.; Schiltenwolf, M.; van Ackern, K.; Flor, H. Central processing of acute muscle pain in chronic low back pain patients: An EEG mapping study. *J. Clin. Neurophysiol.* **2007**, *24*, 76–83. [CrossRef] [PubMed]

70. Reinert, A.; Treede, R.; Bromm, B. The pain inhibiting pain effect: An electrophysiological study in humans. *Brain Res.* **2000**, *862*, 103–110. [CrossRef]

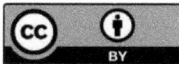

healthcare

MDPI

Review

Surface Electromyographic (SEMG) Biofeedback for Chronic Low Back Pain

Randy Neblett

Productive Rehabilitation Institute of Dallas for Ergonomics (PRIDE) Research Foundation,
5701 Maple Ave. #100, Dallas, TX 75235, USA; randyneblett@pridedallas.com; Tel.: +1-214-351-6600

Academic Editors: Robert J. Gatchel and Sampath Parthasarathy
Received: 8 February 2016; Accepted: 6 May 2016; Published: 17 May 2016

Abstract: Biofeedback is a process in which biological information is measured and fed back to a patient and clinician for the purpose of gaining increased awareness and control over physiological domains. Surface electromyography (SEMG), a measure of muscle activity, allows both a patient and clinician to have direct and immediate access to muscle functioning that is not possible with manual palpation or visual observation. SEMG biofeedback can be used to help "down-train" elevated muscle activity or to "up-train" weak, inhibited, or paretic muscles. This article presents a historical and clinical overview of SEMG and its use in chronic low back pain assessment and biofeedback training.

Keywords: surface electromyography (SEMG); biofeedback; flexion-relaxation; chronic low back pain (CLBP)

1. A Historical Overview of Biofeedback

Biofeedback is a process in which biological information is measured and fed back to a patient and clinician. Though biofeedback technology can be used for diagnostic purposes, it is most often used for self-regulation skills training. The goal of biofeedback training is to teach increased awareness and control over biological process. Due to limitations in the available technology at the time, first generation biofeedback equipment provided only an analogue needle display or a simple sound. As the technology improved in the 1970s, digital numerical displays became available. Biofeedback became computerized in the 1980s with the first Apple computers. Today, biofeedback has become much more sophisticated, allowing computerized multimedia colorful interactive displays and sounds, and allowing detailed recordings and statistical analysis of biological information. Despite these advances, the accuracy and meaningfulness of a biofeedback signal is dependent on the grade of the equipment and the skill of the practitioner, in knowing proper skin preparation, sensor placement, measurement settings, display setup, and signal interpretation [1]. A good source for biofeedback training and certification is the Biofeedback Certification International Alliance [2].

A number of biofeedback modalities are used in chronic pain management and physical rehabilitation, including autonomic nervous system measures (hand temperature, skin conductance, and heart rate), central nervous system measures (electroencephalography (EEG)), and biomechanical measures (force and pressure) [3]. Surface electromyography (SEMG) is one of the oldest biofeedback modalities [4]. It was used in clinical research as early as the 1920s, by Edmond Jacobson, the developer of the progressive muscle relaxation therapeutic technique [5,6]. When speaking with patients, clinicians often describe SEMG as measuring "muscle tension," but it is actually a measure of the electrical activity generated by muscle action potentials, which are rapid electrical signals that travel along the surface of the motor end plate, resulting in a muscle contraction [7]. SEMG allows both a patient and a clinician to have direct and immediate access to muscle functioning that is not possible with manual palpation or visual observation. Three electrodes are required to measure a single muscle area: one positive, one negative, and one reference. In biofeedback terminology, this is called a "placement." When assessing the lumbar muscles, for example, electrodes are most often applied vertically on the erector spinae muscles, with equal distance between the sensors, in two separate placements, on the left and right side of the back [8]. When measuring SEMG with a standard biofeedback instrument, the raw SEMG signal is usually converted to a root mean square, rectified SEMG signal, for easier interpretation [1]. Depending on one's clinical or research purposes, the practitioner can further modify the measurement characteristics of the signal (such as sampling rates and filters) and display characteristics of the signal (such as gain and smoothing) [1]. SEMG biofeedback has been used for general relaxation training, stroke rehabilitation, and treatment of pain. SEMG can be used to help "down-train" elevated muscle activity or to "up-train" weak, inhibited, or paretic muscles [3].

Traditional biofeedback involves an operant conditioning process in which movement toward the desired goal is shaped over time, with minimal therapist instruction [9]. This training methodology works well with autonomic nervous system modalities, in which the training goal is to lower general autonomic nervous system arousal. In fact, it is likely that most biofeedback practitioners who treat chronic pain patients use SEMG in this way. A very common SEMG placement for general relaxation training is to place one active electrode above each eye on the forehead. This Frontalis placement has historically been seen as a good indicator of emotional distress and an indicator of general tension in the rest of the body, although this second assumption has not been shown to be true [10,11]. In fact, early studies of SEMG biofeedback training for pain treatment tended to focus on the Frontalis muscle, regardless of the painful body part that was being treated [12]. Regardless of these old assumptions, stress is well known to exacerbate pain, and many chronic pain patients have poor coping strategies for managing stress, so any skills that patients can learn to help them relax, including SEMG biofeedback training to lower facial tension or other muscle tension in the body, may be found to be beneficial. General relaxation training with a variety of methods, with or without biofeedback assistance, has been shown to be an effective treatment for pain [13].

In contrast to traditional biofeedback, SEMG biofeedback for purposes of muscle re-education lends itself to a more direct coaching methodology [14]. A number of specific SEMG biofeedback protocols for treating pain have been described in the scientific literature [10,14–24]. Although EMG biofeedback is the most widely used and widely reported method of biofeedback in chronic pain treatment and rehabilitation, few clinical SEMG biofeedback training protocols have been scientifically tested and published in peer-reviewed journals [3]. The dearth of randomized control studies is perhaps due, at least in great part, to the difficulty of designing studies with credible sham SEMG feedback, which can be compared with real SEMG feedback, in assessing the efficacy of a defined biofeedback training protocol.

There are generally two goals with SEMG biofeedback training: to increase awareness of the target muscle(s); and to increase control of the muscle(s). A primary concept regarding SEMG biofeedback training with chronic pain patients is that they tend to be very poor at knowing how tense they are when compared with pain-free controls [22]. A seminal study, with chronic low back pain (CLBP) subjects, found a deficit in their ability to discriminate between higher and lower tension levels and a tendency to underestimate tension levels when they were elevated. This difficulty in estimating tension levels was found in both painful and non-painful muscles sites. It was suggested by the study's authors that these deficits may lead patients to believe that elevated muscle tension levels are in a normal range, which may preclude adjustments to lower tension levels [25]. This type of deficit in muscle awareness has been observed in thousands of chronic pain patients by this author.

2. SEMG with Chronic Low Back Pain

Lumbar SEMG measures, in both static and dynamic postures and movements, have been found to be reliable in both normal and CLBP subjects, and both within and between sessions [26–30]. Some studies have found that CLBP patients display lower SEMG levels than controls during certain movements [31–33]. In addition, static left/right asymmetries have been reported in the lumbar musculature [34,35]. Despite the commonly held assumption that muscle bracing can cause increased pain, most studies have found no significant relationship between static SEMG levels and subjective pain reports [36,37]. When comparing low back pain subjects *vs.* control subjects in various static postures, the results have been equivocal, with some studies reporting significant differences, and others not [38]. However, EMG biofeedback training of lumbar muscles in static postures has been found to be associated with significant improvements in cognitive and behavioral indices of CLBP for up to a 2.5 year follow-up [39]. Flor *et al.* (1991) found that SEMG biofeedback of the lumbar muscles in subjects with "mild" chronic back pain was superior to cognitive behavioral counseling (including relaxation without biofeedback) and medical "treatment as usual" in outcome measures of pain, functional interference, and affective distress [12]. A similar study, which replicated aspects of the biofeedback portion of the Flor *et al.* (1991) study, found clinical improvements in both the SEMG biofeedback and cognitive behavioral groups, with no significant differences between the two [40]. In a separate study of CLBP subjects with more severe functional limitations, a combination of cognitive interventions and self-regulation skills training (including SEMG biofeedback) was found to be most efficacious in clinical outcome measures [41]. Correcting muscle imbalances in CLBP subjects have been reported to result in decreased pain, with gains lasting up to four years post-treatment [35]. Interestingly, a comparison group, which was educated on lumbar muscle symmetry, demonstrated similar gains in pain to the SEMG biofeedback group. The addition of SEMG biofeedback to a traditional exercise program for CLBP subjects resulted in a significant increase in lumbar strength measures [42]. Whether the strength improvement was due to an actual change in the muscles or to a reduction of fear avoidance could not be determined.

3. The Flexion-Relaxation Phenomenon

SEMG as an assessment tool has a long history within low back pain research. Beginning in the early 1950s, researchers first began evaluating lumbar muscle activity in different postures and movements [43–46]. This is when the flexion-relaxation (FR) phenomenon was first discovered, in which lumbar muscles relax completely at maximum voluntary flexion. The FR phenomenon is perhaps the most studied pattern of lumbar SEMG activity. It has now been found in many studies that this FR pattern can be reliably measured in most normal subjects, but it is often absent in CLBP patients [26–29,45,47–51]. An extensive meta-analysis of lumbar SEMG found that measures of FR in previous studies have produced a large effect size ($d = -1.71$) in distinguishing between CLBP patients and control subjects [38]. FR deficits in low back pain subjects have also been found to be associated with self-reported disability [52], pain [44,53,54], and fear of pain and re-injury [55]. When assessed as a treatment outcome measure, positive treatment changes in FR with CLBP patients have been found to be associated with clinical improvement in self-efficacy beliefs, fear avoidance beliefs [28], perceived disability, pain intensity, and range-of-motion (ROM) [56].

More recently, attempts have been made to actively modify abnormal FR in CLBP patients with SEMG biofeedback training. A biofeedback training protocol of surface EMG-assisted stretching (SEMGAS) has been described, which teaches CLBP patients how to relax into standing maximum voluntary flexion and achieve FR [57–59]. This procedure was first introduced in the context of an interdisciplinary functional restoration program. The first study on this topic found that a majority of CLBP patients who entered the functional restoration program failed to demonstrate a normal FR pattern or normal flexion ROM. After completion of the program (with SEMGAS as a treatment component), most of them demonstrated a significantly improved FR pattern and associated ROM [29,56]. It was later demonstrated that, compared to functional restoration only, CLBP patients who participated in functional restoration with the addition of SEMGAS were significantly more successful in achieving FR after treatment completion [60]. In fact, most of these treatment patients demonstrated normalization of FR, comparable to a pain-free control group, at treatment completion. A follow-up study compared pre-treatment FR patterns and treatment responsiveness in three groups of CLBP patients: those with previous discectomies, fusions, and no previous surgeries. It was found that patients with prior surgeries initially demonstrated greater SEMG and ROM deficits, but after completing the functional restoration treatment, and participating in SEMGAS, the majority of patients in all three groups demonstrated significantly improved ROM and successfully achieved FR [61]. Two recent pilot studies, using alternative SEMGAS training methodologies than the previously cited studies, have demonstrated modest results in improving FR in groups of CLBP subjects [62,63].

4. Summary and Conclusions

As one can find with a "SEMG biofeedback for low back pain" literature search, the majority of clinical studies on this topic were performed in the 1980s and 1990s. Few clinical outcome studies that focus on SEMG biofeedback for CLBP have appeared in the scientific literature since that time. Perhaps these new studies on SEMGAS indicate a sign of renewed interest in SEMG biofeedback for CLBP. Some other new clinical research avenues may also show relevance for CLBP treatment. Recent studies on the use of real-time muscle monitoring of neck and shoulder muscles with a portable EMG device have been investigated with promising results. In three randomized control trials, portable EMG biofeedback was found to be effective for reducing muscular tension and associated pain and perceived disability in females with chronic neck/shoulder pain who were working in low-impact jobs (including computer work) [64–66]. This same technology may prove helpful for CLBP patients as well. Other new muscle-related biofeedback modalities may also be found to be useful in low back pain rehabilitation, such as real-time ultrasound imaging (RTUS) biofeedback, which provides immediate visual feedback about the shape and length of muscles as they contract and relax [3].

In conclusion, one thing is certain. Chronic pain, including CLBP, is at epidemic proportions. A new report has determined that 100 million people in the United States alone (which is almost one-third of the US population) have some form of chronic pain, and the majority of those have CLBP [67]. Thus, all therapeutic avenues, including SEMG biofeedback, should be considered within a comprehensive treatment plan for CLBP.

Acknowledgments: Thank you to Robert Gatchel and Pedro Cortez for their assistance in the preparation and publication of this article.

Conflicts of Interest: The author declares no conflict of interest.

References

1. Sherman, R.A. Instrumentation methodology for recording and feeding-back surface electromyographic (SEMG) signals. *Appl. Psychophysiol. Biofeedback* **2003**, *28*, 107–119. [CrossRef] [PubMed]
2. Biofeedback Certification Internatioanal Alliance. Become Board Certified. Available online: http://www.bcia.org/i4a/pages/index.cfm?pageid=1 (accessed on 11 May 2016).
3. Giggins, O.M.; Persson, U.M.; Caulfield, B. Biofeedback in rehabilitation. *J. NeuroEngineering Rehabil.* **2013**, *10*, 1–11. [CrossRef] [PubMed]
4. Cram, J.R. The history of surface electromyography. *Appl. Psychophysiol. Biofeedback* **2003**, *28*, 81–91. [CrossRef] [PubMed]
5. Jacobson, E. Electrical measurements of neuromuscular states during mental activities IV: Evidence of contraction of specific muscles during imagination. *Am. J. Physiol.* **1930**, *95*, 703–712.
6. Jacobson, E. Electrical measurement concerning muscular contraction (tonus) and the cultivation of relaxation in man: Relaxation times of individuals. *Am. J. Physiol.* **1934**, *108*, 573–580.
7. Shaffer, F.; Neblett, R. Practical anatomy and physiology: The skeletal muscle system. *Biofeedback* **2010**, *3*, 47–51. [CrossRef]
8. Cram, J.R.; Kasman, G.S. Electrodes and Site Selection Strategies. In *Cram's Introduction to Surface Electromyography*; Cram, J.R., Criswell, E., Eds.; Jones and Bartlett: Sadbury, MA, USA, 2010; pp. 65–73.
9. Tan, G.; Sherman, R.A.; Shanti, B.F. Biofeedback Pain Interventions: New biofeedback therapies—Together with modern technology—Provide viable alternatives in pain management. *Pract. Pain Manag.* **2003**, *17*, 12–18.

10. Alexander, A.B.; Smith, D.D. Clinical Applications of EMG Biofeedback. In *Clinical Application of Biofeedback: Appraisal and Status*; Gatchel, R.J., Price, K.R., Eds.; Pergamon: New York, NY, USA, 1979.

11. Suarez, A.; Kohlenberg, R.; Pagano, R. Is EMG activity from the frontalis site a good measure of general bodily tension in clinical populations? *Biofeedback Self-Regul.* **1979**, *4*, 293–297.

12. Flor, H.; Birbaumer, N. Comparison of the efficacy of electromyographic biofeedback, cognitive-behavioral therapy, and conservative medical interventions in the treatment of chronic musculoskeletal pain. *J. Consult. Clin. Psychol.* **1993**, *61*, 653–658. [CrossRef] [PubMed]

13. Turk, D.C.; Swanson, K.S.; Tunks, E.R. Psychological approaches in the treatment of chronic pain patients—When pills, scalpels, and needles are not enough. *Can. J. Psychiatry* **2008**, *53*, 213–223. [PubMed]

14. Neblett, R. Active SEMG training strategies for chronic musculoskeletal pain: Part 2. *Biofeedback* **2002**, *30*, 39–42.

15. Nouwen, A.; Solinger, J.W. The effectiveness of EMG biofeedback training in low back pain. *Biofeedback Self Regul.* **1979**, *4*, 103–111. [CrossRef] [PubMed]

16. Ettare, D.L.; Ettare, R. Muscle learning therapy—A treatment protocol. In *Clinical EMG for Surface Recordings*; Cram, J.R., Ed.; Clinical Resources: Nevada City, CA, USA, 1990; pp. 197–234.

17. Donaldson, S.; Donaldson, M. Multi-Channel EMG Assessment and Treatment Techniques. In *Clinical EMG for Surface Recordings*; Cram, J.R., Ed.; Clinical Resources: Nevada City, CA, USA, 1990; pp. 143–174.

18. Criswell, E. *Cram's Introduction to Surface Electromyography*, 2nd ed.; Jones and Bartlett Publishers: Sudbury, MA, USA, 2011.

19. Sherman, R.A. *Pain: Assessment & Intervention From a Psychophysiological Perspective*; The Association for Applied Psychophysiology and Biofeedback (AAPB): Denver, CO, USA, 2012.

20. Middaugh, S.J.; Kee, W.G.; Nicholson, J.A. Muscle Overuse and Posture as Factors in the Development and Maintenance of Chronic Musculoskeletal Pain. In *Psychological Vulnerability to Chronic Pain*; Grzesiak, R.C., Ciccone, D.S., Eds.; Springer Publishing Co.: New York, NY, USA, 1994; pp. 55–89.

21. Arena, J.G.; Blanchard, E.B. Biofeedback and Relaxation Therapy for Chronic Pain Disorders. In *Chronic Pain: Psychological Perspectives on Treatment*; Gatchel, R.J., Turk, D.C., Eds.; Guilford Publications, Inc.: New York, NY, USA, 2002; pp. 197–230.

22. Neblett, R. Active SEMG training strategies for chronic musculoskeletal pain: Part 1. *Biofeedback* **2002**, *30*, 28–31.

23. Schwartz, M.S.; Andrasik, F. *Biofeedback: A Practitioner's Guide*, 3rd ed.; Guilford Press: New York, NY, USA, 2003.

24. Taylor, W. Dynamic EMG Biofeedback in Assessment and Treatment Using a Neuromuscular Reeducation Model. In *Clinical EMG for Surface Recordings*; Cram, J.R., Ed.; Clinical REsources: Nevada City, CA, USA, 1990; pp. 175–196.

25. Flor, H.; Fürst, M.; Birbaumer, N. Deficient Discrimination of EMG Levels and Overestimation of Perceived Tension in Chronic Pain Patients. *Appl. Psychophysiol. Biofeedback* **1999**, *24*, 55–66. [CrossRef] [PubMed]

26. Ambroz, C.; Scott, A.; Ambroz, A.; Talbott, E.O. Chronic low back pain assessment using surface electromyography. *J. Occup. Med.* **2000**, *42*, 660–669. [CrossRef]

27. Shihvonen, T.; Partanen, J.; Hanninen, O.; Soimakallio, S. Electric behavior of low back muscles during lumbar pelvic rhythm in low back pain patients and healthy controls. *Arch. Phys. Med. Rehabil.* **1991**, *72*, 1080–1087.

28. Watson, P.J.; Booker, C.K.; Main, C.J.; Chen, A.C.N. Surface electromyography in the identification of chronic low back pain patients: The development of the flexion relaxation ratio. *Clin. Biomech.* **1997**, *12*, 165–171. [CrossRef]

29. Neblett, R.; Mayer, T.G.; Gatchel, R.J.; Keeley, J.; Proctor, T.; Anagnostis, C. Quantifying the lumbar flexion-relaxation phenomenon: Theory, normative data, and clinical applications. *Spine* **2003**, *28*, 1435–1446. [CrossRef] [PubMed]

30. Kippers, V.; Parker, A.W. Posture related to myoelectric silence of erectores spinae during trunk flexion. *Spine* **1984**, *9*, 740–745. [CrossRef] [PubMed]

31. Ahem, D.K.; Follick, M.J.; Council, J.R.; Laser-Wolston, N.; Litchman, H. Comparison of lumbar paravertebral EMG patterns in chronic low back pain patients and non-patient controls. *Pain* **1988**, *34*, 153–160.

32. Wolf, S.L.; Basmajian, J.V.; Russe, C.T.; Kutner, M. Normative data on low back mobility and activity levels. Implications for neuromuscular reeducation. *Am. J. Phys. Med.* **1979**, *58*, 217–229. [PubMed]

33. Wolf, S.L.; Nacht, M.; Kelly, J. EMG feedback training during dynamic movement for low back pain patients. *Behav. Ther.* **1982**, *13*, 395–406. [CrossRef]

34. Cram, J.R.; Steger, J.C. EMG scanning in the diagnosis of chronic pain. *Biofeedback Self Regul.* **1983**, *8*, 229–241. [CrossRef] [PubMed]

35. Donaldson, S.; Romney, D.; Donaldson, M.; Skubick, D. Randomized study of the application of single motor unit biofeedback training to chronic low back pain. *J. Occup. Rehabil.* **1994**, *4*, 23–37. [CrossRef] [PubMed]

36. Arena, J.G.; Sherman, R.A.; Bruno, G.M.; Young, T.R. Electromyographic recordings of low back pain subjects and non-pain controls in six different positions: Effect of pain levels. *Pain* **1991**, *45*, 23–28. [CrossRef]

37. Geisser, M.E.; Robinson, M.E.; Richardson, C.A. A time series analysis of the relationships between ambulatory EMG, pain, and stress in chronic low back pain. *Biofeedback Self Regul.* **1995**, *20*, 339–335. [CrossRef] [PubMed]

38. Geisser, M.E.; Ranavaya, M.; Haig, A.J.; Roth, R.S.; Zucker, R.; Ambroz, C.; Caruso, M. A meta-analytic review of surface electromyography among persons with low back pain and normal, healthy controls. *J. Pain* **2005**, *6*, 711–726. [CrossRef] [PubMed]

39. Flor, H.; Haag, G.; Turk, D.C. Long-term efficacy of EMG biofeedback for chronic rheumatic back pain. *Pain* **1986**, *27*, 195–202. [CrossRef]

40. Newton-John, T.R.O.; Spence, S.H.; Schotte, D. Cognitive-Behavioural Therapy *versus* EMG Biofeedback in the treatment of chronic low back pain. *Behav. Res. Ther.* **1995**, *33*, 691–697. [CrossRef]

41. Vlaeyen, J.W.S.; Haazen, I.W.C.J.; Schuerman, J.A.; Kole-Snijders, A.M.J.; van Eek, H. Behavioural rehabilitation of chronic low back pain: Comparison of an operant treatment, an operant-cognitive treatment and an operant-respondent treatment. *Br. J. Clin. Psychol.* **1995**, *34*, 95–118. [CrossRef] [PubMed]

42. Asfour, S.S.; Khalil, T.M.; Waly, S.M.; Goldberg, M.L.; Rosomoff, R.S.; Rosomoff, H.L. Biofeedback in back muscle strengthening. *Spine* **1990**, *15*, 510–513. [CrossRef] [PubMed]

43. Floyd, W.F.; Silver, P.H.S. Function of erectores spinal in flexion of the trunk. *Lancet* **1951**, *257*, 133–134. [CrossRef]

44. Golding, J.S.R. Electromyography of the erector spinae in low back pain. *Postgrad. Med. J.* **1952**, *28*, 401–406. [CrossRef] [PubMed]

45. Floyd, W.F.; Silver, P.H.S. The function of the erectores spinae muscles in certain movements and postures in man. *J. Physiol.* **1955**, *129*, 184–203. [CrossRef] [PubMed]

46. Morin, F.; Portnoy, H. Electromyographic study of postural muscles in various positions and movements. *Am. J. Physiol.* **1956**, *186*, 122–126. [PubMed]

47. Sihvonen, T.; Partanen, J.; Hanninen, O. Averaged (rms) surface EMG in testing back function. *Electromyogr. Clin. Neurophysiol.* **1988**, *28*, 335–339. [PubMed]

48. Kaigle, A.M.; Wessberg, P.; Hansson, T.H. Muscular and kinematic behavior of the lumbar spine during flexion-extension. *J. Spinal Disord.* **1998**, *11*, 163–174. [CrossRef] [PubMed]

49. Nouwen, A.; van Akkerveeken, P.F.; Versloot, J.M. Patterns of muscular activity during movement in patients with chronic low-back pain. *Spine* **1987**, *12*, 777–782. [CrossRef] [PubMed]

50. Paquet, N.; Malouin, F.; Richards, C.L. Hip-spine movement interaction and muscle activation patterns during sagittal trunk movements in low back pain patients. *Spine* **1994**, *19*, 596–603. [CrossRef] [PubMed]

51. Shirado, O.; Ito, T.; Kaneda, K.; Strax, T.E. Flexion-relaxation phenomenon in the back muscles: A comparative study between healthy subjects and patients with chronic low back pain. *Am. J. Phys. Med. Rehabil.* **1995**, *74*, 139–144. [CrossRef] [PubMed]

52. Triano, J.J.; Schultz, A.B. Correlation of objective measure of trunk motion and muscle function with low-back disability ratings. *Spine* **1987**, *12*, 561–565. [CrossRef] [PubMed]

53. Sihvonen, T.; Huttunen, M.; Makkonen, M.; Airaksinen, O. Functional changes in back muscle activity correlate with pain intensity and prediction of low back pain during pregnancy. *Arch. Phys. Med. Rehabil.* **1998**, *79*, 1210–1212. [CrossRef]

54. Ahem, D.K.; Hannon, D.J.; Goreczny, A.J.; Follick, M.J.; Parziale, J.R. Correlation of chronic low-back pain behavior and muscle function examination of the flexion-relaxation response. *Spine* **1990**, *15*, 92–95.

55. Geisser, M.E.; Haig, A.J.; Wallbom, A.S.; Wiggert, E.A. Pain-related fear, lumbar flexion, and dynamic EMG among persons with chronic musculoskeletal low back pain. *Clin. J. Pain* **2004**, *20*, 61–69. [CrossRef] [PubMed]

56. Mayer, T.G.; Neblett, R.; Brede, E.; Gatchel, R.J. The quantified lumbar flexion-relaxation phenomenon is a useful measurement of improvement in a functional restoration program. *Spine* **2009**, *34*, 2458–2465. [CrossRef] [PubMed]

57. Neblett, R.; Mayer, T.G.; Gatchel, R.J. Theory and rationale for surface EMG-assisted stretching as an adjunct to chronic musculoskeletal pain rehabilitation. *Appl. Psychophysiol. Biofeedback* **2003**, *28*, 139–146. [CrossRef] [PubMed]

58. Neblett, R.; Gatchel, R.J.; Mayer, T.G. A clinical guide to surface-emg-assisted stretching as an adjunct to chronic musculoskeletal pain rehabilitation. *Appl. Psychophysiol. Biofeedback* **2003**, *28*, 147–160. [CrossRef] [PubMed]

59. Neblett, R. Correcting abnormal lumbar flexion relaxation surface electromyography patterns in chronic low back pain subjects. *Biofeedback* **2007**, *35*, 17–22.

60. Neblett, R.; Mayer, T.G.; Brede, E.; Gatchel, R.J. Correcting abnormal flexion-relaxation in chronic low back pain: Responsiveness to a new biofeedback training protocol. *Clin. J. Pain* **2010**, *26*, 403–409. [CrossRef] [PubMed]

61. Neblett, R.; Mayer, T.G.; Brede, E.; Gatchel, R.J. The effect of prior lumbar surgeries on the flexion relaxation phenomenon and its responsiveness to rehabilitative treatment. *Spine J.* **2014**, *14*, 892–902. [CrossRef] [PubMed]

62. Pagé, I.; Marchand, A.; Nougarou, F.; O'Shaughnessy, J.; Descarreaux, M. Neuromechanical responses after biofeedback training in participants with chronic low back pain: An experimental cohort study. *J. Manip. Physiol. Ther.* **2015**, *38*, 449–457. [CrossRef] [PubMed]

63. Moore, A.; Mannion, J.; Moran, R.W. The efficacy of surface electromyographic biofeedback assisted stretching for the treatment of chronic low back pain: A case-series. *J. Bodyw. Mov. Ther.* **2015**, *19*, 8–16. [CrossRef] [PubMed]

64. Dellve, L.; Ahlstrom, L.; Jonsson, A.; Sandsjo, L.; Forsman, M.; Lindegard, A.; Ahlstrand, C.; Kadefors, R.; Hagberg, M. Myofeedback training and intensive muscular strength training to decrease pain and improve work ability among female workers on long-term sick leave with neck pain: A randomized controlled trial. *Int. Arch. Occup. Envion. Health* **2011**, *84*, 335–346. [CrossRef] [PubMed]

65. Ma, C.; Szeto, G.P.; Yan, T.; Wu, S.; Lin, C.; Li, L. Comparing biofeedback with active exercise and passive treatment for the management of work-related neck and shoulder pain: A randomized controlled trial. *Arch. Phys. Med. Rehabil.* **2011**, *92*, 849–858. [CrossRef] [PubMed]

66. Voerman, G.E.; Sandsjo, L.; Vollenbroek-Hutten, M.M.; Larsman, P.; Kadefors, R.; Hermens, H.J. Effects of ambulant myofeedback training and ergonomic counselling in female computer workers with work-related neck-shoulder complaints: A randomized controlled trial. *J. Occup. Rehabil.* **2007**, *17*, 137–152. [CrossRef] [PubMed]

67. The Interagency Pain Research Coordinating Committee. National Pain Strategy: A Comprehensive Population Health Level Strategy for Pain. Available online: http://iprcc.nih.gov/docs/DraftHHSNationalPainStrategy.pdf (accessed on 9 November 2015).

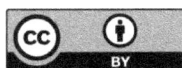

healthcare

MDPI

Article

Person-Centered, Physical Activity for Patients with Low Back Pain: Piloting Service Delivery

Saul Bloxham [1],*, **Phil Barter [2]**, **Slafka Scragg [3]**, **Charles Peers [4]**, **Ben Jane [1]** and **Joe Layden [1]**

[1] Department of Health Sciences, University of St Mark and St John, Plymouth PL11 8BH, UK; bjane@marjon.ac.uk (B.J.); jlayden@marjon.ac.uk (J.L.)
[2] London Sport Institute, Middlesex University, London NW4 4BT, UK; p.barter@mdx.ac.uk
[3] Plymouth Hospitals NHS Trust, Plymouth PL6 8DH, UK; slafka.scragg@nhs.net
[4] Plymouth Community Back Pain Service, Stoke Surgery, Belmont Villas, Stoke, Plymouth PL3 4DP, UK; charles.peers@nhs.net
* Correspondence: sbloxham@marjon.ac.uk; Tel.: +44-01752-636700 (ext. 6526)

Academic Editor: Robert J. Gatchel
Received: 25 February 2016; Accepted: 10 May 2016; Published: 18 May 2016

Abstract: Low back pain (LBP) is one of the most common and costly conditions in industrialized countries. Exercise therapy has been used to treat LBP, although typically using only one mode of exercise. This paper describes the method and initial findings of a person-centered, group physical activity programme which featured as part of a multidisciplinary approach to treating LBP. Six participants (aged 50.7 ± 17 years) completed a six-week physical activity programme lasting two hours per week. A multicomponent approach to physical activity was adopted which included aerobic fitness, core activation, muscular strength and endurance, Nordic Walking, flexibility and exercise gaming. In addition, participants were required to use diary sheets to record physical activity completed at home. Results revealed significant ($p < 0.05$) improvements in back strength (23%), aerobic fitness (23%), negative wellbeing (32%) and disability (16%). Person's Correlation Coefficient analysis revealed significant ($p < 0.05$) relationships between improvement in perceived pain and aerobic fitness ($r = 0.93$). It was concluded that a person-centered, multicomponent approach to physical activity may be optimal for supporting patients who self-manage LBP.

Keywords: low back pain; physical activity; disability; self-management; well-being; physical fitness

1. Introduction

Low back pain (LBP) is a major health concern in Western countries and is associated with high medical expenditure, work absence [1–3] and is the most common musculoskeletal condition [4–6]. Sixty to eighty percent of adults are likely to experience LBP [7,8] with 16% of adults in the United Kingdom (UK) consulting their general practitioner every year [9]. Back pain costs the UK National Health Service £1.3 million every day [1] and results in 12.5% of all work absence in the UK [10]. Low back pain is multifactorial and can have a significant effect on patients' quality of life. Completing routine domestic tasks such as vacuum cleaning, lifting, bending, sitting, twisting, pulling and pushing, repetitive work, static postures and opening doors can become severely restricted [11,12]. Contributory factors to LBP have included heavy physical work, physical fitness, social class, occupation and employment status, drug and alcohol use and smoking history [13,14] yet diagnosing the specific pathological or neurological cause of LBP in individual cases is often not possible [15].

In recent years, exercise therapy has been explored to treat LBP [16–19]. It can be delivered to a group of patients [20] and is more cost effective than individual treatment [21]. The term exercise therapy encompasses a range of different approaches (aerobic, strengthening and flexibility exercises) for which the evidence provides varying degrees of support. Studies suggest that flexibility is not correlated with measures of pain and disability [16], and those that focus upon spine flexibility have often yielded negative results [22]. In contrast, the use of strengthening and stabilising exercises has been shown to be more effective than General Practitioner treatment [23]. A growing body of research has endorsed the use of endurance training to reduce LBP [17–19], as significant reductions in pain intensity, disability and psychological strain have been highlighted.

Previous studies into LBP have focused on specific outcomes of muscular strength or endurance [18], yet few appear to have assessed the effectiveness of LBP exercise programmes which incorporate a range of approaches and outcome measures.

To date, the majority of research into exercise therapy as a treatment for LBP has centered on delivering monodisciplinary interventions that have focused on improving specific outcomes such as strength of the lumbar stabilizing muscles [23], functional range of motion of the lumbar spine [22] or aerobic fitness [18,19]. As approximately 85% of cases are non-specific [15] it is unlikely that one particular approach to exercise therapy can facilitate significant improvements in LBP.

At present, there is a paucity of research that explores the effectiveness of person-centered (bio-psycho-social), multicomponent exercise therapy interventions for the treatment of LBP. This paper describes methods and initial findings from a six week multicomponent physical activity programme aimed at improving physical fitness, physical activity, disability and psychological wellbeing of non-specific LBP patients.

2. Materials and Methods

According to best practice, the Local Health Authority had commissioned a multi-disciplinary team to treat sub-acute and chronic LBP consisting of Osteopathy, Cognitive Behavioral Therapy and exercise. The gym based exercise component had suffered from high drop-out, and as the local University, we were tasked with providing an alternative approach. The brief was to develop a low cost self-management style programme of exercise. We were instructed not to treat the cause of LBP, as specific causes had not been identified and patients had not responded to conventional treatment modalities. This pilot describes our approach taken to maximise adherence and promote self-management of LBP.

Four female and two male patients consented to partake in this pilot (mean age 51 years ± 17). All patients experienced non-specific LBP, and had been expressing symptoms for >3 months. Each patient was medically screened by their general practitioner and Physical Activity Readiness Questionnaire (PAR-Q) and informed consent were obtained. The stature (Leicester Height, Seca Limited, Birmingham, UK) and body mass (Weight Counting Scale, Seca Limited, Birmingham, UK) of the patients were 168.3 cm ± 8.8 cm and 87.7 kg ± 23.1 kg respectively. The instructors explained, demonstrated and supervised all physical activity undertaken by the group with support from student helpers studying for sport and health science related degrees. Each patient was fully informed of their right to withdraw from the programme at any time, or abstain from partaking in prescribed activities. The programme consisted of six weekly sessions lasting up to two hours. The sessions were divided into seven activity blocks to provide regular breaks and cater for patients' needs as documented in Table 1.

Table 1. Summary of programme content.

	Theme	Activity 1	Activity 2	Activity 3	Activity 4	Activity 5	Activity 6	Activity 7
Week One	Introduction & Baseline	Introduction to the programme; Administration	Core activation & posture; chair based warm-up/mobility	Chester step test or alternative & education	Body composition assessment & education	Core flexion extension endurance & education	Flexibility and cool down & education	Pedometer challenge, Personalised goal setting
Week Two	Motion patterns and core activation	Small group discussion of daily diary, pedometers.	Chair based warm-up; sit to stands; calf raises; balance work; glut activation	Back saving motion patterns; hip hinge in context of daily tasks; explore neutral spine	Outside walk focusing on technique, pace, core activation and posture	Introduction to Nordic Walking focusing on co-ordination	Core strengthening; introduction to bird-dog, back saver sit up and side-plank	Flexibility of major muscle groups; Personalised goal setting
Week Three	Aerobic Fitness	Small group discussion of daily diary, pedometers. Larger group sharing as appropriate	Relaxation techniques: Lifestyle integration of learnt skills	Induction to fitness gym and aerobic equipment & education	Explore aerobic equipment; 5-8 min on up to 4 different ergometers	Progressions of bird-dog, back saver sit up and side-plank; glut max and med strengthening	Flexibility of major muscle groups;	Personalised goal setting. Review of achievements since starting the programme
Week Four	Muscular Strength and Endurance	Small group discussion of daily diary, pedometers. Larger group sharing as appropriate. Larger group sharing as appropriate	Introduction to resistance bands for home use	Nutrition and healthy food discussion. Food diary task	Aerobic warm up—patient led based on learnt exercise principles & increased self-efficacy	Introduction to resistance equipment in the fitness gym & education	Patient led core and flexibility exercises. Trouble shooting and adaptations	Personalised goal setting. Reflect on individualised physical activity and lifestyle management
Week Five	Free flow: Water, land & Exergaming	Small group discussion of daily diary, pedometers. Larger group sharing as appropriate	Analysis of food diaries and group comments/observations	Aqua aerobics or land based options: Exercise gaming; aerobic exercise; Pilates; Nordic walking; Resistance exercise; fitness suite; flexibility; Floor based exercises (bird-dog, back saver sit up and side-plank; glut max and med strengthening)			Discussion around exit programme options. Barriers to exercise	Personalised goal setting.
Week Six	Summary & retest	Small group discussion of daily diary, pedometers. Larger group sharing as appropriate	Retest baselines measures Chester step test; Body composition assessment; Core flexion extension; Questionnaires;	Café Group discussion Programme reflections Future plans and back pain management				Finish

2.1. Week One—Introduction

The session commenced with an introduction to the programme, followed by a team building activity and baseline testing. Anthropometric measures such as body mass, stature, body fat and lean muscle mass (Body Stat 1500 Body Composition Measuring Unit, Body Stat, Douglas UK) were obtained. Aerobic capacity was measured using the Chester Step Test (Assist Creative Resources, Wrexham, UK). A back strength dynamometer (Takei Physical Fitness Test, Niigata, Japan) was used to assess back and leg strength, and a hand grip dynamometer (Takei Physical Fitness Test, Niigata, Japan) was used to assess hand grip strength. The prone double straight leg raise test and the plank test were utilised to measure muscular endurance of the low back. Measures of flexibility of the low back, pelvis and hamstrings were recorded using a clinical goniometer (MIE Medical Research Limited, Leeds, UK) and a sit and reach box (Fitech, Southampton, UK). Patients completed a contract outlining the terms and conditions of the programme and Modified Oswestry Low Back Pain Disability (MODQ) and Well-being (WB12-Q) questionnaires. In addition, patients were encouraged to complete a "daily diary" sheet which included an adapted faces pain scale to indicate daily pain levels (1 = feels worst, 6 = feels best). These were subsequently used to inform weekly patient-instructor discussions completed at the start of every session alongside a recap and general introduction.

On the first week, an information booklet was provided to participants to help them complete a programme of home exercise and dietary advice to re-enforce educational themes covered during the sessions. The home exercises followed the weekly theme and the exercise prescription was individualised for each patient. This was informed by the weekly patent-instructor discussion, which encouraged a meaningful dialogue of trial, error and participant feedback. In addition, the context of how the exercises were completed was addressed to promote participant ownership and long-term adherence. For example, some participants wanted to integrate exercise into ADL, whereas others wanted more formal timeslots to complete their exercise. Although imposing a set exercise regime for all participants was avoided, there were daily activities that were encouraged for all participants to complete during the week. These included mild activation of the transverse abdominis, sit-to-stand exercises, the "bird-dog", "back saver sit up", the "side plank" [12] a walking programme and stretches. All these were adapted according to ability, with patients encouraged to set their own weekly goals with support. These were then reviewed at the start of the following week's instructor-patient discussion. All home activities were progressed and adapted over duration of the programme. Participants were encouraged to utilise the back saving techniques when completing ADL and troubleshoot any personal movement difficulties that they encountered (such as lifting, getting into and out of vehicles, vacuuming, occupational tasks). At the end of week one, the group was briefed on the benefits of walking, and each participant was given a "Pedometer Challenge" recording sheet and a pedometer. For the remainder of the programme the patients were asked to record how many steps they completed each day, and new targets were mutually agreed each week.

2.2. Week Two—Motion Patterns and Core Activation

The main focus of this session was core activation and movement motion patterns. After a small group discussion concerning the previous week's activity, an introduction to core activation and chair based activities were completed. These included sit-to-stands, glut activation, calf raises and abdominal bracing. Back saving motion patterns were practiced including the hip hinge and pelvic mobility applied to normal ADL such as lifting, lowering, vacuuming, pushing and pulling, sitting and general domestic tasks. The group was also differentiated into three ability groups (red, amber and green) determined through a combination of patient self-assessment and instructor observation. These sub groups were invited to partake in an outside walk focusing on posture and technique. The patients were then introduced to Nordic Walking, again focusing on mastery of technique, co-ordination and posture. Core strengthening activities were completed at the end of the session. Weekly targets were then personalized for each patient, who were advised to explore places in their local area that could be used for physical activity. Patients were also encouraged to consider significant others to share in these physical activities (spouse, children, grandchildren and friends).

2.3. Week Three—Aerobic Fitness

Session three focused on aerobic exercises and lifestyle management. Following a recap on posture and core activation, relaxation techniques were introduced. Patients were then inducted into the aerobic ergometers in the fitness suit (treadmill, cycle, cross-trainer, rower). Following an extended warm-up, a variety of intensities were explored to enable patients to experience light and moderate intensity exertion. Patients were encouraged to notice their breathing patterns and heart rate as well as ratings of perceived exertion. Exercise bouts were limited to 10 min on each ergometer with an emphasis on mastery, posture, technique and peer-to-peer interaction and enjoyment. The session concluded with core strengthening and a series of lower limb and lumbar stretches. In all activity blocks, patients were encouraged to select the most appropriate activity for them and where appropriate, each was adapted accordingly. Home based tasks and personalized goals were discussed alongside an emphasis on patient achievements and progress.

2.4. Week Four—Muscular Strength and Endurance

Following improvements in group dynamic patients were more inclined to share personal experiences. This session included discussions around diet and nutrition and patients were instructed to keep a week-long food diary for analysis the following week. The group was then introduced to a range of exercises for upper, lower and core exercise that could be completed at home with commercially available resistance bands. The aim was to ensure core stability when completing a series of balanced multi-joint, functional exercises simulating lifting, lowering, pushing and pulling. The group were then tasked with completed their own aerobic warm-up on their desired ergometer in the fitness suit, followed by an induction onto machine based multi-joint resistance equipment. Once again the emphasis was on technique, a selection of balanced exercises and correct breathing. A muscular endurance exercise prescription was adopted. Patients were then encouraged to lead their own core and flexibility activity, based on their prior learning during the programme. A review of home based activities and personalised goal setting concluded the session.

2.5. Week Five—Freeflow

The main purpose of week five was for patients to have a high degree of autonomy and choice. Patients could self-select activities they had already experienced on the programme, participate in an aqua based session, experience exergaming or gentle sporting options such as table tennis. The group shared feedback and comments on their food diaries. The "eat well" plate and other nutritional guidance was discussed with particular emphasis on hydration, dieting and processed food types high in fat, sugar and salt. Further group discussions also focussed on exit progamme opportunities and activities relevant to patient's local area and preferences.

2.6. Week Six—Exit Programme and Post Testing

Post-testing was completed in the final session replicating week one. This enabled patients an opportunity to discuss their progress and exit strategy. The session ended with an informal discussion between the patients and instructors in a café. The patients were encouraged to continue with what they had learned, recognize the progress they had made and adhere to a physically active lifestyle.

2.7. Treatment of Data

All data for pre and post test results were represented as means ± standard deviation. Data were inputted and stored in a Microsoft Office Excel 2007 Spreadsheet (Microsoft Corporation, Reading, UK). Statistical analysis was performed using SPSS Software (SPSSv15 Inc., New York, NY, USA). Differences between means ± standard deviation (SD) were identified using paired sample t-tests where significance was accepted at $p < 0.05$. Pearson's Correlation Coefficient were conducted to represent relationships between the change in physical measures and the MODQ.

3. Results

Analysis of the MODQ as identified in Table 2, revealed improvements in seven of the ten measured categories, with the greatest in sleeping (−50%), employment/homemaking (−27%) and sitting (−27%) with the overall disability rating decreasing by 16%. However none of the categories had statistically improved compared to pre-programme values. There were no improvements in the personal care and walking categories with standing increasing by 11%.

Table 2. Pre-post programme Modified Oswestry Low Back Pain Disability (MODQ) scores (±SD) and percentage changes.

Category	Pre-Programme (±SD)	Post-Programme (±SD)	Change (%)
Pain Intensity	1.6 (1.5)	1.2 (1.6)	−25
Lifting	2.2 (1.8)	1.8 (2.1)	−18
Sitting	2.2 (0.8)	1.6 (0.9)	−27
Personal Care	0.6 (0.9)	0.6 (0.6)	0
Walking	1.2 (1.6)	1.2 (1.6)	0
Standing	1.8 (1.3)	2.0 (1.4)	+11
Sleeping	1.2 (1.3)	0.6 (0.9)	−50
Travelling	2.0 (1.0)	1.8 (0.8)	−10
Social Life	2.0 (1.2)	1.8 (1.1)	−10
Employment/Homemaking	2.2 (0.8)	1.6 (0.9)	−27
Disability Rating	34.0 (22.5)	28.4 (17.6)	−16

The WB12-Q, as reported in Table 3, revealed significant ($p < 0.05$) improvements for negative wellbeing −32% and although not significant ($p > 0.05$), increases in "energy" (35%) and "general wellbeing" (20%) were also identified.

Table 3. Pre-post programme Well-being (WB12-Q) scores (±SD) and percentage changes.

Category	Pre-Programme (±SD)	Post-Programme (±SD)	Change (%)
Negative Wellbeing	5.0 (5.0)	3.4 (3.8)	−32 *
Energy	5.2 (4.2)	7.0 (2.5)	+35
Positive Wellbeing	5.4 (2.7)	5.6 (2.9)	+4
General Wellbeing	17.6 (10.2)	21.2 (8.1)	+20

* Indicates significantly different to pre-programme values ($p < 0.05$).

The value of the trendline identified in Figure 1, demonstrated a small improvement from 3.37 on day one compared to 3.60 on day thirty five. This can be extrapolated to a 7% decrease of pain reported by patients over the duration of the programme.

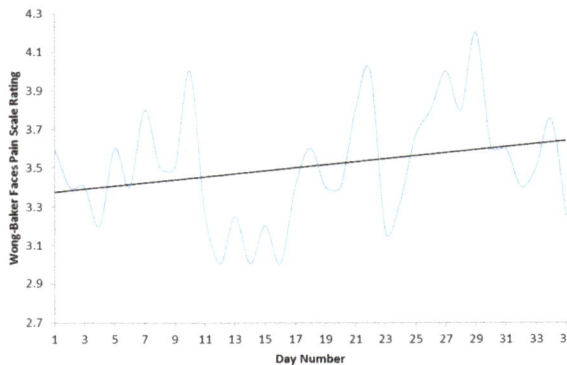

Figure 1. Mean Adapted Faces Pain Scale ratings from day one to day thirty five.

All measures of physical fitness improved during the six-week programme with significant ($p < 0.05$) findings in back (23%), hand grip strength (15%) and aerobic fitness (23%). Improvements in static muscular endurance (33%) and leg strength (29%) were also notable, as identified in Table 4.

Table 4. Pre-post programme physiological performance data.

Measure	Pre-Programme ($\pm$SD)	Post-Programme ($\pm$SD)	Change (%)
Back Strength (kg)	59.0 (51.2)	72.7 (55.0)	+23 *
Leg Strength (kg)	91.6 (45.7)	118.40 (58.4)	+29
Hand Grip Strength—Left (kg)	30.0 (11.6)	34.5 (12.8)	+15 *
Hand Grip Strength—Right (kg)	32.0 (11.9)	34.6 (9.9)	+8
Prone Leg Raise (s)	56.2 (43.0)	49.8 (39.2)	+6
Plank (s)	35.3 (25.5)	53.75 (45.5)	+33
Fluid Goniometer (°)	52.7 (17.1)	62.67 (11.2)	+19
Sit and Reach (cm)	21.7 (9.7)	23.92 (9.0)	+10
Aerobic Capacity (mL $O_2 \cdot kg^{-1} \cdot min^{-1}$)	30.2 (7.60)	37.0 (4.5)	+23 *

* Indicates significantly different to pre-programme values ($p < 0.05$).

The results from the body composition analysis, illustrated in Table 5, revealed significant ($p < 0.05$) 7% increase in lean mass and 13% decrease in body fat mass ($p < 0.05$) whilst body fat percentage also decreased by 9%.

Table 5. Pre and post programme anthropometric measures.

Measure	Pre-Programme ($\pm$SD)	Post-Programme ($\pm$SD)	Change (%)
Body Fat Percentage (%)	32.5 (7.8)	29.6 (10.1)	−9
Body Fat Mass (kg)	27.4 (6.4)	23.8 (7.31)	−13 *
Lean Mass (kg)	54.5 (16.0)	58.1 (17.5)	+7 *
Total Mass (kg)	87.7 (23.1)	88.6 (22.9)	+1

* Indicates significantly different to pre-programme values ($p < 0.05$).

Physical activity levels as measured by daily Pedometer step count increased during the programme (Figure 2). The lowest mean number of steps completed was 5021 on day fourteen, with the greatest mean number of steps, 9281, completed on day twenty nine.

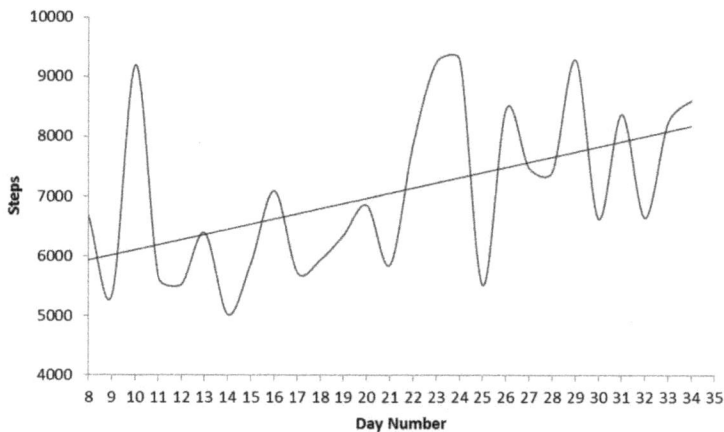

Figure 2. Daily mean step count of the group.

Table 6 shows a significant negative correlation between aerobic fitness and the MODQ. No other variables were related to changes in MODQ.

Table 6. Relationship between the change in MODQ and physiological data.

Mean Change in Physical Measure	*r*-Value
Body mass (Kg)	−0.141
% Body Fat	−0.615
Back Strength (Kg)	0.171
Leg Strength (Kg)	−0.365
Hand Grip (right) (Kg)	−0.107
Hand Grip (left) (Kg)	0.409
Prone Leg Raise (s)	−0.018
Fluid Goniometer (°)	−0.176
Sit and Reach (cm)	−0.614
Aerobic Capacity (mls O_2/Kg/min)	−0.973 *
Walking (steps per day)	−0.179

* Indicates correlation is significant $p < 0.05$ (2-tailed).

4. Discussion

The results from the MODQ indicate that although the disability of the group decreased by 16%, patients disability rating remained classified as moderate. General wellbeing was shown to increase by 20%, however neither of the net improvements in disability or wellbeing were significant ($p > 0.05$). Each patient improved their aerobic fitness, resulting in a significant ($p < 0.05$) group improvement. Data from the pedometers indicated that the group gradually increased their daily mean step count. Improvements occurred in all of the physiological performance measures, with significant ($p < 0.05$) improvements occurring in back and hand grip strength. Daily assessment of pain, using an adapted faces pain scale, highlighted that the group generally experienced less pain (higher score), as the programme progressed. Positive changes were also observed in the body composition of the group with significant ($p < 0.05$) decreases in body fat and increases in lean mass identified.

The results from the MODQ (Table 2) suggest that the intervention programme was effective at decreasing the disability of the group. Prior to the intervention programme, the mean group disability rating of 34 points placed the group closer to the "severely disabled" category (41 points). The 16% decrease in disability over the course of the programme resulted in a post-intervention disability rating of 28.4 points, which placed the group closer to the "minimally disabled" category score (20 points). These findings are encouraging given that the MODQ has been shown to be a reliable LBP questionnaire when detecting changes in disability [24]. However, it should be noted that the overall classification of 'moderately disabled' remained unchanged, and a decrease of less than six points (34−28.4) is at best modest. Perhaps this finding reflects the need to increase the programme's duration to extend beyond six-weeks, the small sample of the pilot and the variable nature of non-specific LBP. An objective of the programme was to improve patient's ability to self-manage back pain and promote exercise as an alternative to prescribed pain medication. Any large reductions in pain are likely to occur over a longer time period, emphasizing the need to conduct a patient follow up.

The overall disability classification includes pain scores from the ten categories within the MODQ. Two of the three areas which showed the greatest improvement were employment/homemaking (−27%) and sitting (−27%). These considerable improvements could be attributed to the educational approach of the programme that was designed to relate to ADL. The programme specifically addressed how to employ good posture and motion patterns such as sitting, vacuuming, opening doors and bending [12].

The only category to reflect an increase in pain was the standing category, which increased by 11%. Throughout the programme, considerable effort was dedicated to increasing overall physical activity, balance work and walking and as such this additional loading may partly explain the 11% increase in "standing pain".

The groups' aerobic fitness improved significantly ($p < 0.05$) over the duration of the intervention from 30.2 mL O$_2 \cdot$ kg$^{-1} \cdot$ min^{-1} at pre-testing to 37.0 mL O$_2 \cdot$ kg$^{-1} \cdot$ min^{-1} at post-testing. Evidence from other studies [17–19] indicates aerobic exercise as one of the most beneficial forms of exercise for people with LBP. Although our pilot intervention was 50% shorter than others [19], the results demonstrated promise. Our pilot recorded a 16% decrease in disability (compared to 31%), a 25% decrease in pain intensity (compared to 41%) and a significant ($p < 0.05$) 32% decrease in negative wellbeing (compared to 35% decrease in psychological strain). A large proportion of this intervention focused on promoting aerobic fitness and physical activity mediated through person-centered lifestyle changes. The "pedometer challenge", prescription of aerobic exercise, educational sessions and self-mediated goal setting are likely to be the reasons for the significant ($p < 0.05$) group improvement in both aerobic fitness and physical activity.

Improvements in each participant's aerobic capacity were negatively correlated ($p < 0.05$) with changes in their MODQ score. Although the sample size in this pilot demand cautious interpretation, the suggestion that greater improvements in aerobic fitness may lead to greater decreases in LBP is consistent with other more substantial studies [25]. The decrease in pain experienced by patients in our pilot was also reflected by 7% improvement identified by the adapted faces pain scale, as highlighted in Figure 1. Upon close scrutiny the lowest scores on the faces pain scale (highest pain) appear to coincide with the lowest pedometer step count (days 11–15 on Figures 1 and 2). Although potentially coincidental, this supports the relationship identified between increased step count and reductions in MODQ disability.

There are various reasons why LBP patients may experience reduced pain following increased aerobic exercise. It is well established that endurance exercise can increase lipid metabolism and if the correct energy balance is established through dietary intake, a reduction in body fat percentage can occur. Our body composition data support this with percentage body fat decreasing by 9%. Excess body fat can add unnecessary loading to the spine, exacerbating pain, which can also further reduce physical activity and thereby create a cycle of deterioration. Therapies that can reduce spinal loading and promote muscle conditioning, in this case as a consequence of increased physical activity, should feature as part of a LBP exercise programme. Moreover it is well documented that aerobic exercise can increase the release of endorphins which can inhibit pain through stimulation of the central and peripheral opiate receptors [26]. Our efforts to promote aerobic physical activities that relate to ADL and functional movement, such as walking, appear justified, particularly as augmented walking programmes have been associated with reduced pain and improvements psychological health [17].

Table 3 shows that the group expressed a significant ($p < 0.05$) 32% decrease in negative wellbeing, which is comparable to the 35% decrease in psychological strain exhibited in other research [19]. Negative wellbeing is a reflection of external factors such as health and social support. The lower the score for negative wellbeing the better the patients feel about their health and the social support available. The significant decrease in negative wellbeing could reflect the effectiveness of the pilot on improving patients' quality of life. Our person-centered approach, willingness of instructors to listen to patient experiences, and patient peer support, were intended to create a comfortable and supportive environment. Nevertheless the lack of improvement in positive wellbeing may also reflect the need for a longer intervention, as the all-encompassing nature of non-specific LBP is notoriously difficult to resolve in a short time.

The greatest improvement represented by the WB12-Q came in the "energy" category, which improved by 35%. This would indicate the group was feeling fresher, more rested and active at the end of the intervention. This finding is supported by the MODQ results for the "sleeping" category which suggest the patients had experienced a 50% improvement in their ability to sleep. These three variables were combined to produce a net 20% increase in "general wellbeing". The "daily diary" provided the patients with the opportunity to comment about each day and the associated impact of LBP. At the start of each session the instructors would review the diaries and discuss key points with the patients. This provided a valuable means of understanding each individual patient need. For example, when planning the skill based activities the instructors used the daily diaries to match pertinent activities for individual patients (such as golf, bowls and netball). Some required personalized support for completing housework activities, yet others required advice for office and computer work. Thereby, the daily diaries enabled instructors to address patient's specific needs and served to monitor and advise on physical activity that they were completing at home. Unpopular or ineffective exercises could also be removed or modified. The diversity of the group with regards to age and severity of LBP was managed through sub-grouping of the patients into ability levels using a traffic light system [27].

Despite the comparatively short six-week time frame, all of the measures of strength, muscular endurance and flexibility improved during the pilot. The greatest improvements were observed in static muscular endurance (33%) and leg strength (29%). Significant improvements ($p < 0.05$) occurred in aerobic fitness, back strength (23%) and hand grip strength of the left hand (15%). The improvements in the fluid goniometer test (19%) and sit and reach test (10%) were not related to MODQ scores which is consistent with other studies [16]. Nevertheless improvements in flexibility to increase the range of motion around the pelvis, hamstrings and low back would intuitively provide improvements in functionality.

The welcome improvements in grip, leg and back strength complemented the back saving techniques taught throughout the programme. The combination of educational and physical training are likely to translate to better patient ability to spare the back during lifts, loads and carrying out ADL more safely. Additionally, the improvements in muscular endurance could delay the onset of fatigue within the muscles associated with the patients' LBP, thereby delaying the symptoms of LBP that hinder functionality during the day.

Patients were complementary about their experience during the programme and although not unexpected, patients reported that the programme was enjoyable and effective. These patient views were perhaps substantiated by the 100% retention and attendance rate recorded during the pilot.

5. Conclusions

The findings of this pilot suggest that our person-centered, multidisciplinary approach to group exercise may be effective at treating LBP, although six weeks may be too short to invoke substantial decreases in disability as measured using the MODQ. Future longitudinal studies, with larger samples are required for these findings to be substantiated. Improvements in aerobic fitness and physical activity may relate to the small decreases in pain (MODQ, adapted faces pain scale), disability (MODQ) and negative wellbeing (WB12-Q).

Acknowledgments: We would like to acknowledge the contribution of students Matt Burgess and Damien Goodall.

Author Contributions: Saul Bloxham is the main author and led the development, delivery and evaluation of the programme with support from Phil Barter, Slafka Scragg and Charles Peers. Ben Jane and Joe Layden support the on-going delivery and editing process associated with the service and scholarship.

Conflicts of Interest: The authors declare no conflict of interest.

Abbreviations

The following abbreviations are used in this manuscript:

MODQ	Modified Oswestry Disability Questionnaire
LBP	Low back pain
WB12-Q	Well-Being 12 Questionnaire
ADL	Activities of Daily Living

References

1. National Health Service (NHS). Backcare Awareness Week. Available online: http://www.nhscareers.nhs.uk/features/2012/october/ (accessed on 16 October 2014).
2. Ricci, J.A.; Stewart, W.F.; Chee, E.; Leotta, C.; Foley, K.; Hochberg, M.C. Back pain exacerbations and lost productive time costs in United States workers. *Spine* **2006**, *26*, 3052–3060. [CrossRef] [PubMed]
3. Van Tulder, M.; Malmivaara, A.; Esmail, R.; Koes, B. Exercise therapy for low back pain: A systematic review within the framework of the cochrane collaboration back review group. *Spine* **2000**, *21*, 2784–2796. [CrossRef]
4. Chan, C.W.; Mok, N.W.; Yeung, E.W. Aerobic exercise training in addition to conventional physiotherapy for chronic low back pain: A randomized controlled trial. *Arch. Phys. Med. Rehabil.* **2011**, *10*, 1681–1685. [CrossRef] [PubMed]
5. Ebadi, S.; Ansari, N.N.; Naghdi, S.; Fallah, E.; Barzi, D.M.; Jalaei, S. A study of therapeutic ultrasound and exercise treatment for muscle fatigue in patients with chronic non specific low back pain: A preliminary report. *J. Back Musculoskelet. Rehabil.* **2013**, *2*, 221–226.
6. Hancock, M.J.; Maher, C.G.; Latimer, J. Spinal manipulative therapy for acute low back pain: A clinical perspective. *J. Man. Manip. Ther.* **2008**, *4*, 198–203. [CrossRef] [PubMed]
7. Kolber, M.J.; Beekhuizen, K. Lumbar stabilization: An evidence-based approach for the athlete with low back pain. *Strength Cond. J.* **2007**, *29*, 26–37. [CrossRef]
8. Lara-Palomo, I.C.; Aguilar-Ferrándiz, M.E.; Matarán-Peñarrocha, G.A.; Saavedra-Hernández, M.; Granero-Molina, J.; Fernández-Sola, C. Short-term effects of interferential current electro-massage in adults with chronic non-specific low back pain: A randomized controlled trial. *Clin. Rehabil.* **2013**, *27*, 439–450. [CrossRef] [PubMed]
9. Thomas, K.J.; MacPherson, H.; Thorpe, L.; Brazier, J.; Fitter, M.; Campbell, M.J. Randomised controlled trial of a short course of traditional acupuncture compared with usual care for persistent non-specific low back pain. *BMJ* **2006**, *333*, 623–626. [CrossRef] [PubMed]
10. Wynne-Jones, G.; Cowen, J.; Jordan, J.; Uthman, O.; Main, C.J.; Glozier, N.; van der Windt, D. Absence from work and return to work in people with back pain: A systematic review and meta-analysis. *Occup. Environ. Med.* **2014**, *6*, 448–456. [CrossRef] [PubMed]
11. May, S. Patients' attitudes and beliefs about back pain and its management after physiotherapy for low back pain. *Physiother. Res. Int.* **2007**, *12*, 126–135. [CrossRef] [PubMed]
12. McGill, S.M. *Low Back Disorders: Evidence Based Prevention and Rehabilitation*, 2nd ed.; Human Kinetics: Champaign, IL, USA, 2007.
13. Andersson, G.B.J. The Epidemiology of Spinal Disorders. In *The Adult Spine, Principles and Practice*; Lippincott-Raven: Philadelphia, PA, USA, 1997.
14. Quittan, M. Management of Back Pain. *Disabil. Rehabil.* **2002**, *8*, 423–434. [CrossRef] [PubMed]
15. Burton, A.K.; Balagué, F.; Cardon, G.; Eriksen, H.R.; Henrotin, Y.; Lahad, A.; Leclerc, A.; Müller, G.; van der Beek, A.J. European guidelines for prevention in low back pain european guidelines for prevention in low back pain. *Eur. Spine J.* **2004**, *15*, 1–53.
16. Kuukkanen, T.; Mälkiä, E. Effects of a three-month therapeutic exercise programme on flexibility in subjects with low back pain. *Physiother. Res. Int.* **2000**, *1*, 46–61. [CrossRef]
17. Hurwitz, E.L.; Morgenstern, H.; Chiao, C. Effects of recreational physical activity and back exercises on low back pain and psychological distress: Findings from the UCLA low back pain study. *Am. J. Public Health* **2005**, *10*, 1817–1824. [CrossRef] [PubMed]
18. Oldervoll, L.M.; Rø, M.; Zwart, J.-A.; Svebak, S. Comparison of two physical exercise programs for the early intervention of pain in the neck, shoulders and lower back in female hospital staff. *J. Rehabil. Med.* **2001**, *33*, 156–161. [CrossRef] [PubMed]
19. Chatzitheodorou, D.; Kabitsis, C.; Malliou, P.; Mougios, V. A pilot study of the effects of high-intensity aerobic exercise *versus* passive interventions on pain, disability, psychological strain, and serum cortisol concentrations in people with chronic low back pain. *Phys. Ther.* **2007**, *87*, 304–312. [CrossRef] [PubMed]
20. UK BEAM Trial Team. United Kingdom Back Pain and Manipulation randomised trial: Effectiveness of physical treatments for back pain in primary care. *BMJ* **2004**, *329*. [CrossRef]

21. Carr, J.L.; Klaber Moffett, J.A.; Howarth, E.; Richmond, S.J.; Torgerson, D.J.; Jackson, D.A.; Metcalfe, C.J. A randomized trial comparing a group exercise programme for back pain patients with individual physiotherapy in a severely deprived area. *Disabil. Rehabil.* **2005**, *27*, 929–937. [CrossRef] [PubMed]

22. Parks, K.A.; Crichton, K.S.; Goldford, R.J.; McGill, S.M.A. Comparison of lumbar range of motion and functional ability scores in patients with low back pain: Assessment for range of motion validity. *Spine* **2003**, *28*, 380–384. [CrossRef] [PubMed]

23. Rackwitz, B.; de Bie, R.; Limm, H.; von Garnier, K.; Ewert, T.; Stucki, G. Segmental stabilizing exercises and low back pain. What is the evidence? A systematic review of randomized controlled trials. *Clin. Rehabil.* **2006**, *20*, 553–567. [CrossRef] [PubMed]

24. Davidson, M.; Keating, J.L. A comparison of five low back disability questionnaires: Reliability and responsiveness. *Phys. Ther.* **2002**, *82*, 8–24. [PubMed]

25. Van der Velde, G.; Mierau, D. The effect of exercise on percentile rank aerobic capacity, pain, and self-rated disability in patients with chronic low-back pain: A retrospective chart review. *Arch. Phys. Med. Rehabil.* **2000**, *8*, 1457–1463. [CrossRef] [PubMed]

26. Constantini, N.; Hackney, A. *Endocrinology of Physical Activity and Sport*, 2nd ed.; Springer: New York, NY, USA, 2013.

27. Brennan, G.P.; Fritz, J.M.; Hunter, S.J.; Thackeray, A.; Delitto, A.; Erhard, R.E. Identifying subgroups of patients with acute/subacute "nonspecific" low back pain: Results of a randomized clinical trial. *Spine* **2006**, *31*, 623–631. [CrossRef] [PubMed]

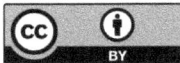

healthcare

MDPI

Article

Biopsychosocial Characteristics, Using a New Functional Measure of Balance, of an Elderly Population with CLBP

Ryan Hulla [1], Michael Moomey [2], Tyler Garner [2], Christopher Ray [3] and Robert J. Gatchel [1,*]

[1] Department of Psychology, University of Texas at Arlington, Arlington, TX 76019, USA; ryanhulla@yahoo.com
[2] Department of Kinesiology, University of Texas at Arlington, Arlington, TX 76019, USA; moomey49@gmail.com (M.M.); tgarner@uta.edu (T.G.)
[3] College of Health Sciences, Texas Woman's University, Denton, TX 76204, USA; chrisray@twu.edu
[*] Correspondence: gatchel@uta.edu; Tel.: +1-817-272-2541

Academic Editor: Sampath Parthasarathy
Received: 30 June 2016; Accepted: 1 August 2016; Published: 23 August 2016

Abstract: This study examined the biopsychosocial characteristics of chronic low back pain (CLBP) in an understudied but increasingly larger part of the population: the elderly (i.e., 65 years and older). A new innovative physical functioning measure (postural control, which is a proxy for the common problem of slips and falls in the elderly) was part of this biopsychosocial evaluation. Also, the National Institutes of Health (NIH)-developed Patient-Reported Outcome Measurement Information System (PROMIS) was also part of this comprehensive evaluation. Two demographically-matched groups of elderly participants were evaluated: one with CLBP (n = 24); and the other without (NCLBP, n = 24). Results revealed significant differences in most of these measures between the two groups, further confirming the importance of using a biopsychosocial approach for future studies of pain and postural control in the elderly.

Keywords: biopsychosocial; chronic low back pain; postural control; PROMIS; elderly patients

1. Introduction

The recent Institute of Medicine Report has documented that musculoskeletal pain is the most common single type of chronic pain; chronic low back pain (CLBP) is the most prevalent in this category [1]. The economic burden of CLBP is also quite large, and continues to grow in the U.S. It should also be kept in mind that, with the "graying of America", this CLBP problem will significantly increase in the future. Currently, there are approximately 35 million Americans 65 years or older, accounting for 12.4% of the total population [2], or about 38 million Americans [3]. By the year 2030, it is projected that about 20% of the population (72 million) will be 65 years of age or older [2]. Awareness of these population trends contributes to increased concern about healthcare issues among older adults, including CLBP. Indeed, the U.S. is in the process of what is known as the "longevity revolution", an occurrence happening as the population of older adults increases. Making up approximately 12% of the population in the US, older adults are more susceptible to falls because of age-associated ailments [4], resulting in roughly one-third of older adults falling annually, with one-fifth of them necessitating medical attention [5]. The monetary burden associated with fall injuries (especially low back pain) is projected to reach $32.4 billion dollars by the year 2020 [6].

Falls and fall-related injuries (such as CLBP) are one of the chief origins of morbidity in older adults, and are a precursor to functional impairment, disability, fractures, pain and, therefore, lower quality of life [7,8]. In more severe cases, falls have been a significant cause of injury-related death in the older adult population [6]. While it is generally accepted that there is an association between falls and chronic pain [9], the relationship between falls and low-back pain from a causal perspective is not entirely understood. This study did not seek to find a causal link. However, a brief overview provides some context for the relationship between fall-risk and CLBP. Rudy, Weiner, Lieber, Slaboda, and Boston found significant differences in physical function, psychosocial function, and severity of medical comorbidity in high functioning community-dwelling older adults with CLBP compared to those who were pain free [10]. Weiner, Rudy, Morrow, Slaboda, and Lieber found a distinct relationship between neuropsychological performance, pain, and physical function [11]. Furthermore, the psychological phenomenon known as "fear of falling" may play a role in increasing the risk for subsequent falls via further limiting physical activity [12] as well as being the catalyst for changes in gait mechanics that lead to inefficient gait characteristics [13], further increasing the risk for falls. The deliberate avoidance of physical activity seen in fear of falling can also lead to muscle atrophy (a marker of physical frailty) [14], which is also seen in older adults with chronic low back pain [15].

Physical activity has been confirmed to improve physiological functions such as balance, flexibility, and muscle tone, thereby reducing the likelihood of sustaining a fall [16]. There is a large body of research that links physical activity, or the lack thereof, to decreased postural control and consequently increased fall risk [17]. Stubbs and colleagues report that sufficient evidence exists to conclude that exercise reduces falls in older adults. Furthermore, evidence suggests impaired physical function also impacts psychosocial well-being [17]. For example, the aging population tends to withdraw from physical activity, increasing fall risk [18]. This withdrawal from physical activity not only negatively affects an elderly individual's postural control, but also disrupts the quality of mental well-being. In fact, Morgan and colleagues concluded that there is a strong relationship between physical activity and mental health, showing that older adults who participate in regular physical being more resistant to experiencing depression, and to having better overall mental health [19]. Overall, a large body of research shows a definite relationship between regular physical activity and improved postural control, and between regular physical activity and improved mental well-being [19], suggesting a relationship could exist between fall risk and psychosocial variables such as anxiety, depression, fatigue, pain and physical function.

In addition, Bradbeer and colleagues found that older adults who exhibit symptoms of depression are more likely to experience chronic pain than those who are not depressed [20]. Osteoarthritis, due to physical inactivity (among other factors), contributes to chronic pain, which is then followed by avoidance of physical activity [21] thus exacerbating the cycle of decreased physical activity, sarcopenia, and osteoporosis. Chronic pain can also decrease participation in ADLs. Decreases in ADLs are seen with aging independent of pain, but pain can initiate a cycle of limited ADLs fostering a fear of movement, further decreasing functional capacity, and then to increased pain [22]. Similar to depression, anxiety is also associated with chronic pain. Older adults tend to have increased anxiety, especially when it comes to fear of falling [23], and this anxiety leads to restricted movement [24], which, as previously discussed, exacerbates pain and impairs postural control. Pain also impacts sleep quality [25], which can also directly impact postural control. One study showed that subjects who reported being "sleepy" had greater postural sway than individuals who were well-rested [26].

Pinpointing easily-measured variables concomitant with fall risk would be advantageous in order to reduce an individual's risk of sustaining a fall. Because experiencing a fall can have a devastating impact on the quality of life in the elderly, it is vital that brief, inexpensive, and easy-to-use tests are available for everyday clinical use [27]. Therefore, as a first step in this process, the present study evaluated what biopsychosocial variables are related to those elderly individuals who have CLBP, and those who do not have NCLBP. Postural control, measured by the NeuroCom Balance System, and other biopsychosocial variables measured by the PROMIS-29, were evaluated.

2. Methods

2.1. Participants

A total of 78 older adults were recruited from the local community from informative presentations about the Center for Healthy Living and Longevity (CHLL) at the University of Texas at Arlington at various places such as churches, retired faculty gatherings, word-of-mouth from friends, and even doctor recommendations. Participants took part in a research project pertaining to postural control and psychosocial assessments through CHLL at the University of Texas at Arlington. All participants had physician approval and provided informed consent to participate per the Institutional Review Board (IRB) at the University of Texas at Arlington. There were 24 participants in the CLBP group and 24 matched participants in the NCLBP group. Participants were also assessed for CLBP with the National Institutes of Health (NIH) definition of CLBP. The definition asks two questions in classifying participants with or without CLBP. They were also matched on demographic variables, which are presented in Table 1.

Table 1. Demographics.

Measure	CLBP	NCLBP	Matched Pair (Total)
Sample size	24	24	48
Mean Age	73.96	74.04	74.00
Male	33.3%	33.3%	33.3%
Female	66.7%	66.7%	66.7%
Previously Exercised (Yes)	58.3%	50.0%	54.2%
Previously Exercised (No)	41.7%	50.0%	45.8%
Education Less than 9th Grade	0.0%	0.0%	0.0%
High School Graduate/GED	4.3%	4.3%	4.3%
Some College	34.86%	26.10%	30.4%
Associates Degree	4.3%	8.7%	6.5%
Bachelors Degree	39.1%	30.4%	34.8%
Graduate/Professional Degree	17.4%	30.4%	23.9%

2.2. Instrumentation

The NeuroCom Smart Balance Master System detects any changes in an individual's balance over time by measuring the participant's ability to control the center of gravity in various sensory and motor conditions. The participant stands on a force plate, facing into a three-sided booth. The force plate and visual surround move in response to the participants' forwards and backwards sway, creating a disturbed proprioceptive or visual input to the brain. This distortion causes the participant to rely heavily on alternative senses to maintain equilibrium. Sway refers to changes in the center of the persons applied force as a result of moving forwards or backwards. Postural control was assessed using the sensory organization test (SOT) and strategy analysis under six conditions with a NeuroCom SOT. The SOT procedure accurately identifies aberrations in the participant's use of the three sensory systems that contribute to postural control: visual, vestibular, and somatosensory [28]. Throughout the assessment, erroneous information is delivered to the participant's feet, eyes, and joints through "sway referencing" of the visual surround and/or the support surface. The participants were fitted with a cushioned vest that was attached to the NeuroCom's system outer structure in order to safeguard him/her from a fall. Each condition was executed three times. Outcome measures for this test included: (1) Equilibrium Score which quantifies the center of gravity (COG) sway or postural stability; (2) Sensory Analysis ratios which are used in conjunction with the participant's equilibrium scores to detect deficiencies of the participant's sensory systems; (3) Strategy Analysis which measures the relative amount of movement of ankle strategy and hip strategy the participant used to maintain balance throughout each trial; and (4) COG Alignment plots the individual's COG position at the beginning of each trial of the SOT, in which each mark determines COG alignment during a single SOT trial, relative to the center of the base of support.

After the participants' postural control was assessed with the NeuroCom Balance System, participants were assessed for the components of physical fitness in upper- and lower-limb muscular strength and endurance, cardiovascular endurance, and upper- and lower-body muscular flexibility. Participants were then questioned on the amount of falls they have had in the past year and 6 months. No measures of physical fitness or fall frequency were used in the current study analysis. All physical fitness scorecards, NIH CLBP definition inventories, and consent forms were stored in file cabinets, and locked in the lab, and later de-identified and coded into SPSS.

The Patient Reported Outcomes Information System (PROMIS 29) is a computer-adaptive test designed to measure the following seven psychosocial constructs: physical function; anxiety; depression; fatigue; sleep disturbance; ability to participate in social roles and activities; and pain interference. The PROMIS-29 has been tested and validated for concurrent and discriminant validity, test-retest reliability, as well as participant preference for measuring health-related quality of life [29].

2.3. Procedures

Participants first consented to the IRB-approved protocol of the current study. After consent, participants filled out the NIH definition of CLBP inventory with paper and pencil. If the participants marked "they have had low-back pain for greater than three months or longer" and also marked "having low-back pain for at least half the days in the past 6 months or more", the participant was classified as having CLBP. Participants who marked "having low-back pain for less than 3 months" or "having it less than half the days for the past 6 months" were classified as NCLBP.

Once consented and the NIH definition of CLBP inventory completed, and demographic information collected, the PROMIS-29 Computer Adaptive Test was administered. The computer-adaptive aspect of the PROMIS proves advantageous in that information is drawn from a large database and is formatted to a specific individual, based on the individual's response to the previous question. The NIH is encouraging its use and have extensively developed it working towards, and achieving, validation among the population. Each participant was assigned a computer, and created a test profile before taking the assessment. When the participants finished the PROMIS-29 CAT, they logged out of their profile and results were saved, to be accessed later in order to be de-identified and transferred and coded into IBM's Statistical Package for Social Science (SPSS). The participants also completed two other inventories on the computer after the PROMIS-29 that were not used in analysis of this present study (the Balance Efficacy Scale, and the Comprehensive Fall Risk Assessment).

2.4. Scoring

During the SOT, participants were tested under 6 conditions, 3 trials per condition, for a total of 18 trials. Each trial lasted 30 s. The force plate and visual surround moved in response to the participant's center of gravity sway. The inclusive composite Equilibrium Score provides a representative score of the individual's' capacity to sustain postural stability throughout all conditions. Effective use of the individual's' sensory inputs is derived from the overall pattern of scores on each of the six conditions. The composite Equilibrium Score is the weighted average encompassing the average scores of conditions 1–6.

The Strategy Analysis score is derived by plotting the data from the force plate and the Equilibrium Scores together to quantify the amount of movement of the ankles or the hips. The Strategy Analysis score reflects the extent of movement concerning the ankles (ankle-dominant strategy) and hips (hip-dominant strategy) used to sustain postural stability throughout each trial. The closer the scores are to 100, the more ankle-dominant strategy was used to maintain stability. Conversely, the closer to 0 score reflects a more hip-dominant strategy used to maintain postural control. Typically, as stability is sustained, individuals utilize an ankle-dominant strategy primarily, shifting to a more hip-dominant strategy under conditions where postural control is more difficult to maintain [30].

The constructs of the PROMIS-29 item banks have been individually developed using patients' representative of the 2000 US Census [29]. The subsequent question pool contrasts between each domain (anxiety, depression, fatigue, pain-interference, sleep disturbance, and physical function). There are 29 questions each in the anxiety and anger domains, 28 questions with respect to depression, 95 questions pertaining to fatigue, 41 in the pain-interference bank, 39 questions with regards to pain-behavior, 27 questions about sleep disturbances, 124 questions regarding physical function, 16 questions in the sleep impairment domain, 12 and 14 in the social impairment and social roles domains, respectively. The CAT selects a group of questions from the item pool for the participants to answer, generally 4–12 questions per domain. The CAT presents the first question and, based on the participant's answer, selects subsequent questions from the question bank, until the responses satisfy the precision criteria of 80% reliability [29]. The resultant outcome is a t-score and standard deviation based on the standardized US population. The mean t-score is 50 and the standard deviation is 10. An individual score is given per each domain. Each domain provides a total score, a score compared with the general US population, a score compared with patients in the same age group, and a score compared with non-patients in the same age group. Each score is reported as either better or worse than norms [29].

2.5. Data Analyses

SPSS version 22.0 statistical software was used to conduct all statistical analyses.

3. Results

The PROMIS data for each of the two groups are presented in Table 2. Multivariate statistical analysis of these data yielded a significant Pillai's Trace Statistic of $V = 0.40$ $F_{(6, 41)} = 4.59$, $p = 0.001$, $\eta_p^2 = 0.40$. As can be seen, CLBP and NCLBP groups significantly differed (based on separate analyses of variance) for: perception of pain interference, $F_{(1, 46)} = 24.89$, $p < 0.001$, $\eta_p^2 = 0.35$; perception of physical function, $F_{(1, 46)} = 10.26$, $p = 0.002$, $\eta_p^2 = 0.18$; and fatigue $F_{(1, 46)} = 5.01$, $p = 0.03$, $\eta_p^2 = 0.10$. Sleep disturbance approached significance $F_{(1, 46)} = 3.01$, $p = 0.089$, $\eta_p^2 = 0.06$. It should be noted that all of the above had medium-large effect sizes (large: >0.14; medium: >0.05; small: >0.009). No significant differences were found between groups for anxiety and depression.

Table 2. Patient-Reported Outcome Measurement Information System (PROMIS) data descriptives.

Measure	CLBP		NCLBP	
	M	SD	M	SD
Anxiety	51.38	6.63	50.25	7.30
Depression	49.08	5.33	46.54	6.29
Fatigue	53.00	7.60	48.71	5.53
Pain Interference	59.17	7.15	49.08	6.85
Physical Function	40.96	4.91	46.29	6.51
Sleep Disturbance	48.38	5.82	45.33	631

The NeuroCom data for each of the two groups are presented in Table 3. Multivariate statistical analysis of the data did not yield statistical significant results between CLBP and NCLBP groups' overall equilibrium, strategy (ankle-dominant or hip-dominant strategy), or composite balance scores. However, for differentiating between CLBP versus NCLBP groups, the following measures taken together were significant: NeuroCom average equilibrium scores in conditions four, five, and six; NeurCom average strategy scores in condition three and six; overall average NeuroCom somatic system score; and PROMIS scores on pain inference and sleep disturbance, $R^2 = 0.56$, $F_{(8, 39)} = 6.15$, $p < 0.001$. Results of this regression model yielded individual significant relationships, reported as individual beta-weight t tests, for: average scores of equilibrium NeuroCom condition four ($\beta = -0.29$, $t(39) = -2.02$, $p = 0.05$); equilibrium average score in NeuroCom condition five, ($\beta = 0.50$, $t(39) = 2.39$, $p = 0.022$); NeuroCom overall somatic system score ($\beta = -0.25$, $t(39) = -2.26$, $p = 0.029$); sleep disturbance ($\beta = 0.31$, $t(39) = 2.45$, $p = 0.019$); and pain interference ($\beta = 0.45$, $t(39) = 3.56$,

$p = 0.001$). Average strategy score on NeuroCom condition three approached statistical significance ($\beta = -0.28$, $t(39) = -1.98$, $p = 0.054$).

Table 3. Neurocom data descriptives.

Measure	CLBP		NCLBP	
	M	**SD**	**M**	**SD**
Strategy	81.85	6.55	84.88	4.96
Equilibrium	77.32	5.34	79.14	5.41
Composite Balance	73.96	6.53	76.00	6.99

4. Discussion

The purpose of this present study was to determine whether or not a relationship exists between a new functional measure of balance (postural control as assessed using the NeuroCom Balance System), and the PROMIS psychosocial variables, in elderly individuals with or without CLBP. A number of significant findings were revealed. Most importantly, there were differences found between the two groups on various psychosocial measures and newer postural control functioning indices. To date, there has been little to no research conducted to establish whether or not a relationship exists between postural control and mental health and well-being, especially in the elderly. Moreover, the logistic regression model independently replicated a number of previous studies that assessed only one or two of the measures evaluated in the present more comprehensive biopsychosocial investigation. For example, Bradbeer and colleagues have found that older adults who experience symptoms of depression are more likely to exhibit chronic pain than older adults who are not depressed [20]. A number of other studies have independently confirmed some of the individual associations revealed in the present investigation. For example, Messier and colleagues found osteoarthritis contributed to chronic pain, avoidance of physical activity, sarcopenia, and osteoporosis [21]. Mossey and Gallagher reported that pain initiated a decreased ADL, fostering a fear of movement, and decreasing functional capacity [22]. Howland and colleagues showed that older adults tend to have increased anxiety, particularly in regards to fear of falling [23], van Haastregt and colleagues reported that anxiety leads to limited movement [24]. Lautenbacher, Kundermann, and Krieg found that pain impaired sleep quality [25]. Finally, Jorgensen and colleagues revealed that being "more sleepy" resulted in greater postural sway [26]. The great significance of the present investigation is that it is the only one in the scientific literature to evaluate the majority of the measures reported in the aforementioned studies together as a whole in an elderly population, and differentiating those participants who either had CLBP or NCLBP.

The field of biopsychosocial clinical research views the importance of the interaction among biological, psychological and social factors in pain, and the need in taking all of these into consideration when evaluating the "whole" person [31,32]. The significance of the present study was the use of a relatively new physical measure of postural control, and its relationship to pain and other psychosocial measures (as assessed by the PROMIS) in an elderly community-dwelling population. Taken as a whole in the regression model, it was revealed that there were greater levels of perceived pain inference, sleep disturbance, and fatigue (in the CLBP sufferers) compared to their NCLP counterparts. Also, there were significantly lower scores on perceived physical function and strategy of balance in the CLBP group, relative to the NCLBP group. Moreover, the CLBP group had greater scores on depression and anxiety, with lower scores in equilibrium and composite balance compared to the NCLBP group.

Of course, it should be noted that in any clinical research study of this type, there could be some potentially confounding factors that may or may not have played a role in influencing the findings. For example, the selection process of the participants in the sample could be a source of bias [32] due to the sample not being representative of the population in terms of education level and income level, history of diseases among participants, and medication influence. In the total matched paired sample of the current study, 73.1% of the participants had a college degree, and 38.5% of the total sample had a graduate or professional degree. It has been reported that individuals with lower levels of education are more likely to have a sedentary lifestyle, relative to those with a higher education. There are many health-risk factors and unhealthy habits associated with a sedentary lifestyle [22]. The sample of participants in the current study were more educated than the normal population and, therefore, may not have been totally representative of the population as a whole. Nevertheless, as reviewed above, many novel and important statistically significant findings were revealed, and the study provided the first comprehensive biopsychosocial results in the scientific literature, using different outcome measures, in the under-studied elderly population with CLBP. These results warrant further investigation.

5. Conclusions

The results of the study yielded significant differences between elderly individuals with CLBP and NCLBP, with the CLBP participants scoring higher in the psychosocial dimensions of pain interference, fatigue, and the approaching significance in regards to the dimension of sleep disturbance. Physical function scores were also significantly different between groups, with the CLBP group scoring lower than the NCLBP group. No significant differences were found between groups in regards to balance variables measured by the NeuroCom balance system, although the variables of condition four results of the NeuroCom (participant balance on a tilting force plate from sway with eyes closed), equilibrium average scores on condition five (force plate and surroundings move in regard to participants sway), NeuroCom overall somatic scores, along with sleep disturbance and pain interference measures, significantly predicted CLBP among participants, with strategy scores on condition three of the NeuroCom approaching significance as a predictor of CLBP. The results suggest that it is imperative that a biopsychosocial approach is used when investigating future constructs for the manifestation and management of pain and fall prevention in the geriatric population, and suggest a treatment to address the psycho-social and balance aspects of CLBP.

Acknowledgments: No funding was received for this study.

Author Contributions: Ryan Hulla: Contributed in data collection, data analysis, and writing of the manuscript. Michael Moomey: Contributed in data collection and writing of the manuscript. Tyler Garner: Contributed in data collection and writing of the manuscript. Chris Ray: Contributed to the conceptualization and writing of the manuscript; Robert Gatchel also contributed to the conceptualization and writing of the manuscript.

Conflicts of Interest: The authors declare no conflict of interest.

References

1. Institute of Medicine of the National Academy of Science. *Relieving Pain in America: A Blueprint for Transforming Prevention, Care, Education, and Research*; National Academies Press (US): Washington, DC, USA, 2011.
2. U.S. Census Bureau. *The 65 Years and over Population: 2000*; U.S. Census Bureau: Washington, DC, USA, 2001.
3. U.S. Census Bureau. *Population Projections of the United States by Age, Sex, Race, Hispanic Origin, and Nativity: 1999 to 2000*; U.S. Census Bureau: Washington, DC, USA, 2000.
4. DePasquale, L. Fall Prevention: Current Perspectives, Tools with Evidence. *Phys. Tehrapy Prod.* **2014**, *25*, 16. Avaliable online: https://www.physicaltherapist.com/articles/fall-prevention-current-perspectives-tools-with-evidence/ (accessed on 20 July 2016).
5. Lee, D.A.; Day, L.; Finch, C.F.; Hill, K.; Clemson, L.; McDermott, F.; Haines, T.P. Investigation of older adults' participation in exercises following completion of a state-wide survey targeting evidence-based falls prevention strategies. *J. Aging Phys. Act.* **2015**, *23*, 256–263. [CrossRef] [PubMed]
6. Englander, F.; Hodson, T.J.; Terregrossa, R.A. Economic dimensions of slip and fall injuries. *J. Forensic Sci.* **1996**, *41*, 733–746. [CrossRef] [PubMed]

7. Halvarsson, A.; Franzén, E.; Ståhle, A. Balance training with multi-task exercises improves fall-related self-efficacy, gait, balance performance and physical function in older adults with osteoporosis: A randomized controlled trial. *Clin. Rehabil.* **2015**, *29*, 365–375. [CrossRef] [PubMed]

8. D'Arcy, Y.M. *How to Manage Pain in the Elderly*; Sigma Theta Tau International: Indianapolis, IN, USA, 2010.

9. Leveille, S.G.; Jones, R.N.; Kiely, D.K.; Hausdorff, J.M.; Shmerling, R.H.; Guralnik, J.M.; Bean, J.F. Chronic musculoskeletal pain and the occurrence of falls in an older population. *JAMA* **2009**, *302*, 2214–2221. [CrossRef] [PubMed]

10. Rudy, T.E.; Weiner, D.K.; Lieber, S.J.; Slaboda, J.; Boston, J.R. The impact of chronic low back pain on older adults: A comparative study of patients and controls. *Pain* **2007**, *131*, 293–301. [CrossRef] [PubMed]

11. Weiner, D.K.; Rudy, T.E.; Morrow, L.; Slaboda, J.; Lieber, S. The Relationship Between Pain, Neuropsychological Performance, and Physical Function in Community-Dwelling Older Adults with Chronic Low Back Pain. *Pain Med.* **2006**, *7*, 60–70. [CrossRef] [PubMed]

12. Boyd, R.; Stevens, J. Falls and fear of falling: Burden, beliefs and behaviours. *Age Ageing* **2009**, *38*, 423–428. [CrossRef] [PubMed]

13. Toebes, M.J.; Hoozemans, M.J.; Furrer, R.; Dekker, J.; van Dieën, J.H. Associations between measures of gait stability, leg strength and fear of falling. *Gait Posture* **2015**, *41*, 76–80. [CrossRef] [PubMed]

14. Petrella, R.J.; Payne, M.; Myers, A.; Overend, T.; Chesworth, B. Physical function and fear of falling after hip fracture rehabilitation in the elderly. *Am. J. Phys. Med. Rehabil.* **2000**, *79*, 154–160. [CrossRef] [PubMed]

15. Hanada, E.Y.; Johnson, M.; Hubley-Kozey, C. A comparison of trunk muscle activation amplitudes during gait in older adults with and without chronic low back pain. *PM R J. Inj. Funct. Rehabil.* **2011**, *3*, 920–928. [CrossRef] [PubMed]

16. Pike, E.C.J. The Active Aging Agenda, Old Folk Devils and a New Moral Panic. *Sociol. Sport J.* **2011**, *28*, 209–225. [CrossRef]

17. Stubbs, B.; Brefka, S.; Denkinger, M.D. What Works to Prevent Falls in Community-Dwelling Older Adults? Umbrella Review of Meta-analyses of Randomized Controlled Trials. *Phys. Ther.* **2015**, *95*, 1095–1110. [CrossRef] [PubMed]

18. Arfken, C.L.; Lach, H.W.; Birge, S.J.; Miller, J.P. The prevalence and correlates of fear of falling in elderly persons living in the community. *Am. J. Public Health* **1994**, *84*, 565–570. [CrossRef] [PubMed]

19. Morgan, A.J.; Parker, A.G.; Jimenez, M.A.; Jorm, A.F. Exercise and Mental Health: An Exercise and Sports Science Australia Commissioned Review. *J. Exerc. Physiol.* **2013**, *16*, 64–73.

20. Bradbeer, M.; Helme, R.D.; Yong, H.H.; Kendig, H.L.; Gibson, S.J. Widowhood and other demographic associations of pain in independent older people. *Clin. J. Pain* **2003**, *19*, 247–254. [CrossRef] [PubMed]

21. Messier, S.P.; Royer, T.D.; Craven, T.E.; O'Toole, M.L.; Burns, R.; Ettinger, W.H. Long-Term Exercise and its Effect on Balance in Older, Osteoarthritic Adults: Results from the Fitness, Arthritis, and Seniors Trial (FAST). *J. Am. Geriatr. Soc.* **2000**, *48*, 131–138. [CrossRef] [PubMed]

22. Mossey, J.M.; Gallagher, R.M. The Longitudinal Occurrence and Impact of Comorbid Chronic Pain and Chronic Depression over Two Years in Continuing Care Retirement Community Residents. *Pain Med.* **2004**, *5*, 335–348. [CrossRef] [PubMed]

23. Howland, J.; Peterson, E.W.; Levin, W.C.; Fried, L.; Pordon, D.; Bak, S. Fear of Falling among the Community-Dwelling Elderly. *J. Aging Health* **1993**, *5*, 229–243. [CrossRef] [PubMed]

24. Van Haastregt, J.C.; Zijlstra, G.R.; van Rossum, E.; van Eijk, J.T.M.; Kempen, G.I. Feelings of anxiety and symptoms of depression in community-living older persons who avoid activity for fear of falling. *Am. J. Geriatr. Psychiatry* **2008**, *16*, 186–193. [CrossRef] [PubMed]

25. Lautenbacher, S.; Kundermann, B.; Krieg, J. Sleep deprivation and pain perception. *Sleep Med. Rev.* **2006**, *10*, 357–369. [CrossRef] [PubMed]

26. Jorgensen, M.G.; Rathleff, M.S.; Laessoe, U.; Caserotti, P.; Nielsen, O.B.F.; Aagaard, P. Time-of-day influences postural balance in older adults. *Gait Posture* **2012**, *35*, 653–657. [CrossRef] [PubMed]

27. Swanenburg, J.; Mittaz Hager, A.G.; Nevzati, A.; Klipstein, A. Identifying fallers and nonfallers with the maximal base of support width (BSW): A one-year prospective study. *J. Aging Phys. Act.* **2015**, *23*, 200–204. [CrossRef] [PubMed]

28. Ritchie, R.F.; Palomaki, G. Selecting clinically relevant populations for reference intervals. *Clin. Chem. Lab. Med.* **2004**, *42*, 702–709. [CrossRef] [PubMed]

29. Bajaj, J.S.; Thacker, L.R.; Wade, J.B.; Sanyal, A.J.; Heuman, D.M.; Sterling, R.K.; Revicki, D.A. PROMIS computerised adaptive tests are dynamic instruments to measure health-related quality of life in patients with cirrhosis. *Aliment. Pharmacol. Ther.* **2011**, *34*, 1123–1132. [CrossRef] [PubMed]

30. Biggan, J.R.; Melton, F.; Horvat, M.A.; Ricard, M.; Keller, D.; Ray, C.T. Increased load computerized dynamic posturography in prefrail and nonfrail community-dwelling older adults. *J. Aging Phys. Act.* **2014**, *22*, 96–102. [CrossRef] [PubMed]

31. Gatchel, R.J.; Peng, Y.; Peters, M.L.; Fuchs, P.N.; Turk, D.C. The Biopsychosocial Approach to Chronic Pain: Scientific Advances and Future Directions. *Psychol. Bull.* **2007**, *133*, 581–624. [CrossRef] [PubMed]

32. Gatchel, R.J. *Clinical Essentials of Pain Management*; American Psychological Association: Washington, DC, USA, 2005.

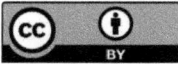

healthcare

MDPI

Article

Treatment of Lower Back Pain—The Gap between Guideline-Based Treatment and Medical Care Reality

Andreas Werber [1] and Marcus Schiltenwolf [2,*]

[1] Department of Orthopedics and Orthopedic Surgery, University Hospital Giessen, Klinikstr. 33, 35392 Giessen, Germany; andreas.werber@ortho.med.uni-giessen.de
[2] Department of Orthopedics and Traumatology, University Hospital Heidelberg, Schlierbacher Landstr. 200a, 69118 Heidelberg, Germany
* Correspondence: marcus.schiltenwolf@med.uni-heidelberg.de; Tel.: +49-6221-56-26323

Academic Editor: Robert J. Gatchel
Received: 3 June 2016; Accepted: 12 July 2016; Published: 15 July 2016

Abstract: Despite the fact that unspecific low back pain is of important impact in general health care, this pain condition is often treated insufficiently. Poor efficiency has led to the necessity of guidelines addressing evidence-based strategies for treatment of lower back pain (LBP). We present some statements of the German medical care reality. Self-responsible action of the patient should be supported while invasive methods in particular should be avoided due to lacking evidence in outcome efficiency. However, it has to be stated that no effective implementation strategy has been established yet. Especially, studies on the economic impact of different implementation strategies are lacking. A lack of awareness of common available guidelines and an uneven distribution of existing knowledge throughout the population can be stated: persons with higher risk suffering from LBP by higher professional demands and lower educational level are not skilled in advised management of LBP. Both diagnostic imaging and invasive treatment methods increased dramatically leading to increased costs and doctor workload without being associated with improved patient functioning, severity of pain or overall health status due to the absence of a functioning primary care gate keeping system for patient selection. Opioids are prescribed on a grand scale and over a long period. Moreover, opioid prescription is not indicated properly, when predominantly persons with psychological distress like somatoform disorders are treated with opioids.

Keywords: low back pain; guideline-based treatment; somatisation

1. Introduction

The onset of chronic lower back pain (cLBP) is based upon various factors. A former history of LBP is the most consistent risk factor for transition from a baseline of a pain-free state [1]. LBP is marked as chronic if the pain occurs on more than half of the days of the last half-year. In a broader sense, cLBP is defined as the final point of a chronification process including the following characteristics: generalization of pain, changing areas of pain, other complaints that cannot be explained merely somatically (buzzing in one's ears, digestive disorders, insomnia). Furthermore, changes in behaviour are concomitant, for instance increasing consumption of medication, alternating presentation of different symptoms, avoidance of exercises and social withdrawal [2].

The risk of suffering from LBP differs significantly within the general population. Especially psychological distress in terms of dysfunctional behaviour plays a decisive role in the development process [2]. In less than 10% of the cases LBP can solely be explained somatically. In fact, LBP is often an alternative expression of physical stress symptoms of which the patients are seldom aware. LBP is rather a medical condition than a complete medical entity. In combination with other symptoms like depression or anxiety disorders, cLBP is an expression of distress [3].

Several countries developed guidelines in order to provide a systematic approach for treatment of cLBP with similar procedures both for diagnosis and treatment [4,5]. However, both patients and physicians are seldom aware of how to deal properly with LBP according to recommendations of common available guidelines [5]. Monomodal therapy often leads to insufficient therapeutic response, hence it is important to identify the distinct factors of causing pain and treat them properly in terms of a multidisciplinary (=multimodal) therapeutic approach [6].

The aim of this article is to outline the medical care reality in Germany in terms of diagnosis and treatment of LBP by presenting processed statistical data of German insitute for tarification system for hospital care. Despite increasing numbers of diagnostic and therapeutical procedures, the effectiveness of treatment is still poor. Lacking awareness of common available guidelines of how to cope with LBP leads both to an increasing dependency of the patient from the therapist due to insufficient perception of self-effectiveness of a therapy and furthermore to outdated treatment approaches heavily influenced by the habits of the therapist.

1.1. Epidemiology

Life time prevalence for acute LBP (aLBP) varies between 58% and 85% (in Western industrial nations), one-year prevalence varies between 20% and 40% and point prevalence for Germany is 8% for men and 14% for women. The biggest incidence is found in the fourth decade of life [7,8]. The resulting costs (both direct costs for medical treatment and indirect costs for stoppage and/or retirement pay) varies between €400 and €7000 per patient and year. In total, costs of over 50 Billion Euros occur solely in Germany each year. Six percent of all direct costs for medical treatment, 15% of all incapacity for work and 18% of all early retirements are associated with LBP [8]. Education and appearance of LBP correlate significantly [5]. A representative study of how to coop with available guidelines proved that higher education is a protecting factor for suffering from LBP. A total of 82.9% of the participants with lower education levels suffered from lower back pain at least once in their lifetime compared to only 62.4% of people with university degrees. Especially women with lower education had a significantly higher risk of suffering from LBP. In contrast to this, participants with an university-entrance degree had a 70% lower risk, those with completed academic studies had a 60% lower risk of developing LBP [5].

1.2. Data Source

Our data analysis was based upon free availabe health care data provided by the German insitute for tarification system for hospital care—InEK (http://www.g-drg.de). To ensure compensation for general hospital services in Germany, a consistent performance-oriented remuneration system was established according to the Hospital Finance Act (KHG). Basis for this is the G-DRG-system (German-Diagnosis Related Groups-System), in which every treatment case is compensated by flat-rate payment depending upon the according DRG. Duties associated with the implementation, further development and maintenace of the payment system were assigned by the German Hospital Federation and health insurance associations to the InEK GmbH as the German DRG institue. All provided in-patient and out-patient data was analysed and classified in terms of procedures and body region to allow statements of common diagnosis and treatment procedures.

2. Diagnostics

According to the German insitute for tarification system for hospital care—InEK—the number of MRIs of the lumbar spine rose from 40,000 in 2004 to more than 75,000 in 2007 and to more than 385,000 in 2015 (inpatient treatment). An analysis of six random trials with a total of 1084 patients showed that with diagnostic assessment neither in short-term nor in medium-term improved clinical outcome could be achieved, provided the fact that there was no evidence for serious underlying conditions, so-called "red flags" (Table 1) [9].

Table 1. "Red Flags"—specific causes of back pain symptoms.

Anamnesis	Specific Cause
history of fall and/or accident	fracture
drug abuse	spondylodiscitis
malignant primary disease	metastasis, pathological fracture
immunosupression (e.g., AIDS)	spondylodiscitis
chronic infection	spondylodiscitis
long-term cortisone intake	cortisone-induced osteoporosis
involuntary urination and defecation	conus-cauda-syndrome
paresis	nerve root compression

Psychosocial risk factors, so-called "yellow flags", gained importance as predictors of chronification and extent of subjective impairment (Table 2). The underlying tendency for chronification occurs on several levels: typical somatic factors like heavy labor are eclipsed by a converse behavior as a result of a sedentary lifestyle leading to a degradation of the musculoscelettal system, influenced by psychosocial risk factors like depressiveness and acquired helplessness in terms of coping strategies [10].

Table 2. "Yellow Flags"—risk factors of chronification of back pain symptoms.

Risk Factor
low work satisfaction
low social status
stress
age
female sex
possibility of morbid gain
passive lifestyle
nicotine, alcohol, drug abuse
obesity
insufficient self-regulation
little physical and psychological resources

3. Therapy

3.1. Monomodal Therapy

Subjective impairment with inability to participate in terms of activities of daily-living due to LBP lead to physician consultation. Since chronification factors from psychosocial co-morbidity are by definition not relevant for aLBP, the usual therapy approach is merely a medical treatment with analgesia [11]. Another aspect is a physician's recommendation of avoidance of any physical strain despite the fact being counterproductive in terms of a chronification process. Actually, bed rest should be avoided with LBP, except for ischialgia where no distinct recommendation is stated; however, an active lifestyle should be advised [12].

3.1.1. Medical Therapy

According to the pain ladder of the WHO, NSAID medication is used for mild pain. For moderate to severe pain, mild and strong opioids are usually prescribed. Co-Analgesia like antidepressants and antiepileptic drugs augment the analgesic effect of the basic medication. An Australian study showed that for aLBP neither diclofenac nor spinal manipulative therapy appreciably reduced the number of days until recovery compared with placebo drug or placebo manipulative therapy [11]. During the transition from acute to chronic LBP it is pretty common to escalate pain medication from NSAIDs to opioid medication. Both in the USA and in Germany, the number of prescriptions of opioids increased by more than 100% between 1997 and 2004 [13]. However, in the long term, no difference in pain relive can be stated for NSAIDs or opioids. Hence, an interdisciplinary guideline for long-term opioid application for nun-tumor pain was published in Germany in 2010 (LONTS) [14] and revised in 2015 [15]. Continuous application of opioid medication is inconsistent with the strict indication considering contraindications of the guideline. For instance, an application of opioids for more than 12 weeks is only recommended if an essential and comprehensible pain relief is achieved without dosage escalation. Patients with intermittent pain episodes (for instance trigeminus neuralgia), continuous headaches with physical not sufficiently explainable symptoms as well as patient's with depressive or anxiety disorders should not be treated with opioids. Continuously decreasing analgesic effects result in a paradox hyperalgesia and cognitive impairment, thus leading to abusive intake of opioids. An evaluation of health insurance data of a German statutory health insurance company between 2006 and 2010 showed that the number of prescriptions of opioid prescriptions increased virtually linearly. Prescriptions of mild opioids were decreasing for non-tumor pain, but increasing for tumor pain, while the number of prescriptions of strong opioids was increasing both for tumor and non-tumor pain. Differences occurred in terms of duration and kind of the preferred substances, including the considerations of common contraindications (e.g., somatoform disorders). The majority of strong opioids being prescribed for non-tumor pain were fentanyl pain patches for 40 to 45 year old males with average annual costs of 1833 Euros per patient. Out of 21,000 patients with somatoform pain disorder, 44.4% were treated with opioids (20.7% with mild, 23.7% with strong opioids). Prescribing behavior was often not consistent with common indications and contraindications.

3.1.2. Interventional Therapy

During the last few years, a massive increase of spinal injections in the lumbar region from 778,362 in 2006 to 1,197,302 in 2009 (inpatient and outpatient treatment) was observed, a trend similar both in the USA and in Germany [16]. Effects of injections can be stated, but only last for a limited period of time [17]. Beside the doubtful effectiveness of those therapies, the risk of side-effects like infection and/or vascular lesions are considerably increased leqading to problematic cost-benefit-ratio [18].

3.1.3. Surgical Therapy

In Germany, the number of lumbar spinal surgery increased from 165,000 in 2006 to 250,000 in 2009 an to more than 705,000 in 2015 (inpatient treatment), comparable to the development in the USA (Table 3). Although leading to considerable costs and complications by an increasing number of spinal surgeries, a verifiable benefit of quality of life cannot bet stated [18]. Several studies showed that less than half of the patients with spinal surgery became pain free, independent from the applied surgical technique [9,17,18].

3.1.4. Synopsis of Monomodal Therapy

Considering present studies, monomodal strategies—conservative, interventional or operative—show only little effects in terms of treatment of cLBP. In a recent meta-analysis with a total of 76 trials reporting on 34 treatments it was observed that only 50% of the investigated treatments had statistically significant effects and for most the effects were small or moderate [19]. This meta-analysis revealed that the analgesic effects of many treatments for non-specific low back pain are small and that they do not differ in populations with acute or chronic symptoms. A main reason for this outcome is that cLBP has a multifactorial pathogenesis which is not covered sufficiently with a monomodal therapy approach. Pointless therapeutical action (due to unfulfilled patient's desires and physician's increasing readiness to act) leads to a medicalization of a common pain phenomenon, ignores patient's own resources and replaces theses resources by ongoing escalation of therapeutical approaches. Since the patient's resources are hereby ignored paternalistically, a sustainability of a therapeutical approach is not reachable [2,5,13].

Table 3. Number of procedures of inpatient treatment between 2014 and 2015 according to the German Procedure Classification System (OPS) [1].

OPS Code	Procedure Definition	Number of Cases
3-802	MRI of the vertebral column and spinal cord	280,631
3-823	MRI of the vertebral column and spinal cord with application of contrast media	92,779
3-841	MRT myelography	12,418
		385,828
5-83 (5.836)	surgical procedures of the spine (spondylodesis)	706,666 (64,812)
8-020.7	therapeutical injections of the intervertebral disc	9860
8-914	injections of nerve roots and injections near the spine for pain therapy	127,678
8-915	injections of peripheral nerves for pain therapy	136,700
8-916	injections of the sympathetic nervous system for pain therapy	2592
8-917	injections of vertebral joints for pain therapy	4452
		281,282

[1] The German procedure classification (Operationen- und Prozedurenschlüssel-OPS) is the official classification for the encoding of operations, procedures and general medical measures in the inpatient sector and for surgical procedures in the outpatient sector. The German Institute of Medical Documentation and Information (DIMDI) publishes the OPS classification on behalf of the Federal Ministry of Health. Its use in inpatient care is laid down in § 301 Volume V of the German Social Security Code (SGB V) and for surgical procedures in the outpatient sector in § 295 SGB V (www.dimdi.de).

3.2. Multidisciplinary Therapy

This is understood as the application of different kinds of body therapy (exercises for strength, endurance and mobility as well as body perception) and coequally psychotherapy (cognitive behavioural therapy or psychodynamic therapy) in the presence of chronified pain syndromes. The objective is an active somatic and psychological therapeutical approach. Passive methods should be avoided. All therapies should be in a group setting with a maximum of 8 participants, seldom as an individual therapy. The key aspect of a multidisciplinary therapy is the collaboration of all involved persons under an individual dysfunctional concept of each patient. At least once a week, the patient's individual progress and drawback is discussed in a team and the patient's treatment focus is adjusted accordingly. It could be shown that only intensive (more than 100 h) multidisciplinary biopsychosocial rehabilitation with functional restoration reduces pain and improves function in patients with CLBP chronic low back pain, while less intensive interventions did not show improvements in clinically relevant outcomes [20].

3.2.1. National Disease Management Guideline Recommendations

National disease management guidelines (NVL) incorporate medical guiding decisions and criteria regarding diagnosis, management, and treatment of chronic diseases based upon systematic developed and evaluated therapy strategies. In Germany, the German Agency for Quality in Medicine (ÄZQ) coordinates a national program for disease management guidelines, similar to the National Guideline Clearinghouse in the USA [5].

In terms of acute lower back pain, extensive diagnostic and therapeutical interventions should be avoided and the mainly harmless natural history of the condition should be monitored [21]. However, it is important that distinct warning signs, so-called "red flags", of serious physical illness are excluded reliably and at an early stage. In case of a red flag, a target-oriented therapy should be pursued including appropriate diagnostic and therapeutical instruments, for example MRI and laboratory diagnostics. After the exclusion of red flags, imaging diagnostic should be avoided completely for at least 4 weeks since the information yield is negligible. It is important to explain this approach to the patient, taking his complaints seriously. In case of persisting pain (pain reduction less than 50% after 4 weeks), a reevaluation of the clinical findings should be carried out, including imaging diagnostics, preferably MRI. A short-term administration of medicatio—without recommendation of a distinct substance—can be considered, even if a relevant benefit is not verifiable [22]. In fact, active exercises under the patient's own authority should be encouraged while passive therapies (including physiotherapy) should be avoided. Long-term certificates of incapacity should not be prescribed since with the continuation of inability to work the demands of the working place increase as as the demands of the labor market in case of job loss. With increasing inability to work and the loss of physical and psychological strength, the probability of occupational reintegration decreases accordingly.

Due to psychosocial risk factors, so-called "yellow flags", of chronification of LBP, a merely somatically based therapeutical approach is to be considered only partially promising. According to current studies, the cost-benefit-ratio of surgical approaches (for instance disc prostheses or mono-segmental fusions) is inconsistent, hence being not recommended [16,23]. A multidisciplinary therapy including psychotherapy for treating CLBP is not just equal to a surgical approach in terms of pain reduction but also more cost-effective and less risky. Multidisciplinary pain therapy is the central therapy recommendation of the NVL encapsulating a combination of medical and psychotherapeutical methods as well as movement therapy addressing a patient's individual dysfunctional concept [24]. The patient's own capabilities should be encouraged while fears and conflicts should be overcome to achieve greatest possible self-effectiveness. One mandatory requirement for a therapy's sustainability is the movativation of the patient for self-responsible acting. The degree of chronification as a substantial prognostic factor includes a generalization of pain areas from local to widely spread pain and other complaints that cannot be explained merely somatically (buzzing in one's ears, digestive disorders, insomnia). The effects of a multidisciplinary pain therapy are inversely proportional to the number of pain areas [25]. With persisting pain after 12 weeks of proper treatment (according to common guidelines) and relevant activity limitations, a multidisciplinary therapy should be evaluated. In the presence of psychological risk factors, a multidisciplinary therapy should be considered after 6 weeks of unsuccessful treatment.

3.2.2. Synopsis of Multidisciplinary Therapy

The treatment of LBP is characterized by a large number of acute medical oriented methods, for instance diagnostic imaging, injection therapy or chiropractic therapy. Due to only little additional information yield, diagnostic imaging should be reduced to a minimum, hence treatment is usually not affected.

Psychosocial risk factors of chronification are only respected sparsely. In particular, the number of interventional procedures increased significantly with limited evidence for efficiency as well as increased costs for treatment and increased risk of complications in the healing process.

Based on the recommendations of the national disease management guideline for LBP, four aspects of treatment should be taken into account:

1. exclusion of specific causes of the complaints, red flags, by considering the medical history and a thorough clinical and neurological examination.
2. identification of psychosocial risk factors, yellow flags, and adjusting the treatment accordingly including psychological assistance.
3. workflow for patients with unspecific lower back pain according to the suggestions of the National Disease Management Guidelines (NVL) (Figure 1).
4. interdisciplinary diagnosis: Due to the increasing relevance of psychosocial risk factors in case of persisting pain, a transition to chronic pain syndromes has to be expected. Hence, further treatment of subacute or even chronic pain syndromes must be accompanied by an interdisciplinary diagnostic approach. In case of persisting pain after 12 weeks (or 6 weeks with psychosocial risk factors), both re-evaluation with regard to specific causes of the pain syndromes and diagnostic imaging (preferably by MRI) should be carried out. If no specific cause can be verified, a chronification of the LBP is very likely. Therefore, an early activating and self-effective therapy is of high significance. Interventional and surgical procedures, especially in terms of

cost-benefit ratio, are negligible. With larger distance to re-integration to work and daily life, the patient's morbid gain will increase, therefore the patient's motivation will be presumably be impaired. Furthermore, the outcome of the therapy will be affected as well, hence it is of great significance to include the patient into self-effective therapeutical possibilities.

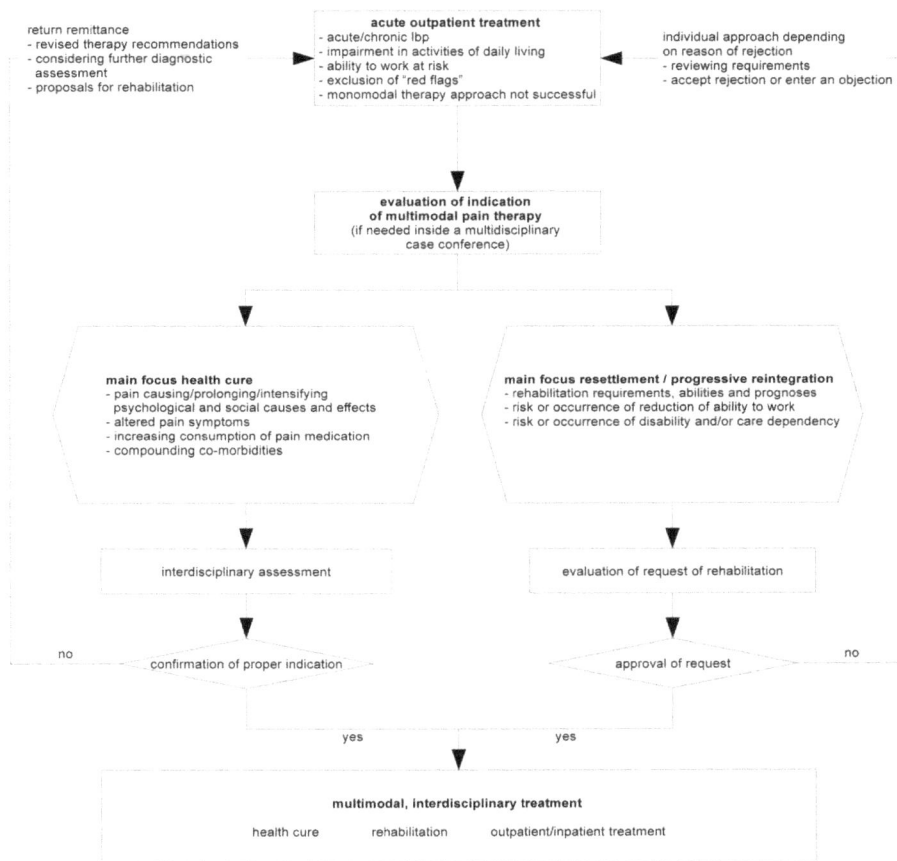

Figure 1. Algorithm for treatment of patients with unspecific LBP according to the suggestions of the National Disease Management Guidelines (NVL).

4. Discussion

The increasing number of diagnostic and therapeutical procedures (medical imaging, interventional and surgical procedures) with no verification of effectiveness and high expectations of the patients for successful treatment using technical solutions demonstrate that LBP is not merely a medical, but rather a social phaenomenon. Despite lacking evidence, both patients and service providers agree that a massive medicalisation of the phenomenon back pain is indispensable. However, this view leads to a further passiveness of the patient in terms of self-effectiveness of any therapeutical approach and an increasing level of dependence of the patient from the therapist.

A lack of awareness of common available guidelines how to cope with LBP can be stated with an uneven distribution of existing knowledge throughout the population. Passive coping strategies like taking pain medication or ointment therapy are favored over active coping strategies like gymnastics, physical activities, and relaxation exercises. Respondents with a higher level of education suffer significantly less often from LBP and tend toward active treatment strategies. Respondents with lower levels of education more often demand passive treatment strategies. The general population, especially those with lower education, is not sufficiently aware of behavioral strategies for managing LBP, as proposed in available guidelines.

The option of an active self-effective acting is ignored. The national medical guidelines for unspecific LBP establish a therapeutical concept at different stages offering evidence-based recommendations. Small effects of common treatment approaches for LBP yielded to the necessity of interdisciplinary created, generally accepted and evidence-based recommendations for treatment.

However, one major problem is the focus of the guideline on unspecific LBP, because every monomodal therapeutical approach (for instance interventional and surgical procedures) can be legitimized by arguing that a specific cause for the pain syndrome is present. Because of the insufficient distinctiveness between specific and unspecific pain syndromes, it will be possible to skip the recommendations of the guideline by referring to a specific cause devaluing the concept of a multidisciplinary therapeutical approach.

5. Conclusions

Knowledge of treatment guidelines for LBP is not sufficiently available in the general population. Physicians should address the knowledge of patients about the rightful treatment behavior and should provide guideline-oriented treatment strategies. Active rules of management should be emphasized while the importance of passive rules of management should be downgraded.

Acknowledgments: We thank Bernhard Arnold, Multidisciplinary Pain Therapy Center, Helios Amper-Clinic in Dachau, Germany, for calculating the number of MRI of the lumbar spine, the number of surgical procedures of the back and the number of injections using data provided by the German tarification system for hospital care—InEK for the years 2007 und 2009.

Author Contributions: A.W. analyzed data and wrote the paper; M.S. proofread the paper.

Conflicts of Interest: The authors declare no conflict of interest.

References

1. Taylor, J.B.; Goode, A.P.; George, S.Z.; Cook, C.E. Incidence and risk factors for first-time incident low back pain: A systematic review and meta-analysis. *Spine J.* **2014**, *14*, 2299–2319. [CrossRef] [PubMed]
2. Werber, A.; Schiltenwolf, M. Chronified back pain. *MMW Fortschr. Med.* **2012**, *154*, 39–43. (In German) [CrossRef] [PubMed]
3. Henningsen, P. The psychosomatics of chronic back pain. Classification, aetiology and therapy. *Orthopade* **2004**, *33*, 558–567. (In German) [CrossRef] [PubMed]
4. Krismer, M.; van Tulder, M.; Low Back Pain Group of the Bone and Joint Health Strategies for Europe Project. Strategies for prevention and management of musculoskeletal conditions. Low back pain (non-specific). *Best Pract. Res. Clin. Rheumatol.* **2007**, *21*, 77–91. [CrossRef] [PubMed]
5. Werber, A.; Zimmermann-Stenzel, M.; Moradi, B.; Neubauer, E.; Schiltenwolf, M. Awareness of the German population of common available guidelines of how to cope with lower back pain. *Pain Physician* **2014**, *17*, 217–226. [PubMed]
6. Bishop, A.; Foster, N.E.; Thomas, E.; Hay, E.M. How does the self-reported clinical management of patients with low back pain relate to the attitudes and beliefs of health care practitioners? A survey of UK general practitioners and physiotherapists. *Pain* **2008**, *135*, 187–195. [CrossRef] [PubMed]
7. Henningsen, P.; Jakobsen, T.; Schiltenwolf, M.; Weiss, M.G. Somatization revisited: Diagnosis and perceived causes of common mental disorders. *J. Nerv. Ment. Dis.* **2005**, *193*, 85–92. [CrossRef] [PubMed]
8. Schneider, S.; Schmitt, H.; Zoller, S.; Schiltenwolf, M. Workplace stress, lifestyle and social factors as correlates of back pain: A representative study of the German working population. *Int. Arch. Occup. Environ. Health* **2005**, *78*, 253–269. [CrossRef] [PubMed]

9.   Chou, R.; Fu, R.; Carrino, J.A.; Deyo, R.A. Imaging strategies for low-back pain: Systematic review and meta-analysis. *Lancet* **2009**, *373*, 463–472. [CrossRef]

10. Von Korff, M. Studying the natural history of back pain. *Spine* **1994**, *19*, 2041S–2046S. [CrossRef] [PubMed]

11. Hancock, M.J.; Maher, C.G.; Latimer, J.; McLachlan, A.J.; Cooper, C.W.; Day, R.O.; Spindler, M.F.; McAuley, J.H. Assessment of diclofenac or spinal manipulative therapy, or both, in addition to recommended first-line treatment for acute low back pain: A randomised controlled trial. *Lancet* **2007**, *370*, 1638–1643. [CrossRef]

12. Dahm, K.T.; Brurberg, K.G.; Jamtvedt, G.; Hagen, K.B. Advice to rest in bed versus advice to stay active for acute low-back pain and sciatica. *Cochrane Database Syst. Rev.* **2010**. [CrossRef]

13. Werber, A.; Marschall, U.; L'Hoest, H.; Hauser, W.; Moradi, B.; Schiltenwolf, M. Opioid therapy in the treatment of chronic pain conditions in Germany. *Pain Physician* **2015**, *18*, E323–E331. [PubMed]

14. Reinecke, H.; Sorgatz, H.; German Society for the Study of Pain (DGSS). S3 guideline LONTS. Long-term administration of opioids for non-tumor pain. *Schmerz* **2009**, *23*, 440–447. (In German) [CrossRef] [PubMed]

15. Hauser, W.; Bock, F.; Engeser, P.; Hege-Scheuing, G.; Huppe, M.; Lindena, G.; Maier, C.; Norda, H.; Radbruch, L.; Sabatowski, R.; et al. Recommendations of the updated LONTS guidelines. Long-term opioid therapy for chronic noncancer pain. *Schmerz* **2015**, *29*, 109–130. (In German) [PubMed]

16. Deyo, R.A.; Mirza, S.K.; Turner, J.A.; Martin, B.I. Overtreating chronic back pain: Time to back off? *J. Am. Board Fam. Med.* **2009**, *22*, 62–68. [CrossRef] [PubMed]

17. Chou, R.; Atlas, S.J.; Stanos, S.P.; Rosenquist, R.W. Nonsurgical interventional therapies for low back pain: A review of the evidence for an American Pain Society clinical practice guideline. *Spine* **2009**, *34*, 1078–1093. [CrossRef] [PubMed]

18. Chou, R.; Loeser, J.D.; Owens, D.K.; Rosenquist, R.W.; Atlas, S.J.; Baisden, J.; Carragee, E.J.; Grabois, M.; Murphy, D.R.; Resnick, D.K.; et al. Interventional therapies, surgery, and interdisciplinary rehabilitation for low back pain: An evidence-based clinical practice guideline from the American Pain Society. *Spine* **2009**, *34*, 1066–1077. [CrossRef] [PubMed]

19. Machado, L.A.; Kamper, S.J.; Herbert, R.D.; Maher, C.G.; McAuley, J.H. Analgesic effects of treatments for non-specific low back pain: A meta-analysis of placebo-controlled randomized trials. *Rheumatology* **2009**, *48*, 520–527. [CrossRef] [PubMed]

20. Guzman, J.; Esmail, R.; Karjalainen, K.; Malmivaara, A.; Irvin, E.; Bombardier, C. Multidisciplinary rehabilitation for chronic low back pain: Systematic review. *BMJ* **2001**, *322*, 1511–1516. [CrossRef] [PubMed]

21. Jarvik, J.G.; Hollingworth, W.; Heagerty, P.J.; Haynor, D.R.; Boyko, E.J.; Deyo, R.A. Three-year incidence of low back pain in an initially asymptomatic cohort: Clinical and imaging risk factors. *Spine* **2005**, *30*, 1541–1548. [CrossRef] [PubMed]

22. Keller, A.; Hayden, J.; Bombardier, C.; van Tulder, M. Effect sizes of non-surgical treatments of non-specific low-back pain. *Eur. Spine J.* **2007**, *16*, 1776–1788. [CrossRef] [PubMed]

23. Deyo, R.A. Back surgery—Who needs it? *N. Engl. J. Med.* **2007**, *356*, 2239–2243. [CrossRef] [PubMed]

24. Mirza, S.K.; Deyo, R.A. Systematic review of randomized trials comparing lumbar fusion surgery to nonoperative care for treatment of chronic back pain. *Spine* **2007**, *32*, 816–823. [CrossRef] [PubMed]

25. Moradi, B.; Zahlten-Hinguranage, A.; Barie, A.; Caldeira, F.; Schnatzer, P.; Schiltenwolf, M.; Neubauer, E. The impact of pain spread on the outcome of multidisciplinary therapy in patients with chronic musculoskeletal pain—A prospective clinical study in 389 patients. *Eur. J. Pain* **2010**, *14*, 799–805. [CrossRef] [PubMed]

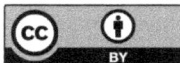

healthcare

MDPI

Article

Differences in the Association between Depression and Opioid Misuse in Chronic Low Back Pain *versus* Chronic Pain at Other Locations

Arpana Jaiswal [1], Jeffrey F. Scherrer [1,*], Joanne Salas [1], Carissa van den Berk-Clark [1], Sheran Fernando [1] and Christopher M. Herndon [1,2]

[1]   Department of Family and Community Medicine, Saint Louis University School of Medicine, St. Louis, MO 63104, USA; jaiswala@slu.edu (A.J.); salasj@slu.edu (J.S.); cvanden1@slu.edu (C.B.-C.); fernandos@slu.edu (S.F.); cherndo@siue.edu (C.M.H.)
[2]   Department of Pharmacy Practice, School of Pharmacy, Southern Illinois University Edwardsville, Edwardsville, IL 62026, USA
*   Correspondence: scherrjf@slu.edu; Tel.: +1-314-977-8486

Academic Editor: Robert J. Gatchel
Received: 8 March 2016; Accepted: 12 June 2016; Published: 16 June 2016

Abstract: Patients with chronic pain and depression are more likely to develop opioid abuse compared to patients without depression. It is not known if this association differs by pain location. We compared the strength of association between depression and opioid misuse in patients with chronic low back pain (CLBP) *vs.* chronic pain of other location (CPOL). Chart abstracted data was obtained from 166 patients seeking care in a family medicine clinic. Depression was measured by the PHQ-9 and opioid misuse was measured using the Current Opioid Misuse Measure. Pain severity and interference questions came from the Brief Pain Inventory. Cross-tabulations were computed to measure the association between depression and opioid misuse stratified on pain location. Exploratory logistic regression modeled the association between depression and opioid misuse after adjusting for pain location and pain severity and interference. Depression was significantly associated with opioid misuse in CPOL but not in CLBP. Regression results indicate pain interference partly accounts for the depression–opioid misuse association. These preliminary results from a small patient sample suggest depression may co-occur with opioid misuse more often in CPOL than in CLBP. Further research is needed to compare this comorbidity in specific pain diagnoses such as arthritis, fibromyalgia and CLBP.

Keywords: chronic pain; pain location; depression; opioid misuse

---

1. Introduction

Patients with comorbid chronic pain and depression are more likely to receive a longer duration of opioid treatment at higher doses and are more likely to develop opioid abuse compared to non-depressed patients [1,2]. To our knowledge, it is not known if the link between depression and opioid abuse is similarly present in all types of chronic pain or is more common in chronic low back pain (CLPB). We are aware of one study of pain location and opioid misuse which found prevalence of opioid misuse was 82.8% in CLBP, 76.8% in those with arthritis, and 87.9% in neck/joint pain diagnosis suggesting some variation in opioid misuse by pain location [3]. The association between opioid misuse and depression could be stronger in CLBP given some evidence from patient populations that this pain location is associated with more depression than other pain types such as migraine and nerve root pain [4]. Comparison of fibromyalgia to other pain diagnostic groups found prevalence of the personality profile for neuroticism was greatest in fibromyalgia (46.2%) followed by 29.2% for lumbar, 20.5% for lower extremity and 15.4% for thoracic [5]. These results indicate that back pain patients have higher neuroticism compared to patients with other pain diagnoses with the exception of fibromyalgia. Significantly greater psychological distress and higher geriatric depression measures were reported for geriatric patients with CLBP compared to those with joint pain [6]. Data from survey studies indicate the prevalence and incidence of depression varies by pain location [7–9].

Thus, this limited literature provides some evidence that CLBP is associated with more depression and psychological distress than other pain types with the exception of fibromyalgia when data are obtained from patient populations. Given the strong association between opioid misuse and depression, we hypothesized that patients with CLBP would have a higher prevalence of depression and opioid misuse and this association would be stronger in CLBP than in patients with Chronic Pain of Other Location (CPOL).

We computed exploratory analysis to determine if: (1) the prevalence of depression and risk of opioid misuse differed among patients with CLBP *vs.* those with CPOL; and (2) the association between depression and risk of opioid misuse differed in patients with CLBP *vs.* those with CPOL.

2. Materials and Methods

2.1. Study Design and Population

Data for this cross-sectional study were obtained from a retrospective chart review of 166 chronic pain patients receiving pain management services at an academic family medicine clinic between January 2013 and December 2014. As part of routine care, patients presenting to the service completed the Brief Pain Inventory (BPI), Patient Health Questionnaire-9 (PHQ-9) and the Current Opioid Misuse Measure (COMM) at each visit. Data from initial clinical encounters were abstracted into an anonymized data set for the present study. After removing patients with missing data on any variable, the analytic data file contained 122 patients.

Pain conditions: From 22 primary pain diagnoses, we created a binary variable indicating the patient had CLBP, (n = 61) or CPOL (n = 61). Conditions among the CPOL group were osteoarthritis (n = 18), cervicalgia (n = 10), fibromyalgia (n = 7), migraine (n = 6), rheumatoid arthritis (n = 4), neuropathic pain (n = 4), HIV neuropathy (n = 2), avascular necrosis of the hip (n = 2), temporomandibular joint pain (n = 1), osteogenesis imperfecta (n = 1), lymphedema (n = 1), lower extremity trauma (n = 1), diffuse idiopathic skeletal hyperostosis (n = 1), complex regional pain syndrome (n = 1), chronic post stroke pain (n = 1) and abdominal pain (n = 1).

2.2. Measures

The three main measures assessed in this study were depression, risk of opioid misuse and pain interference.

2.2.1. Depression

The PHQ-9 questionnaire was utilized to assess depression. PHQ-9 is a self-report tool used in screening, diagnosing, monitoring and measuring severity of depression. The tool measures Diagnostic and Statistical Manual of Mental Disorders—4th Edition (DSM-IV) depression symptoms with nine items. Scores range from 0–27 and suggested thresholds are 5 (mild), 10 (moderate), 15 (moderately severe) and 20 (severe depression) [10]. Due to sample size, we used a binary indicator of depression with a threshold of at least 15 for depression. We used this threshold to ensure patients had clinically relevant depression associated with seeking care and receiving treatment.

2.2.2. Opioid Misuse

The Current Opioid Misuse Measure (COMM) questionnaire was used to measure risk of opioid misuse [11]. This questionnaire reflects patient's risk of medication-related aberrant behavior among chronic pain patients using prescription opioids. The COMM includes 17-items ranging from 0–4.

A summative score more than 9 is considered an elevated risk for opioid misuse. For ease of presentation, we refer to patients with this score as positive for risk of opioid misuse.

2.2.3. Pain Severity and Interference

We used the Brief Pain Inventory (BPI) short form [12] as a tool for measuring pain severity and pain interference. Pain severity had four questions measuring least pain, worst pain, average pain and current pain score, with each item measured on a 0–10 Likert scale (10 being the worst). Pain interference contained seven questions measuring interference with: activity, mood, walking, work, relationships, sleep, and joy using the same 0–10 Likert scale. Following BPI scoring instructions, we created the average pain severity score by averaging all four pain scores (least pain, worst pain, average pain and current pain score) and similarly created an average pain interference score by averaging the seven interference components.

2.2.4. Demographic Variables

Demographic data available from chart abstraction included age, gender and race. Due to small numbers of minority groups other than African-Americans (AA) we created a binary white/non-white race variable.

This study was approved by the IRBs of participating institutions.

2.3. Statistical Analysis

Frequencies, means and associations were computed using SPSS 23 [13]. Differences between CPOL and CLBP in demographics, pain indicators, depression, and opioid misuse risk were assessed using chi-square tests for categorical variables and independent samples t-tests for continuous variables. Also, chi-square and independent samples t-tests were conducted and stratified on pain location, to determine if there were differences in the association between depression and no depression with opioid misuse risk and pain. Similarly, the associations between pain characteristics and depression with opioid misuse risk were computed after stratifying by pain location. To assess whether there were any differential effects of depression or opioid misuse on other variables based on pain location strata, the interaction term in an ANOVA (for continuous variables) and the Breslow-Day test (categorical variables) were conducted. Last, a hierarchical logistic regression was conducted to calculate odds ratios and 95% confidence intervals by first adding pain characteristics and then adding depression, pain location, and the interaction of pain location and depression in successive blocks. All tests were conducted at $p < 0.05$.

3. Results

Table 1 displays the characteristics of the 122 pain patients included in our study sample. On average, patients were 49.6 ($\pm$ 12.6) years of age, 56.6% female and nearly 80% white. One-fourth were positive for opioid misuse risk and 35.2% met the criteria for depression. The average total pain score was 6.3 ($\pm$ 1.7) and average pain interference was 6.7 ($\pm$ 2.4). Comparisons between CPOL and CLBP indicated that those with CLBP had lower average pain severity, lower average least pain and lower average pain than those with CPOL.

Table 2 shows the association between opioid misuse and pain characteristics by depression, stratified by pain location. Among CPOL patients, 66.7% of depressed patients were positive for opioid misuse compared to 7.5% of non-depressed CPOL patients ($p < 0.001$). Among CLBP patients, depression was not related to positive opioid misuse ($p = 0.19$). A Breslow-Day test showed that depression and opioid misuse were more strongly associated among CPOL than among CLBP patients ($p = 0.019$). Average COMM score was significantly greater among depressed compared to non-depressed CPOL ($p < 0.0001$) and CLBP ($p < 0.01$) patients; however the difference between depressed and non-depressed was larger (interaction p-value = 0.016) among CPOL (difference = 13.0) patients than CLBP patients (difference = 5.8). Among CPOL, but not among CLBP patients, average pain severity was significantly higher among depressed *vs.* non-depressed patients. Pain interference was significantly greater among depressed *vs.* non-depressed patients in both CPOL and CLBP patients. The relationship of BPI measures and depression were similar across pain location strata.

Table 1. Characteristics of family medicine pain clinic patients, n = 122.

Variables, Mean (sd)	Total (n = 122)	CPOL (n = 61) [1]	CLBP (n = 61) [1]	*p*-value
Age	49.6 ($\pm$ 2.6)	50.4 ($\pm$ 11.5)	48.8 ($\pm$ 13.0)	0.485
Gender, n(%)				0.100
Female	69 (56.6%)	39 (63.9%)	30 (49.2%)	
Male	53 (43.4%)	22 (36.1%)	31 (50.8%)	
Race, n(%)				0.501
White	97 (79.5%)	47 (77.0%)	50 (82.0%)	
Non-white	25 (20.5%)	14 (23.0%)	11 (18.0%)	
Positive opioid misuse (COMM [2] > 9), n(%)	30 (24.6%)	17 (27.9%)	13 (21.3%)	0.400
COMM score [2]	9.2 ($\pm$ 9.1)	9.5 ($\pm$ 9.8)	8.9 ($\pm$ 8.5)	0.639
Depression (PHQ-9 [3] > 14), n(%)	43 (35.2%)	21 (34.4%)	22 (36.1%)	0.850
PHQ-9 [3] score	11.0 ($\pm$ 6.7)	11.0 ($\pm$ 6.8)	11.0 ($\pm$ 6.7)	0.989
BPI [4] mean, (sd)				
Total Average pain index	6.3 ($\pm$ 1.7)	6.6 ($\pm$ 1.8)	5.9 ($\pm$ 1.7)	0.035
Worst pain level	7.7 ($\pm$ 1.7)	7.9 ($\pm$ 1.7)	7.4 ($\pm$ 1.6)	0.112
Least pain level	5.0 ($\pm$ 2.2)	5.4 ($\pm$ 2.2)	4.5 ($\pm$ 2.1)	0.029
Pain level on average	6.3 ($\pm$ 1.8)	6.7 ($\pm$ 1.8)	6.0 ($\pm$ 1.7)	0.039
Pain level right now	6.2 ($\pm$ 2.3)	6.5 ($\pm$ 2.3)	5.9 ($\pm$ 2.2)	0.115
Total Average pain interference	6.7 ($\pm$ 2.4)	6.7 ($\pm$ 2.6)	6.7 ($\pm$ 2.2)	0.900
General activity	7.2 ($\pm$ 2.3)	7.2 ($\pm$ 2.5)	7.2 ($\pm$ 2.2)	0.957
Mood	6.5 ($\pm$ 2.8)	6.4 ($\pm$ 2.9)	6.6 ($\pm$ 2.7)	0.713
Walking ability	6.7 ($\pm$ 2.8)	6.7 ($\pm$ 2.9)	6.7 ($\pm$ 2.6)	0.987
Normal work	7.5 ($\pm$ 2.6)	7.4 ($\pm$ 2.7)	7.5 ($\pm$ 2.5)	0.755
Relations with others	5.2 ($\pm$ 3.4)	5.3 ($\pm$ 3.6)	5.1 ($\pm$ 3.3)	0.762
Sleep	6.8 ($\pm$ 2.8)	6.8 ($\pm$ 2.8)	6.8 ($\pm$ 2.8)	0.987
Enjoyment of life	7.0 ($\pm$ 2.9)	6.9 ($\pm$ 3.2)	7.1 ($\pm$ 2.7)	0.658

Note: *p*-value is for chi-square tests for categorical variables and independent samples *t*-tests for continuous variables. [1] CPOL: Chronic pain of other location, CLBP: Chronic low back pain; [2] COMM= Chronic Opioid Misuse Measure (0–68); [3] PHQ-9 = Depression scale (0–27); [4] BPI = Brief Pain Inventory (Average Severity and interference: 0–10, Individual BPI items: 0–10).

Table 2. Distribution of patient opioid misuse risk and pain characteristics by depression, stratified by pain location (n = 122).

Variables, Mean(sd)	CPOL [1] (n = 61)			CLBP [1] (n = 61)			Interaction *p*-value [4]
	Not depressed (n = 40)	Depressed (n = 21)	*p*-value	Not depressed (n = 39)	Depressed (n = 22)	*p*-value	
Positive opioid misuse (COMM [2] > 9), n(%)	3 (7.5%)	14 (66.7%)	<0.001	6 (15.4%)	7 (31.8%)	0.19	0.019
COMM [2]	5.1 ($\pm$ 5.1)	18.1 ($\pm$ 10.9)	<0.001	6.8 ($\pm$ 7.5)	12.6 ($\pm$ 9.1)	0.01	0.016
BPI [3]							
Total average pain index	6.1 ($\pm$ 1.8)	7.6 ($\pm$ 1.2)	<0.001	5.8 ($\pm$ 1.7)	6.3 ($\pm$ 1.6)	0.25	0.143
Total average pain interference	5.7 ($\pm$ 2.6)	8.5 ($\pm$ 0.9)	<0.001	6.1 ($\pm$ 2.1)	7.8 ($\pm$ 1.9)	0.004	0.151

Note: *p*-value is for chi-square tests for categorical variables and independent samples *t*-tests for continuous variables. [1] CPOL: Chronic Pain of Other Location, CLBP: Chronic Low Back Pain; [2] COMM = Current Opioid Misuse Measure (0–68); [3] BPI = Brief Pain Inventory (Average Severity and interference: 0–10); [4] *p*-value for interaction term of pain location x depression, ANOVA for continuous variables and Breslow-Day test for dichotomous variables.

Table 3 shows the association between PHQ-9 score and pain characteristics by opioid misuse, stratified by pain location. The average PHQ-9 scores were significantly higher among COMM positive CPOL patients compared to COMM negative CPOL patients. The association between COMM status and PHQ-9 score was not significant in the CLBP group. There were marginally significant between strata differences in the relationship of opioid misuse and PHQ-9 score (interaction *p*-value = 0.050). Both pain severity and pain interference were positively related to COMM positive status among CPOL patients. Conversely, only pain interference was higher among COMM positive CLBP patients compared to COMM negative CLBP patients. There were no between strata differences in the relationship of opioid misuse and pain characteristics.

Table 3. Distribution of depression score and pain characteristics by opioid misuse, stratified by pain location (n = 122).

Variables, mean (sd)	CPOL [1] (n = 61)			CLBP [1] (n = 61)			Interaction *p*-value [5]
	COMM [2] negative (n = 44)	COMM [2] positive (n = 17)	*p*-value *	COMM [2] negative (n = 48)	COMM [2] positive (n = 13)	*p*-value *	
PHQ-9 [3]	8.6 (± 5.6)	17.4 (± 5.2)	<0.001	10.3 (± 6.8)	13.9 (± 5.7)	0.08	0.050
BPI [4]							
Total Average pain index	6.3 (± 1.8)	7.5 (± 1.3)	0.017	5.8 (± 1.7)	6.6 (± 1.6)	0.101	0.638
Total Average pain interference	5.9 (± 2.6)	8.6 (± 1.0)	<0.001	6.3 (± 2.2)	8.2 (± 1.2)	0.005	0.384

Note: *p*-value is for chi-square tests for categorical variables and independent samples *t*-tests for continuous variables. [1] CPOL: Chronic Pain of Other Location, CLBP: Chronic Low Back Pain; [2] COMM = Current Opioid Misuse Measure (0–68); [3] PHQ-9 = Depression scale (0–27); [4] BPI = Brief Pain Inventory (Average Severity and interference: 0–10); [5] *p*-value for interaction term of pain location * COMM Opioid Misuse, ANOVA for continuous variables and Breslow-Day test for dichotomous variables.

Table 4 shows results of a hierarchical logistic regression. In model 1, pain severity and interference explain 32.0% of the variance in the likelihood of opioid misuse risk, with each unit increase in pain interference having over twice the likelihood of opioid misuse risk (OR = 2.25; 95% CI: 1.45–3.48); however, pain severity was unrelated to opioid misuse risk. Adding depression explained an additional 5.2% (*p* = 0.019) of the variance in opioid misuse risk and increased the odds of opioid misuse risk by over 3-fold (OR = 3.32; 95% CI: 1.20–9.16). Pain location did not significantly explain any additional variance in opioid misuse risk; however, adding an interaction term of pain location and depression in a final model explained an additional 4.5% of the variance (*p* = 0.025). The significant interaction term showed that the odds ratio for the relationship of depression and opioid misuse risk increased by over a factor of 10 comparing CPOL to CLBP (depression OR: 10.57 *vs.* 1.04, respectively).

Table 4. Logistic regression models for opioid misuse risk (COMM [1]) (n = 122).

Predictor Variables	Model 1. Pain severity and interference	Model 2. Add depression	Model 3. Add pain location	Model 4.Add depression * pain location
Variables	OR (95% CI)	OR (95% CI)	OR (95% CI)	OR (95% CI)
Total average pain severity [2]	0.88 (0.60–1.29)	0.92 (0.61–1.37)	0.87 (0.58–1.31)	0.81 (0.52–1.26)
Total average pain interference [2]	2.25 (1.45–3.48)	1.91 (1.21–3.01)	1.95 (1.23–3.09)	2.09 (1.26–3.47)
Depression (Yes *vs.* No)		3.32 (1.20–9.16)	3.32 (1.19–9.23)	
Pain Location [3]				
CPOL			1.00	-
CLBP			0.64 (0.23–1.77)	-
Depression * Pain Location [4]				
CPOL: Depression (Yes *vs.* No)				10.57 (2.21–50.49)
CLBP: Depression (Yes *vs.* No)				1.04 (0.25–4.41)
Chi-square change (df, *p*-value)	29.58 (2, <0.0001)	5.48 (1, 0.019)	0.74 (1, 0.390)	5.00 (1, 0.025)
Nagelkerke R-square	0.320	0.372	0.378	0.423

Note: OR = odds ratio; CI = confidence interval; [1] COMM = Chronic opioid Misuse Measure; [2] Brief Pain Inventory (Average Severity and interference: 0–10), odds ratio represents the change in odds of opioid misuse risk given one unit increase in average pain severity or interference; [3] CPOL: Chronic pain other location, CLBP: Chronic low back pain; [4] Wald Chi-square $p = 0.031$.

4. Discussion

In patients seeking treatment at a family medicine pain clinic, we observed evidence that the association between depression and opioid misuse differed in patients with CLBP compared to CPOL. Results of bivariate analysis stratified on pain location revealed that depression was more strongly associated with opioid misuse among CPOL patients than in patients with CLBP. This observation is not explained by pain interference which showed similar significant associations with depression in both CPOL and CLBP. Exploratory hierarchical logistic regression found that depression increases the odds of opioid misuse after adjusting for pain location and pain characteristics (severity and interference) and that this relationship is over 10 times stronger in CPOL than in CLBP. While pain severity was not significantly associated with opioid misuse risk in adjusted analysis, results suggest that pain interference independently contributes to opioid misuse risk after accounting for depression.

Our data expand on the existing literature on the prevalence of depression among different pain types [4–9] and the prevalence of opioid misuse across different pain types [3] by showing prevalence estimates of both opioid misuse and depression in groups stratified by pain location. Additional studies are warranted to determine if the frequent depression—opioid misuse comorbidity varies in CLBP compared to other specific types of pain such as arthritis, migraine, fibromyalgia, *etc.*

Because neuroticism is thought to be more common in CLBP [5] we expected CLBP patients to have more depression and subsequently more opioid misuse. However our results indicate the prevalence of depression does not differ by pain location. We did not expect to find a stronger association of depression and opioid misuse among CPOL patients. Though speculative, these results may be due to evidence from Morasco *et al.* [3] that neck and joint pain patients are more likely to have a history of substance use disorder compared to CLBP patients (94.4% *vs.* 83.3%).

One potential explanation for the stronger association between depression and opioid misuse in CPOL patients could be the significantly higher BPI score, higher average least pain and higher average pain level among CPOL *vs.* CLBP. In addition BPI scores were significantly greater in the depressed CPOL compared to non-depressed CPOL patients but did not differ by depression status in the CLBP patients. BPI scores were also higher in COMM positive *vs.* COMM negative patients in the CPOL patients but not CLBP patients. Greater pain severity in CPOL may lead to both depression and opioid misuse in patients with CLBP. Although pain severity was not significant when modeled with pain interference in regression analysis, this does not preclude the possibility that pain severity leads to greater pain interference which then increases depression and opioid misuse. Longitudinal data collection is needed to confirm this possibility.

There are several biological mechanisms proposed for the association between pain and depression. Common vulnerability due to past psychopathology or trauma leads to chronic pain via changes in catecholamines, substance P and cytokine activity and less responsive opioid receptors that may perpetuate or worsen depression [14]. Another biological underpinning for the pain-depression relationship is inflammatory processes and oxidative stress [15]. Studies of memantine, an NMDA receptor antagonist improves both pain and depression via reduction in glutamate activity and thereby reducing inflammatory factors related to pain and depression [16].

Limitations include small sample size which limits the precision of our conclusions. We did not have enough subjects to compare CLBP to specific types of CPOL such as arthritis or fibromyalgia; however, sensitivity analysis removing fibromyalgia which is often comorbid with depression, did not change our conclusions. We also lacked sample size to conduct stratified multivariable logistic regression models. The data did not contain type of opioid or co-medication which may bias results if CLBP or CPOL systematically differed in morphine equivalent dose because higher daily opioid morphine equivalent dose is associated with depression [17,18] and opioid misuse [19]. Comorbid conditions such as specific co-occurring pain conditions and anxiety disorders, were not available to improve control of confounding. The results may not apply to other geographic locations or to pain patients seeking care in other settings.

5. Conclusions

We found depression was more strongly associated with opioid misuse in patients with CPOL compared to patients with CLBP. The well-established association between depression and opioid misuse may be less prominent in CLBP than in other pain types. Further research with larger samples should compare this association in CLBP, arthritis, fibromyalgia and neuralgia. Refining which pain patients are most likely to develop comorbid depression and opioid misuse can inform clinical care and target limited resources to patients at greatest risk for this comorbidity.

Acknowledgments: Arpana Jaiswal and Sheran Fernando were supported by a training fellowship. No funds were received to cover the costs to publish in open access.

Author Contributions: Arpana Jaiswal and Jeffrey F. Scherrer conceived and designed the experiments; Arpana Jaiswal and Jeffrey F. Scherrer and Joanne Salas analyzed the data; Christopher M. Herndon contributed data. Jeffrey F. Scherrer, Arpana Jaiswal, Carissa van den Berk-Clarkand Joanne Salas wrote the paper. All authors contributed to revisions and approval of the final manuscript.

Abbreviations

The following abbreviations are used in this manuscript:

CLBP	Chronic low back pain
CPOL	Chronic pain of other location
COMM	Current Opioid Misuse Measure
PHQ-9	Patient Health Questionnaire-9
BPI	Brief Pain Inventory

References

1. Edlund, M.J.; Martin, B.C.; Fan, M.Y.; Devries, A.; Braden, J.B.; Sullivan, M.D. Risks for opioid abuse and dependence among recipients of chronic opioid therapy: Results from the Troup study. *Drug Alcohol Depend.* **2010**, *112*, 90–98. [CrossRef] [PubMed]

2. Sullivan, M.D.; Edlund, M.J.; Zhang, L.; Unützer, J.; Wells, K.B. Association between mental health disorders, problem drug use, and regular prescription opioid use. *Arch. Intern. Med.* **2006**, *166*, 2087–2093. [CrossRef] [PubMed]

3. Morasco, B.J.; Dobscha, S.K. Prescription medication misuse and substance use disorder in VA primary care patients with chronic pain. *Gen. Hosp. Psychiatry* **2008**, *30*, 93–99. [CrossRef] [PubMed]

4. Makovec, M.; Vintar, N.; Makovec, S. Self-reported depression, anxiety and evaluation of own pain in clinical sample of patients with different location of chronic pain. *Zdrav Var.* **2015**, *54*, 1–10.

5. Porter-Moffit, S.; Gatchel, R.J.; Robinson, R.C.; Deschner, M.; Posamentier, M.; Polatin, P.; Lou, L. Biophysical profile of different pain diagnostic groups. *J. Pain* **2006**, *7*, 308–318. [CrossRef] [PubMed]

6. Morone, N.E.; Karp, J.F.; Lynch, C.; Bost, J.E.; El Khoudhry, S.R.; Weiner, D.K. Impact of chronic musculoskeletal pathology on older adults: A study of differences between knee OA and low back pain. *Pain Med.* **2009**, *4*, 693–701. [CrossRef] [PubMed]

7. de Heer, E.W.; Gerrits, M.M.; Beekman, A.T.; Dekker, J.; van Marwijk, H.W.; de Waal, M.W.; Spinhoven, P.; Penninx, B.W.; van der Feltz-Cornelis, C.M. The association of depression and anxiety with pain: A study from NESDA. *PloS ONE* **2014**, *9*, e106907.

8. Gerritis, M.M.; van Oppen, P.; van Marwijk, H.W.; Penninx, B.W.; van der Horst, E.H. Pain and the onset of depressive and anxiety disorders. *Pain* **2014**, *155*, 53–59. [CrossRef] [PubMed]

9. Baune, B.T.; Caniato, R.N.; Garcia-Alcaraz, M.A.; Berger, K. Combined effects of major depression, pain and somatic disorders on general functioning in the general adult population. *Pain* **2008**, *138*, 310–317. [CrossRef] [PubMed]

10. Kroencke, K.; Spitzer, R.; Williams, J. The PHQ-9: Validity of a brief depression severity measure. *J. Gen. Intern. Med.* **2001**, *16*, 606–613. [CrossRef]

11. Butler, S.F.; Budman, S.H.; Fernandez, K.C.; Houle, B.; Benoit, C.; Katz, N.; Jamison, R.N. Development and validation of the current opioid misuse measure. *Pain* **2007**, *130*, 144–156. [CrossRef] [PubMed]

12. Cleeland, C.S. The Brief Pain Inventory. Available online: https://www.mdanderson.org/education-and-research/departments-programs-and-labs/departments-and-divisions/symptom-research/symptom-assessment-tools/BPI_UserGuide.pdf (accessed on 1 March 2016).

13. Statistical package for the social sciences. Available online: http://www.ibm.com/analytics/us/en/technology/spss/ (accessed on 1 March 2015).

14. Leo, R.J. Chronic pain and comorbid depression. *Curr. Treat. Options Neurol.* **2005**, *7*, 403–412. [CrossRef] [PubMed]

15. Moura, F.A.; Queiroz de Andrade, K.; dos Santos, J.C.; Araujo, O.R.; Goulart, M.O. Antioxidant therapy for treatment of inflammatory bowel disease: Does it work? *Redox Biol.* **2015**, *6*, 617–639. [CrossRef] [PubMed]

16. Olivan-Blazquez, B.; Herrera-Mercadal, P.; Puebla-Guedea, M.; Perez-Yus, M.C.; Andres, E.; Fayed, N.; Lopez-Del-Hoyo, Y.; Magallon, R.; Roca, M.; Carcia-Campayo, J. Efficacy of memantine in the treatment of fibromyalgia: A double-blind, randomised, controlled trial with 6-month follow-up. *Pain* **2014**, *155*, 2517–2525. [CrossRef] [PubMed]

17. Merrill, J.O.; Von Korff, M.; Banta-Green, C.J.; Sullivan, M.D.; Saunders, K.W.; Campbell, C.I.; Weisner, C. Prescribed Opioid difficulties, depression and opioid dose among chronic opioid therapy patients. *Gen. Hosp. Psychiatry* **2012**, *24*, 581–587. [CrossRef] [PubMed]

18. Scherrer, J.F.; Salas, J.; Lustman, P.J.; Burge, S.; Schneider, F.D. Residency Research network of Texas (RRNeT) Investigators. *Pain* **2015**, *156*, 348–355. [CrossRef] [PubMed]

19. White, A.G.; Birnbaum, H.G.; Schiller, M.; Tang, J.; Katz, N.P. Analytic models to identify patients at risk for prescription opioid abuse. *Am. J. Manag. Care* **2009**, *15*, 897–906. [PubMed]

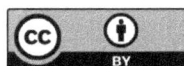

healthcare

MDPI

Article

The Relationship between Pain Beliefs and Physical and Mental Health Outcome Measures in Chronic Low Back Pain: Direct and Indirect Effects

Andrew Baird * and David Sheffield

Centre for Psychological Research, Kedleston Road Campus, University of Derby, Derby DE22 1GB, UK; d.sheffield@derby.ac.uk
* Correspondence: A.Baird@derby.ac.uk; Tel.: +44-13-3259-3042

Academic Editor: Robert J. Gatchel
Received: 22 May 2016; Accepted: 11 August 2016; Published: 19 August 2016

Abstract: Low back pain remains a major health problem with huge societal cost. Biomedical models fail to explain the disability seen in response to reported back pain and therefore patients' beliefs, cognitions and related behaviours have become a focus for both research and practice. This study used the Pain Beliefs Questionnaire and had two aims: To examine the extent to which pain beliefs are related to disability, anxiety and depression; and to assess whether those relationships are mediated by pain self-efficacy and locus of control. In a sample of 341 chronic low back pain patients, organic and psychological pain beliefs were related to disability, anxiety and depression. However, organic pain beliefs were more strongly related to disability and depression than psychological pain beliefs. Regression analyses revealed that these relationships were in part independent of pain self-efficacy and locus of control. Further, mediation analyses revealed indirect pathways involving self-efficacy and, to a lesser extent chance locus of control, between organic pain beliefs, on the one hand, and disability, anxiety and depression, on the other. In contrast, psychological pain beliefs were only directly related to disability, anxiety and depression. Although longitudinal data are needed to corroborate our findings, this study illustrates the importance of beliefs about the nature of pain and beliefs in one's ability to cope with pain in determining both physical and mental health outcomes in chronic low back pain patients.

Keywords: low back pain; pain beliefs; disability; pain self-efficacy; anxiety; depression; locus of control

---

1. Introduction

Despite considerable attention, low back pain remains one of medicine's most enigmatic problems, particularly in its chronic form. The majority of people will experience back pain at some point in their lives [1], but only a minority will receive a definitive diagnosis [2,3]. Most low back pain is largely non-specific in nature, but nevertheless has a societal cost greater than that for cancer, coronary artery disease and AIDS combined [4]. A systematic review by Dagenais, Caro and Haldeman [5] showed inconsistencies in the calculation of costs but found all studies to indicate back pain to be a substantial burden on society. In terms of healthcare costs, a recent study from the UK indicates that costs associated with chronic low back pain sufferers were twice that of matched controls [6]. The situation has been described in terms of an "epidemic" [7] and as a "20th Century medical disaster" [8] and is still perhaps one of the greatest examples of the failure of biomedical approaches. Biopsychosocial perspectives now dominate the literature, with psychosocial factors recognized as being fundamental in both assessment [9,10] and treatment/management [11,12]. Key to understanding the psychosocial influence is the consideration of individuals' beliefs, cognitions and behaviours.

Therefore, addressing patients' pain beliefs, cognitions and associated behaviours has become a major issue in pain management, particularly in chronic pain. Beliefs and associated behaviours have been associated with: The level of activity interference [13]; the frequency of pain behaviour [14]; the severity of pain experienced [15]; and levels of associated depression [16]. Two of the most important constructs in this area, which are driven by beliefs and which influence subsequent cognition and behaviour, are fear and catastrophising. These overlapping constructs impact upon vigilance to pain which can in turn also lead to increases in perceived pain severity [17]. A recent meta-analysis showed the relationship between fear and disability to be moderate to large in magnitude [18].

Ultimately, pain-related fear is more disabling than pain itself [19] as fear motivates avoidance behaviours [20,21]. In turn, avoidance behaviour affects activities of daily living and has a role in the transition from acute to chronic pain [22]. One of the key elements of fear is that of fear of further injury and re-injury [23], which can be a major barrier to recovery. In addition, expectancy beliefs are also a key factor in chronic pain. Ashari and Nicholas [24] showed pain self-efficacy beliefs to be an important determinant of pain behaviours and the disability associated with pain. More recently, Denison et al.'s [25] findings suggest that self-efficacy beliefs are even more important determinants of disability than fear avoidance beliefs in primary health care patients with musculoskeletal pain. Pain self-efficacy can mediate the relationship between clinical predictors and outcome measures. Pain self-efficacy mediates the relationship between pain severity and associated disability [26,27] and between pain related fear and disability [28]. It also mediates the relationship between fear and pain intensity [28] and between pain intensity and related depression [26]. Internal pain control can mediate reduction in levels of depression and pain behaviour following treatment [29].

Addressing problematic beliefs and related cognitions and behaviours can however, bring improvement in function [30]. Modern back pain management programmes are frequently grounded in the proven effectiveness of cognitive behavioural approaches [31–33] and exercise [34,35].

In the current study, participants were from a programme that explicitly addresses pain beliefs with participants [36], particularly the erroneous notion that "hurt = harm" and "more hurt = more harm". Addressing these "organic" pain beliefs has been shown to be associated with improvements in function following a rehabilitation programme [37] and the strength of these beliefs has been shown to clearly differentiate patients with chronic low back pain from the general population [38]. This study aims to assess the extent to which pain related physical and mental outcome measures can be explained by individuals' pain beliefs as measured with the Pain Beliefs Questionnaire (PBQ) [39]. Furthermore, it aims to assess the extent to which the relationship between pain beliefs and physical and mental outcome measures is mediated by pain self-efficacy and locus of control.

2. Materials and Methods

2.1. Sample

The sample comprised 341 individuals who had been referred to the Nottingham Back Team programme located in Nottinghamshire, England. It is multi-disciplinary back pain management programme for individuals with chronic low back pain, delivered using 7 half day sessions on consecutive weeks. It is undertaken in community settings, i.e., utilising facilities at leisure centres as an alternative to requiring participants to visit a hospital site. The programme takes a cognitive behavioural approach and patients were informed that each session would incorporate, education, exercise, relaxation and discussions with a key worker (including goal setting). The sessions are delivered by a combination of physiotherapists, occupational therapists and nurses, with additional input from a clinical psychologist. The authors are independent of the programme and have no clinical role within it. Participants completed the standard battery of tests used within the programme together with the Pain Beliefs Questionnaire. Every patient that attended for assessment during the research period consented for their data to be used in the research, but not all responses were complete (n = 290). All data was gathered at assessment, before commencement of the programme.

2.2. Measures

The PBQ consists of 12 items representing two scales, which the authors described as "organic" (8 items) and "psychological" (4 items) [37]. One advantage of this questionnaire is that it is designed such that it is not necessary for the completer to be in pain or suffering from a specific condition (i.e., it is condition independent). The PBQ has previously been used successfully in research investigating chronic back pain [37–40] and with a UK general population [38]. On this occasion, the original 6 point ("always" to "never") scale response was modified to a 5 point scale fit better with other questionnaires it was being used with, as part of the broader research [38]. The five items were "All of the time", "Most of the time", "Some of the time", "A little of the time", "None of the time". In their study with patients experiencing chronic low back pain, Walsh and Radcliffe also describe using a 5-point scale [37]. The PBQ organic and psychological sub-scales are scored using the sum of the items for each scale respectively.

The Roland-Morris Disability Questionnaire (RDQ) [41] is one of the most widely used measures of back pain related disability and was originally derived from the Sickness Impact Profile (SIP). Twenty-four items that related to physical functions potentially affected by back pain were selected from the SIP. Each item was then qualified with the phrase "because of my back pain" to differentiate back pain disability from disability due to other causes [42]. Patients are asked to indicate which of the series of statements applies to them on the day of completing the questionnaire. The RDQ provides a single score which is calculated by summing the number of items selected. The items are not weighted in any way. The scores therefore range from 0 (no disability) to 24 (maximum disability). The RDQ is short, easy to understand and simple to complete [42].

The Pain Self-efficacy Questionnaire [43] is a ten item questionnaire, with each item assessed on a scale from 0 to 6 where 0 indicates no confidence and 6 indicates complete confidence. The 10 items are designed to cover a range of factors relating to activities of daily living. The items are not weighted and the questionnaire provides a single scale. The scores therefore range from 0, indicating no confidence in carrying out activities of daily living, to 60, indicating complete confidence in carrying out normal activities of daily living.

The Hospital Anxiety and Depression Scale (HADS) [44] is a 14 item screening tool comprising two seven item scales—anxiety and depression. To ensure a focus on anxiety and depression, symptoms which could also be associated with somatic disorders were excluded as were those indicative of more complex/serious psychiatric conditions. It is a widely used instrument in both clinical practice and research. A review by Bjellanda et al. [45] identified over seven hundred papers reporting use of HADS. It has been found to have good psychometric properties and performed well in assessing the general severity and 'caseness' of both anxiety disorders and depression. It has been widely used in trials relating to back pain including the large STarT Back trial [46].

The Multi-Dimensional Health Locus of Control Questionnaire [47] is an 18 item questionnaire comprising 3 scales—internal, chance and powerful others. The measure has been used for several decades and the scales are considered reliable and valid [48]. It is a general measure; not specific to particular symptoms or conditions. The measure has been used in back pain research in the past [49] and it was used during the development of the Pain Beliefs Questionnaire [39].

2.3. Analytic Strategy and Scoring

Initial analyses focused on examining differences in age and gender between those who completed the questionnaires and those that did not. Gender data was not available from one completer and one non-completer of all questionnaires. Then attention focused on correlations between beliefs, self-efficacy, locus of control, and depression, anxiety and disability. Next, regression analysis was used to examine the independent contributions that beliefs, self-efficacy, and locus of control variables make to the prediction of depression, anxiety and disability. Finally, a bootstrapped mediation model tested the conceptual model outlined in Figure 1. For each belief-mental or physical outcome relationship hypotheses were tested simultaneously using the "Process" macro for SPSS [50], with

5,000 bootstrapping re-samples and bias-corrected 95% confidence intervals (CIs) for each indirect effect. In bootstrapping analyses, bias corrected CIs that do not contain 0 signify a significant indirect effect [51,52]. Direct effects estimate how much two cases differing on the independent variable (organic or psychological belief) also differ on the dependent variable (disability, anxiety, or depression) independent of the effect of the mediator variables (self-efficacy and locus of control variables) on the dependent variable. Total effects are the sum of the indirect and direct effects of the independent variables on the dependent variable [50]. Alternate models were tested and these are presented in the Appendix. Analysis was conducted using IBM SPSS 22 for Windows with an alpha = 0.05. No participants were excluded from the analysis.

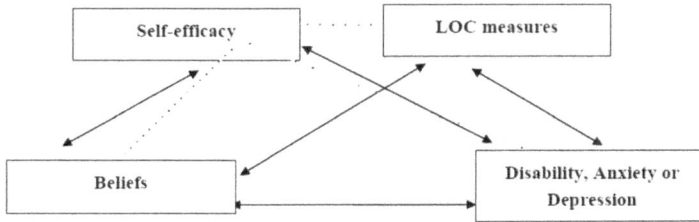

Figure 1. Conceptual Model of Bootstrapped Mediation Model.

2.4. Ethics

Ethical approval for the study was provided through the Nottingham Back Team via National Health Service processes. Participants received both written and verbal explanation during their assessment before informed consent was sought for their data to be used for the purposes of this research.

3. Results

3.1. Gender and Age Differences

Individuals who completed all questionnaires were significantly older (mean ± S.D. = 45.35 ± 13.14 vs. 48.02 ± 13.61 years) and more likely to be men (43.8% vs. 31.8%) than those who did not, $p < 0.05$.

3.2. Demographics

Examination of the mean and standard deviations suggested that participants were similar to previous low back pain samples [46]; see Table 1.

Table 1. Bivariate correlations and Means (SDs).

Variables	2	3	4	5	6	7	8	9	Mean (SD)
1. Disability	0.41 ***	0.57 ***	0.56 ***	0.21 ***	−0.70 ***	−0.19 ***	0.14 *	0.12 *	9.58 (5.34)
2. Anxiety	–	0.58 ***	0.34 ***	0.26 ***	−0.45 ***	−0.03	0.35 ***	0.21 ***	8.22 (3.97)
3. Depression	0.58 ***	- -	0.50 ***	0.15 **	−0.70 ***	−0.13 **	0.26 ***	0.17 **	5.96 (3.54)
4. Organic Beliefs	0.34 ***	0.50 ***	- -	0.13 **	−0.59 ***	−0.22 ***	0.27 ***	0.18 **	25.91 (4.90)
5. Psychological Beliefs	0.26 ***	0.15 **	0.13 **	- -	−0.08	0.17 **	0.00	0.02	11.28 (3.50)
6. Self-efficacy	0.45 ***	−0.70 ***	−0.59 ***	−0.08	- -	0.22 ***	−0.19 ***	−0.19 ***	34.09 (13.39)
7. LOC—Internal	−0.03	−0.13 **	−0.22 ***	0.17 **	0.22 ***	- -	−0.01	0.06	26.58 (4.75)
8. LOC—Chance	0.35 ***	0.26 ***	0.27 ***	0.00	−0.19 ***	−0.01	- -	0.39 ***	19.02 (5.27)
9. LOC—Other	0.21 ***	0.17 **	0.18 **	0.02	−0.19 ***	0.06	0.39 ***	- -	20.07 (6.23)

LOC: locus of control; * $p < 0.05$; ** $p < 0.01$; *** $p < 0.001$; -- There is perfect correlation between the same variable/s.

3.3. Bivariate Correlations

There were no gender differences in any predictor or outcome measures, $p > 0.1$. Age was negatively related to anxiety, $r = -0.15$, $p < 0.01$, and internal locus of control, $r = -0.13$, $p < 0.05$.

Accordingly, age was entered in subsequent regression analyses. Pearson's correlations revealed that disability, anxiety and depression were strongly inter-related but as the proportion of shared variance was less than 50% regression models with each as an outcome variable were calculated. Disability was strongly related to organic pain beliefs and self-efficacy, and more weakly, but significantly, related to psychological pain beliefs and locus of control measures. Anxiety was related to organic and psychological pain beliefs and self-efficacy, and more weakly, but significantly, related to internal and other locus of control measures; it was unrelated to chance locus of control. Depression was strongly related to organic pain beliefs and self-efficacy and more weakly related to psychological pain beliefs and locus of control measures. Fisher transformations revealed that organic pain beliefs were more strongly related to disability and depression than psychological pain beliefs ($p < 0.05$); correlations between organic and psychological pain beliefs and anxiety were not different. Organic pain beliefs were strongly related to self-efficacy and more weakly related to locus of control measures. Psychological pain beliefs were related to internal locus of control, but were not related to self-efficacy or chance and other locus of control (see Table 1).

3.4. Regression Analyses: Disability

After testing for multi-collinearity (all VIF < 2; all tolerances > 0.5), analysis revealed that the regression model was significant ($F(7, 333) = 56.82$, $p < 0.001$), with 54% of the variance in the outcome being explained by the predictors ($R^2 = 0.544$, adjusted $R^2 = 0.535$). There were significant positive relationships between organic pain beliefs and disability and between psychological pain beliefs and disability, and a significant negative relationship between pain self-efficacy and disability; there were no other significant relationships (see Table 2).

Table 2. Beta (standard deviation) and *t*-values for Regression Models.

Variables	Disability Beta (SD)	T	Anxiety	t	Depression	t
Age	0.011 (0.016)	0.71	−0.046 (0.014)	−3.24 **	−0.014 (0.011)	−1.33
Organic Beliefs	0.222 (0.052)	4.26 ***	0.035 (0.046)	0.76	0.071 (0.035)	2.01 *
Psychological Beliefs	0.229 (0.058)	3.94 ***	0.259 (0.052)	5.02 ***	0.086 (0.039)	2.19 *
Self-efficacy	−0.225 (0.019)	−12.31 ***	−0.103 (0.017)	−6.24 ***	−0.163 (0.013)	−12.93 ***
LOC—Internal	−0.041 (0.044)	−0.93	−0.003 (0.040)	−0.07	0.002 (0.030)	0.07
LOC—Chance	−0.015 (0.043)	−0.34	0.170 (0.038)	4.47 ***	0.074 (0.029)	2.55 *
LOC—Other	−0.021 (0.036)	−0.57	0.048 (0.032)	1.49	−0.001 (0.024)	−0.06

* $p < 0.05$; ** $p < 0.01$; *** $p < 0.001$.

Results of the mediation analyses indicated that there was a significant indirect effect of organic pain beliefs on disability through self-efficacy, $b = −0.23$, $p < 0.01$, BCa CI (−0.27, −0.19), which explained 36% of the total effect. In contrast, there were no significant indirect effects of organic pain beliefs on disability through LOC measures. The direct effect of organic pain beliefs on disability was also significant, $b = 0.25$, $t = 4.79$, $p < 0.0001$. In contrast, there was no significant indirect effect of organic pain beliefs on disability through LOC measures. For psychological pain beliefs on disability, there were no significant indirect effects through self-efficacy or LOC measures. The direct effect of psychological pain beliefs on disability was significant, $b = 0.26$, $t = 4.35$, $p < 0.0001$. Analyses with belief and locus of control measures as mediators of the self-efficacy-disability relationship were also examined. These suggest that the model is less parsimonious than the one proposed; these are presented in the Appendix.

3.5. Regression Analyses: Anxiety

The regression model was significant ($F(7, 333) = 25.39$, $p < 0.001$), with 35% of the variance in the outcome being explained by the predictors ($R^2 = 0.348$, adjusted $R^2 = 0.334$). There were significant positive relationships between psychological pain beliefs and anxiety and between chance locus of control and anxiety, and significant negative relationships between age and anxiety and pain self-efficacy and anxiety; there were no other significant relationships (see Table 2).

Results of the mediation analyses indicated that there was a significant indirect effect of organic pain beliefs on anxiety through self-efficacy, $b = -0.11$, $p < 0.0001$, BCa CI $(-0.15, -0.07)$, which explained 18% of the total effect, and through chance locus of control, $b = 0.19$, $p < 0.0001$, BCa CI $(0.11, 0.27)$, which explained 5% of the total effect. There were no significant indirect effects of organic pain beliefs on anxiety through other LOC measures and there was no direct effect of organic pain beliefs on anxiety, $b = 0.05$, $t = 1.06$, $p = 0.29$. For psychological pain beliefs on anxiety, there were no significant indirect effects through self-efficacy or LOC measures. The direct effect of psychological pain beliefs on anxiety was significant, $b = 0.26$, $t = 4.70$, $p < 0.0001$.

3.6. Regression Analyses: Depression

The regression model was significant ($F(7, 333) = 52.23$, $p < 0.001$), with 52% of the variance in the outcome being explained by the predictors ($R^2 = 0.523$, adjusted $R^2 = 0.513$). There were significant positive relationships between organic pain beliefs and depression, psychological pain beliefs and depression, and between chance locus of control and depression, and a significant negative relationship between pain self-efficacy and depression; there were no other significant relationships (see Table 2).

Results of the mediation analyses indicated that there was a significant indirect effect of organic pain beliefs on depression through self-efficacy, $b = -0.17$, $p < 0.0001$, BCa CI $(-0.19, -0.14)$, which explained 27% of the total effect, and through chance locus of control, $b = 0.08$, $p < 0.005$, BCa CI $(-0.02, 0.13)$, which explained 2% of the total effect. There were no significant indirect effects of organic pain beliefs on depression through other LOC measures. There was a direct effect of organic pain beliefs on depression, $b = 0.07$, $t = 2.20$, $p = 0.03$. For psychological pain beliefs on depression, there were no significant indirect effects through self-efficacy or LOC measures. The direct effect of psychological pain beliefs on depression was significant, $b = 0.10$, $t = 2.42$, $p = 0.01$.

4. Discussion

This study had two aims: To examine the extent to which pain beliefs are related to disability, anxiety and depression; and to assess whether those relationships are mediated by pain self-efficacy and locus of control. In a sample of 341 low back pain patients, organic and psychological pain beliefs were related to disability, anxiety and depression. However, organic pain beliefs were more strongly related to disability and depression than psychological pain beliefs. Regression analyses revealed that these relationships were in part independent of pain self-efficacy and locus of control. Further, mediation analyses revealed indirect pathways involving self-efficacy and, to a lesser extent chance locus of control, between organic pain beliefs, on the one hand, and disability, anxiety and depression, on the other. In contrast, psychological pain beliefs were only directly related to disability, anxiety and depression.

The gender split of the 341 participants included in the study was comparable with other studies of chronic low back pain [46,53]. Consideration of the descriptive statistics for the commonly taken measures—RMDQ, PSEQ and HADS—shows a pattern fairly typical of chronic low back pain patients. A mean disability of 9.6 is similar to that found by Hill et al. within the STarT Back trial [46] (9.8), though slightly higher than in the large study by Foster et al. [53] (8.6). The PSEQ mean of 34.1 was similar to that found by Foster et al. [53] (37.8). This is higher than reported by Nicholas [54] (25.8), but lower than reported by Costa et al. [55] (44.4) in chronic low back pain patients, so it appears to be in the range reported for chronic low back pain patients. A mean anxiety score of 8.2 was again similar to that reported by Foster et al. [53] (8.3) albeit slightly higher than that reported by Hill et al. [46] (7.5). Depression scores were lower than anxiety scores as is consistent within the literature and the mean of 6.0 is in line with that reported by Foster et al. [53] (6.5) and Hill et al. [46] (5.9). Overall, therefore this could be said to be an 'unremarkable' sample of chronic low back pain patients.

Organic pain beliefs deal with both the perceived cause of an individual's pain ("hurt = harm") and its management (issues of control and exercise/activity). As such, they could be considered a measure of 'biomedical thinking' [38]. These organic beliefs are associated with the outcome measures of disability, anxiety and depression. Higher organic pain beliefs are associated with higher levels of disability, depression and anxiety. On its own it could interpreted to be a good predictor of these outcomes, but mediation analyses show that much of the effect (all in the case of anxiety) is indirect through self-efficacy and to a lesser extent chance locus of control. The cross-sectional nature of the data is such that different mediation models could be described, but the defined model is in keeping with the literature on pain self-efficacy [26–28] and was the most parsimonious one (see Appendix).

Psychological pain beliefs are concerned with the impact of anxiety, depression, attention to pain and the issue of relaxation. These beliefs are also associated with the outcome measures, but the strength of the belief was much lower than for the organic beliefs. Higher levels of psychological pain beliefs are associated with higher levels of disability, depression and anxiety, but the relationship is relatively weak. Moreover, the mediation analyses showed that none of the effects were indirect through self-efficacy or locus of control measures. Thus, psychological pain beliefs are directly related to disability, depression and anxiety. Moreover, they appear to relate to markedly different constructs than other commonly used belief measures, such as fear avoidance beliefs, which like organic beliefs are mediated by self-efficacy [28]. Baird and Haslam [38] found that psychological beliefs differentiated between chronic low back pain patients and a non-clinical sample, but unlike with organic beliefs, there was no difference within the non-clinical sample between those who experienced frequent pain and those who did not. It was suggested that this may indicate that psychological pain beliefs are uniquely influenced by chronicity and not simply the presence of pain.

The PBQ has been used successfully with chronic low back pain samples [37,38,40] and this study supports the value of the measure. The scales illustrate both direct and mediated effects on key physical and mental health outcome measures. The measure has utility in both research and practice as it taps into clinically relevant beliefs that are amenable to change and are the focus of many rehabilitation programmes. Indeed, efforts to reduce the strength of these beliefs about the origins, nature and treatment of pain, particularly the 'biomedical' beliefs, should yield positive results in chronic low back pain rehabilitation [37,40].

This study supports the view that self-efficacy is an important predictor of disability [24,25,53]. It has a strong relationship with disability in bivariate analysis and its importance as an independent predictor of disability is confirmed in the regression models. Self-efficacy also has a strong association with mental health outcome measures, particularly depression. Further, the findings support previous studies indicating a role for self-efficacy as mediator between beliefs and outcomes [26–28]. Although Schiphorst Preuper et al. [56] questioned the impact of psychological variables, including self-efficacy, in a study in which psychological variables explained only 19% of the variance in self-reported disability, it was noticeable that the research used a general measure of self-efficacy and not a pain-specific measure as used in the current study and in previous studies mentioned above [24,28,53]. Pain self-efficacy may represent one of the most influential and most valuable psychological constructs in chronic low back pain [53] and it may be wise to measure this construct in both practice and research. These beliefs may be the target of clinical intervention via cognitive-behavioural, exercise-based programmes using both education and graded exposure.

The Multidimensional Health Locus of Control (MHLC) measure is a generic measure rather than a pain-specific questionnaire like the other scales used within the study. As such it may lack a degree of sensitivity with this patient population. The MHLC was used in the development of the Pain Beliefs Questionnaire [39] but it is noticeable that the correlations found in this study are weaker than those found by Edwards et al. [39]. The PBQ developers found no relationship between internal locus of control and organic pain beliefs, but this study indicated a negative relationship, albeit a relatively weak one. The regression analyses in this study illustrate that internal and powerful other locus of control are not predictors of any of the outcomes. Chance locus of control does however predict anxiety and, to a lesser extent, depression. Mediation analyses showed that there was some effect of organic pain beliefs on anxiety and depression which was indirect, through chance locus of control. Overall MHLC appears to have limited utility in relation to chronic low back pain.

This study utilises a suitably large sample whose characteristics indicate it to be a fairly typical chronic low back pain population. However, there were differences between questionnaire battery completers and non-completers. Failure to fully complete the questionnaire battery was perceived to be a consequence of time pressures during the assessment process. The difference in age (mean of 45 v 48 years) was not large however, given the nature of the sample. It was surprising that a higher proportion of men completed the battery than did not. Given the time pressure at initial assessment, men, who tend to be less conscientious than women [57], may have attempted the battery more quickly and so completed it.

Finally, the study is cross-sectional so causal inferences cannot be made from this data. The mediation models tested do reflect the literature, but it must be recognized that alternative models could be produced which could also fit with the available data, for example beliefs may mediate the relationships observed between self-efficacy and outcomes however this was a less good fit. Alternatively, unmeasured variables such as pain catastrophizing, may play a role in these relationships. Future longitudinal studies using the Pain Beliefs Questionnaire could further assess the usefulness of the measure in predicting and explaining variations in disability, anxiety and depression following low back pain rehabilitation programmes. In addition, controlled trials would help provide causal information about the role of beliefs in pain rehabilitation.

5. Conclusions

Overall, this study illustrates the importance of beliefs about the nature of pain and beliefs in one's ability to cope with pain in determining both physical and mental health outcomes amongst chronic low back pain patients. The pain beliefs questionnaire is a simple measure that is independent of condition or the presence of pain, but nevertheless provides two scales that are useful in predicting disability and mental health outcomes. Pain self-efficacy is an excellent predictor of physical and mental pain-related outcomes and can act indirectly in the relationship between organic ('biomedical') beliefs about pain and disability, anxiety and depression.

Acknowledgments: The authors would like to acknowledge the generous support offered by all staff at the Nottingham Back Team.

Author Contributions: Andrew Baird conceived, designed and undertook the study. Andrew Baird and David Sheffield analyzed the results and wrote the paper.

Conflicts of Interest: The authors declare no conflicts of interest.

Appendix

The main body of the paper describes the most parsimonious model, but further analyses were undertaken to consider alternatives in relation to disability, anxiety and depression as described below:

Disability: In order to test the possibility that a third unmeasured variable may account for these relationships, further mediation analysis was conducted, with belief and LOC measures as mediators of the self-efficacy-disability relationship. There was a significant indirect effect of self-efficacy on disability through organic pain beliefs, $b = -0.23$, $p < 0.0001$, BCa CI $(-0.07, -0.03)$, which explained 5% of the total effect. The direct effect of self-efficacy on disability was also significant, $b = -0.22$, $t = -12.13$, $p < 0.0001$.

Anxiety: In order to test the possibility that a third unmeasured variable may account for these relationships, further mediation analysis was again conducted, with belief and LOC measures as mediators of the self-efficacy-anxiety relationship. There was a significant indirect effect of self-efficacy on anxiety through chance LOC, $b = -0.20$, $p < 0.0001$, BCa CI $(-0.03, -0.01)$, which explained 1% of the total effect. The direct effect of self-efficacy on anxiety was also significant, $b = -0.11$, $t = -6.50$, $p < 0.0001$.

Depression: Again, to test the possibility that a third unmeasured variable may account for these relationships, further mediation analysis was conducted, with belief and LOC measures as mediators of the self-efficacy-depression relationship. There was a significant indirect effect of self-efficacy on depression through chance LOC, $b = -0.08$, $p < 0.005$, BCa CI $(-0.01, 0.00)$, which explained 1% of the total effect. The direct effect of self-efficacy on depression was also significant, $b = -0.16$, $t = -13.11$, $p < 0.0001$.

References

1. Balague, F.; Manion, A.F.; Pellise, F.; Cedraschi, C. Non-specific low back pain. *Lancet* **2012**, *379*, 482–491. [PubMed]
2. Snook, S. Work-related low back pain: Secondary intervention. *J. Electromyogr. Kinesiol.* **2004**, *14*, 153–160. [CrossRef] [PubMed]
3. Deyo, R.; Weinstein, J. Low back pain. *N. Engl. J. Med.* **2001**, *344*, 363–370. [CrossRef] [PubMed]
4. Thomsen, A.; Sorenson, J.; Sjorgen, P.; Eriksen, J. Chronic non-malignant pain patients and health economic consequences. *Eur. J. Pain* **2002**, *6*, 341–352. [PubMed]
5. Dagenais, G.; Caro, J.; Haldeman, S. A systematic review of low back pain cost of illness studies in the United States and internationally. *Spine J.* **2008**, *8*, 8–20. [CrossRef] [PubMed]
6. Hong, J.; Reed, C.; Novick, D.; Happich, M. Costs associated with treatment of chronic low back pain: An analysis of the UK General Practice Research Database. *Spine* **2013**, *38*, 75–82. [CrossRef] [PubMed]
7. Lidgren, L. The Bone and Joint Decade and the global economic and healthcare burden of musculoskeletal disease. *J. Rheumatol.* **2003**, *67*, 4–5.
8. Waddell, G. *The Back Pain Revolution*, 2nd ed.; Churchill Livingstone: Edinburgh, UK, 2004.
9. Waddell, G.; Burton, A.K. Occupational health guidelines for the management of low back pain at work: Evidence review. *Occup. Med. (Lond.)* **2001**, *51*, 124–135. [CrossRef] [PubMed]
10. Main, C.J.; George, S.Z. Psychologically informed practice for management of low back pain: Future directions in practice and research. *Phys. Ther.* **2011**, *91*, 820–824. [CrossRef] [PubMed]
11. Burton, A.K.; Balague, F.; Cardon, G.; Eriksen, H.R.; Henrotin, Y.; Lahad, A.; Leclerc, A.; Müller, G.; van der Beek, A.J. Chapter 2. European guidelines for prevention in low back pain. *Eur. Spine J.* **2006**, *15*, S136–S168. [CrossRef] [PubMed]
12. Chou, R.; Qaseem, A.; Snow, V.; Casey, D.; Cross, J.T.; Shekelle, P.; Owens, D. Diagnosis and treatment of low back pain: A joint clinical practice guideline from the American College of Physicians and the American Pain Society. *Ann. Intern. Med.* **2007**, *147*, 478–491. [CrossRef] [PubMed]
13. Turner, J.; Dworkin, S.; Mancl, L.; Huggins, K.; Truelove, E. The roles of beliefs, catastrophizing, and coping in the functioning of patients with temporomandibular disorders. *Pain* **2001**, *92*, 41–51. [CrossRef]
14. Jensen, M.; Romano, J.; Turner, J.; Good, A.; Wald, L. Patient beliefs predict patient functioning: Further support for a cognitive-behavioural model of chronic pain. *Pain* **1999**, *81*, 95–104. [CrossRef]
15. Vowle, K.E.; Gross, R.T. Work-related beliefs about injury and physical capability for work in individuals with chronic pain. *Pain* **2003**, *101*, 291–298. [CrossRef]
16. Turner, J.; Jensen, M.; Romano, J. Do beliefs, coping, and catastrophizing independently predict functioning in patients with chronic pain? *Pain* **2000**, *85*, 115–125. [CrossRef]
17. Goubert, L.; Crombez, G.; Van Damme, S. The role of neuroticism, pain catastrophizing and pain-related fear in vigilance to pain: A structural equations approach. *Pain* **2004**, *107*, 234–241. [CrossRef] [PubMed]
18. Zale, E.L.; Lange, K.L.; Fields, S.A.; Ditre, J.W. The relation between pain-related fear and disability: A meta-analysis. *J. Pain* **2013**, *14*, 1019–1030. [CrossRef] [PubMed]
19. Crombez, G.; Vlaeyen, J.W.; Heuts, P.; Lysens, R. Pain-related fear is more disabling than pain itself: Evidence on the role of pain-related fear in chronic back pain disability. *Pain* **1999**, *80*, 329–339. [CrossRef]
20. Vlaeyen, J.W.; Linton, S.J. Fear-avoidance and its consequences in chronic musculoskeletal pain: A state of the art. *Pain* **2000**, *85*, 317–332. [CrossRef]

21. Pfingsten, M.; Leibing, E.; Harter, W.; Kroner-Herwig, B.; Hempel, D.; Kronshage, U.; Hildebrandt, J. Fear-avoidance behavior and anticipation of pain in patients with chronic low back pain: A randomized controlled study. *Pain Med.* **2001**, *2*, 259–266. [CrossRef] [PubMed]

22. Buer, N.; Linton, S.J. Fear-avoidance beliefs and catastrophizing: Occurrence and risk factor in back pain and ADL in the general population. *Pain* **2002**, *99*, 485–491. [CrossRef]

23. Shaw, W.S.; Main, C.J.; Johnston, V. Addressing occupational factors in the management of low back pain: Implications for physical therapist practice. *Phys. Ther.* **2011**, *91*, 777–789. [CrossRef] [PubMed]

24. Ashari, A.; Nicholas, M.K. Pain self-efficacy beliefs and pain behaviour. A prospective study. *Pain* **2001**, *94*, 85–100. [CrossRef]

25. Denison, E.; Asenlof, P.; Lindberg, P. Self-efficacy, fear avoidance, and pain intensity as predictors of disability in subacute and chronic musculoskeletal pain patients in primary health care. *Pain* **2004**, *111*, 245–252. [CrossRef] [PubMed]

26. Amstein, P.; Caudill, M.; Mandler, C.; Norris, A.; Beasley, R. Self-efficacy as a mediator of the relationship between pain intensity, disability and depression in chronic pain patients. *Pain* **1999**, *80*, 483–491.

27. Arnstein, P. The mediation of disability by self-efficacy in different samples of chronic pain patients. *Disabil. Rehabil.* **2000**, *22*, 794–801. [CrossRef] [PubMed]

28. Woby, S.; Urmston, M.; Watson, P. Self-efficacy mediates the relation between pain-related fear and outcome in chronic low back pain patients. *Eur. J. Pain* **2007**, *11*, 711–718. [CrossRef] [PubMed]

29. Spinhoven, P.; ter Kuile, A.; Mansfeld, M.H.; den Ouden, D.J.; Vlaeyen, J.W.S. Catastrophizing and internal pain control as mediators of outcome in the multidisciplinary treatment of chronic low back pain. *Eur. J. Pain* **2004**, *8*, 211–219. [CrossRef] [PubMed]

30. Woby, S.; Watson, P.; Roach, N.; Urmston, M. Are changes in fear-avoidance beliefs, catastrophizing, and appraisals of control, predictive of changes in chronic low back pain and disability? *Eur. J. Pain* **2004**, *8*, 201–210. [CrossRef] [PubMed]

31. Morley, S.; Eccleston, C.; Williams, A. Systematic review and meta-analysis of randomized controlled trials of cognitive behaviour therapy and behaviour therapy for chronic pain in adults, excluding headache. *Pain* **1999**, *80*, 1–13. [CrossRef]

32. van Tulder, M.; Ostelo, R.; Vlaeyen, J.; Linton, S.; Morley, S.; Assendelft, W. Behavioral treatment for chronic low back pain: A systematic review within the framework of the Cochrane Back Review Group. *Spine* **2000**, *25*, 2688–2699. [CrossRef] [PubMed]

33. Linton, S.J.; Ryberg, M. A cognitive-behavioral group intervention as prevention for persistent neck and back pain in a non-patient population: A randomized controlled trial. *Pain* **2001**, *90*, 83–90. [CrossRef]

34. Abenhaim, L.; Rossignol, M.; Valat, J.P.; Nordin, M.; Avouac, B.; Blotman, F.; Charlot, J.; Dreiser, R.; Legrand, E.; Rozenberg, S.; et al. The role of activity in the therapeutic management of back pain. Report of the International Paris Task Force on Back Pain. *Spine* **2000**, *25*, 1S–33S. [CrossRef] [PubMed]

35. Liddle, S.; Baxter, G.; Gracey, J. Exercise and chronic low back pain: What works? *Pain* **2004**, *107*, 176–190. [CrossRef] [PubMed]

36. Baird, A.; Worral, L.; Haslam, C.; Haslam, R. Evaluation of a multi-disciplinary back pain rehabilitation programme—-Individual and group perspectives. *Qual. Life Res.* **2008**, *17*, 357–366. [CrossRef] [PubMed]

37. Walsh, D.A.; Radcliffe, J.C. Pain beliefs and perceived physical disability of patients with chronic low back pain. *Pain* **2002**, *97*, 23–31. [CrossRef]

38. Baird, A.J.; Haslam, R.A. Exploring differences in pain beliefs within and between a large nonclinical (workplace) population and a clinical (chronic low back pain) population using the pain beliefs questionnaire. *Phys. Ther.* **2013**, *12*, 1615–1624. [CrossRef] [PubMed]

39. Edwards, L.; Pearce, S.; Turner-Stokes, L.; Jones, A. The Pain Beliefs Questionnaire: An investigation of beliefs in the causes and consequences of pain. *Pain* **1992**, *51*, 267–272. [CrossRef]

40. Sloan, T.; Gupta, R.; Zhang, W.; Walsh, D. Beliefs about the causes and consequences of pain in patients with chronic inflammatory or non-inflammatory low back pain and in pain-free individuals. *Spine* **2008**, *33*, 966–972. [CrossRef] [PubMed]

41. Roland, M.; Morris, R. A study of the natural history of low back pain. Part 1: Development of a reliable and sensitive measure of disability in low-back pain. *Spine* **1983**, *8*, 141–144. [CrossRef] [PubMed]

42. Roland, M.; Fairbank, J. The Roland–Morris Disability questionnaire and the oswestry disability questionnaire. *Spine* **2000**, *25*, 3115–3124. [CrossRef] [PubMed]

43. Nicholas, M.K. Self-efficacy and Chronic Pain. In Proceedings of the Annual Conference of the British Psychological Society, St. Andrews, Scotland, 1 April 1989.
44. Zigmond, A.S.; Snaith, R.P. The Hospital Anxiety and Depression Scale. *Acta. Psychiatr. Scand.* **1983**, *67*, 361–370. [CrossRef] [PubMed]
45. Bjellanda, I.; Dahlb, A.A.; Tangen Haugc, T.; Neckelmann, D. The validity of the Hospital Anxiety and Depression Scale: An updated literature review. *J. Psychosom. Res.* **2002**, *52*, 69–77. [CrossRef]
46. Hill, J.C.; Whitehurst, D.G.T.; Lewis, M.; Dunn, K.M.; Foster, N.E.; Konstantinou, K.; Main, C.J.; Mason, E.; Somerville, S.; Sowden, G.; Vohora, K.; Hay, E.M. Comparison of stratified primary care management for low back pain with current best practice (STarT Back): A randomised controlled trial. *Lancet* **2011**, *378*, 1560–1571. [CrossRef]
47. Wallston, K.A.; Wallston, B.S.; DeVellis, R. Development of the multidimensional health locus of control (MHLC) scales. *Health Educ. Monogr.* **1978**, *6*, 160–170. [CrossRef] [PubMed]
48. Wallston, K.A. The Validity of the Multidimensional Health Locus of Control Scales. *J. Health Psychol.* **2005**, *10*, 623–631. [CrossRef] [PubMed]
49. Harkapaa, K.; Jarvikovski, A.; Mellin, G.; Hurri, H.; Luoma, J. Health locus of control beliefs and psychological distress as predictors for treatmeant outcome in low-back pain patients: Results of a 3-month follow-up of a controlled intervention study. *Pain* **1991**, *46*, 35–41. [CrossRef]
50. Hayes, A.F. PROCESS: A versatile computational tool for observed variable mediation, moderation, and conditional process modelling. Available online: http://afhayes.com/public/process2012.png (accessed on 10 April 2015).
51. Preacher, K.J.; Hayes, A.F. SPSS and SAS procedures for estimating indirect effects in simple mediation models. *Behav. Res. Methods Instrum. Comput.* **2004**, *36*, 717–731. [CrossRef] [PubMed]
52. Preacher, K.J.; Hayes, A.F. Asymptotic and resampling strategies for assessing and comparing indirect effects in multiple mediator models. *Behav. Res. Methods* **2008**, *40*, 879–891. [CrossRef] [PubMed]
53. Foster, N.E.; Thomas, E.; Bishop, A.; Dunn, K.M.; Main, C.J. Distinctiveness of psychological barriers to recovery in low back pain patients in primary care. *Pain* **2010**, *148*, 398–406. [CrossRef] [PubMed]
54. Nicholas, M.K. The pain self-efficacy questionnaire: Taking pain into account. *Eur. J. Pain* **2007**, *11*, 153–163. [CrossRef] [PubMed]
55. Costa, L.D.C.M.; Maher, C.G.; McAuley, J.H.; Hancock, M.J. Self-efficacy is more important than fear of movement in mediating the relationship between pain and disability in chronic low back pain. *Eur. J. Pain* **2011**, *15*, 213–219. [CrossRef] [PubMed]
56. Schiphorst Preuper, H.R.; Reneman, M.F.; Boonstra, A.M.; Dijkstra, P.U.; Versteegen, G.J.; Geertzen, J.H.B.; Brouwer, S. Relationship between psychological factors and performance-based and self-reported disability in chronic low back pain. *Eur. Spine J.* **2008**, *17*, 1448–1456. [CrossRef] [PubMed]
57. Vianello, M.; Schnabel, C.; Sriram, N.; Nosek, B. Gender differences in implicit and explicit personality traits. *Pers. Individ. Dif.* **2013**, *55*, 994–999. [CrossRef]

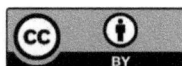

healthcare

MDPI

Article

Associations between Trunk Extension Endurance and Isolated Lumbar Extension Strength in Both Asymptomatic Participants and Those with Chronic Low Back Pain

Rebecca Conway [1], Jessica Behennah [1], James Fisher [1], Neil Osborne [2] and James Steele [1,*]

[1] School of Sport, Health and Social Sciences, Southampton Solent University, East Park Terrace, Southampton SO14 0YN, UK; 0conwr69@solent.ac.uk (R.C.); 0behej96@solent.ac.uk (J.B.); james.fisher@solent.ac.uk (J.F.)
[2] AECC Clinic, Anglo European College of Chiropractic, Bournemouth BH5 2DF, UK; NOsborne@aecc.ac.uk
* Correspondence: james.steele@solent.ac.uk; Tel.: +44-787-8127785

Academic Editor: Robert J. Gatchel
Received: 27 May 2016; Accepted: 8 September 2016; Published: 19 September 2016

Abstract: *Background:* Strength and endurance tests are important for both clinical practice and research due to the key role they play in musculoskeletal function. In particular, deconditioning of the lumbar extensor musculature has been associated with low back pain (LBP). Due to the relationship between strength and absolute endurance, it is possible that trunk extension (TEX) endurance tests could provide a proxy measure of isolated lumbar extension (ILEX) strength and thus represent a simple, practical alternative to ILEX measurements. Though, the comparability of TEX endurance and ILEX strength is presently unclear and so the aim of the present study was to examine this relationship. *Methods:* Thirty eight healthy participants and nineteen participants with non-specific chronic LBP and no previous lumbar surgery participated in this cross-sectional study design. TEX endurance was measured using the Biering–Sorensen test. A maximal ILEX strength test was performed on the MedX lumbar-extension machine. *Results:* A Pearson's correlation revealed no relationship between TEX endurance and ILEX strength in the combined group ($r = 0.035$, $p = 0.793$), the chronic LBP group ($r = 0.120$, $p = 0.623$) or the asymptomatic group ($r = -0.060$, $p = 0.720$). *Conclusions:* The results suggest that TEX is not a good indicator of ILEX and cannot be used to infer results regarding ILEX strength. However, a combination of TEX and ILEX interpreted together likely offers the greatest and most comprehensive information regarding lumbo-pelvic function during extension.

Keywords: strength; endurance; isolated lumbar extension; trunk extension; low back pain

1. Introduction

Low back pain (LBP) is one of the most common medical disorders in today's society [1], affecting both the Western developed world [2] and less economically developed countries [3–7]. This results in a considerable economic burden worldwide and includes the costs of healthcare, indemnity payment, staff training and productivity loss [8,9]. With over 100 million work days lost per year in the UK [10] and an estimated yearly total cost of £10.6 billion [11], LBP not only affects the individual, but places a great strain on families, industries and governments [3,12]. A further financial strain is also placed on institutions as accurate clinical assessments of musculoskeletal function often rely on specialist, expensive equipment.

An estimated 60%–80% of the population report back pain at some time in their life, with it often being recurrent and persistent [13]. However, only 5%–15% of this population have attributed LBP to a specific cause. The remaining 85% cannot be given a precise patho-anatomical diagnosis, and so is referred to as "non-specific" LBP [14]. Although many sufferers will recover in the acute stages without intervention, approximately 40% of individuals will develop chronic LBP [15]. This is defined as pain in the area between the inferior margin of the twelfth rib and the inferior gluteal fold [3,16], with the duration of symptoms longer than twelve weeks [17,18].

Due to the symptoms experienced, people suffering with chronic LBP tend to restrict movement, avoiding using their low back in everyday situations because of fear of pain [19]. Research suggests that this reduction in physical activity may cause muscle atrophy, as a result of disuse of the lumbar extensors [20]. However, several researchers have reported no difference in physical activity levels of chronic LBP participants compared with asymptomatic controls [21–23]. Therefore, the relationship may in fact be bidirectional, in which deconditioning itself is seen as a factor contributing to the intolerance of physical activity [24]. Whichever the case, one of the multi-factorial dysfunctions consistently reported in the literature is the deconditioning of the lumbar extensor musculature, i.e., thoracic and lumbar erector spinae, multifidus and quadratus lumborum [25–27]. One role of the lumbar extensor musculature is to provide stability to the lumbar spine [28]. As such deconditioning in these muscles has been speculated to lead to spinal instability and contribute to the high recurrence rate in CLBP (chronic low back pain) [29].

This diminished function has invited research into the association between back strength and endurance and LBP. Numerous testing methods exist to examine the function of the lumbo-pelvic complex in extension. Broadly though they can be generalised into tests to either examine trunk extension (TEX) or isolated lumbar extension (ILEX).

During dynamic actions, TEX utilises both the paraspinal muscle group and the hip extensors in order to extend the low back and the pelvis through a range of motion (ROM) of approximately 180 degrees [30]. ILEX function, which isolates the lower back muscles through the prevention of pelvic rotation, is responsible for a ROM of approximately 72 degrees [31]. Therefore, TEX might best be considered a compound movement that results in additional backward rotation of the pelvis as the hip extensors contract. As a result, it is not possible to conclude specifically whether differences occur due to contribution from the hip extensors or the lumbar extensors. In contrast, since ILEX involves stabilising the pelvis to isolate the lumbar spine and remove torque produced by the hip extensors, this allows for a more precise measurement of the smaller and weaker lumbar extensor muscles [32].

However, as it does at least partly involve contributions from the paraspinal musculature, and that there is a well evidenced relationship between muscular strength and absolute muscular endurance [33], results obtained from TEX endurance methods of testing may be potential indicators of lumbar extension strength. As such these tests could be utilised in both prospective studies of risk factors for LBP in addition to cross sectional studies. In previous research, a number of studies implementing the Biering-Sorensen test as a measure of TEX endurance have reported significantly reduced holding times in the CLBP groups [19,34–40]. This suggests that chronic LBP is associated with decreased endurance of the trunk extensor muscles. In addition, studies implementing ILEX methods of testing have also reported chronic LBP participants to be significantly weaker than asymptomatic participants [26,41–45]. Therefore, the aim of this study was to investigate whether there is a relationship between TEX and ILEX to determine the necessity of adequate pelvic restraints. A correlation between the two methods would suggest that TEX could in fact be conducted instead of ILEX and represent a cheaper and more practical alternative.

2. Materials and Methods

2.1. Research Design

A cross sectional study design was adopted with one asymptomatic control group and one chronic LBP group, in order to investigate whether a correlation exists between the two methods of testing (TEX absolute endurance and ILEX strength). The study was approved by the Centre for Health,

Exercise and Sport Science ethics committee at the first author's institution, and was conducted within the Sport Science Laboratories. Prior to testing, all subjects were provided with a participant information sheet, detailing what would be asked of them as well as their right to withdraw and were then required to sign an informed consent form.

2.2. Participants

Thirty eight asymptomatic participants (23 males and 15 females) and 19 participants with non-specific chronic LBP (10 males and 9 females) aged between 19 and 57 years were recruited. The participants in this study were staff or undergraduate students studying at a UK higher education institution. This was a sample of convenience, with participants being recruited via email, adverts, social media and word of mouth. Inclusion criteria for participants with chronic LBP were as follows: lumbar or lumbosacral pain occurring almost daily for at least twelve weeks [46], and no medical conditions for which a maximal effort test is contraindicated. Exclusion criteria for the asymptomatic control group was back pain exceeding one week in the preceding year. General exclusion criteria were: pregnancy, sciatica, pain radiating below the knee, disc herniation, vertebral fractures, other major structural abnormalities [47] and surgery of the pelvis or spinal column. All chronic LBP participants received physiotherapist/chiropractic consultation to confirm suitability, as well as referral, prior to inclusion.

2.3. Instrumentation

Stature was measured using a stadiometer (Holtan ltd, Crymych, Dyfed, UK) and body mass was measured using scales (Seca, Hamburg, Germany), from this body mass index was calculated. Age, mass, stature and body mass index were similar in both asymptomatic and symptomatic participants (Table 1). Isometric strength testing for ILEX was performed using the MedX Lumbar Extension Machine (MedX, Ocala, FL, USA; Figure 1). This equipment has been found to be highly reliable through a 72 degree range of motion of lumbar extension in asymptomatic participants ($r = 0.81$–0.97; [31]) and LBP symptomatic participants ($r = 0.57$–0.93; [48]). TEX endurance was measured using the Biering–Sorensen test (Figure 2) and has been shown to produce reliable results when testing asymptomatic (ICC, 0.83) and symptomatic participants (ICC, 0.88; [49]). The Oswestry Disability Index (ODI) version 2.0 was used to assess disability and has been shown to be a valid and rigorous measure of condition-specific disability [50]. A 100-mm Visual Analogue Scale (VAS) was used to measure pain rating in chronic LBP participants [51].

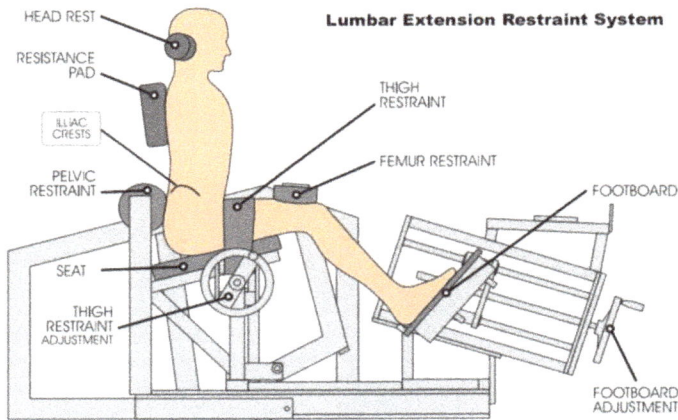

Figure 1. MedX schematic demonstrating the restraint system, thus isolating lumbar extensors [44].

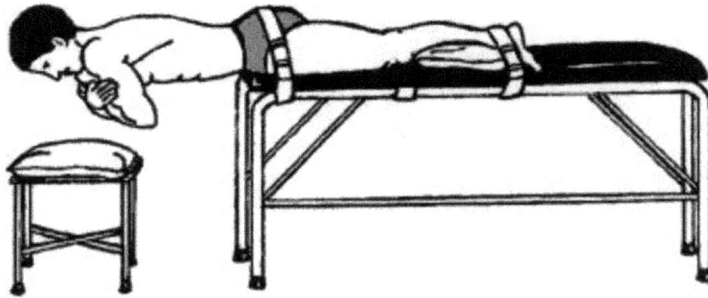

Figure 2. Biering-Sorensen schematic demonstrating body position and restraining belts [52].

2.4. Procedures

A Physical Activity Readiness Questionnaire (PARQ) was completed to screen for contraindications and confirm suitability based on inclusion and exclusion criteria. The participants visited the laboratory for testing on two separate occasions. These test days were separated by at least 72 h to allow the participants to recover from any residual fatigue or soreness that might have been associated with the testing [31]. The first testing day included the collection of anthropometric data, followed by TEX using the Biering-Sorensen and finally, a familiarisation session for ILEX testing. The Biering-Sorensen test was performed according to the following prescription. The participant was positioned prone on a treatment couch with the upper edge of the iliac crests aligned with the edge of the couch. The lower body was fixed to the couch by two straps, located at the level of the greater trochanter of the femur and at the ankles as close to the malleoli as possible [50]. The straps were tightened securely, whilst causing minimal discomfort to the participant. Whilst the participants were secured into position they were allowed to rest their upper body on a stool for comfort and to minimise fatigue. At the start of the test, the participants placed their arms diagonally across their chest and maintained a neutral position for as long as possible. The time the position could be held was measured using a stopwatch. Termination of the test occurred as follows: excessive fatigue, downward sloping of the trunk by more than 10° (as observed by visual inspection), unendurable pain or when 240 s was reached [52]. If the participant's horizontal position dropped, they were asked to regain horizontal alignment until it could no longer be successfully performed. Participants were verbally encouraged to hold the position for as long as possible.

The familiarisation session on the MedX was performed as follows in order to produce reliable results [31]. The participants were seated in the lumbar extension machine, with their thighs parallel to the seat and their toes slightly inverted. A thigh restraint was placed over the lap and tightened securely, limiting movement at the thigh and pelvis. A femur restraint was placed above the flexed knees and the feet were pressed against the foot boards, which were then tightened securely. This drives the femurs towards the pelvis, thus securing the pelvis against the lumbar pad. Tests were carried out to ensure there was limited rotation of the lumbar pad and limited movement at the femur restraints; this ensures isolation of the lumbar extensors. The headrest was adjusted to the level of the occipital bone for comfort, support and positional standardisation [31]. Participants were asked to maintain a light grip on the handles during testing procedures to maintain standardisation.

After the participant had been seated, initial testing was carried out to check for any limitations in their range of lumbar motion between 0° and 72° of flexion and to adjust the counterweight to neutralise the gravitational forces of head, torso and upper extremities [31]. A slow, controlled dynamic warm-up was administered, lasting for approximately one minute. For the maximal test, the movement arm was locked into place at each specified angle (0, 12, 24, 36, 48, 60, 72 degrees if full ROM was achieved) and the participant was instructed to gradually build up tension to a maximal effort over a 3 s period. The movement arm of this testing device is attached to a load cell that is interfaced to an IBM microcomputer [30], which allows for torque to be calculated. Between each isometric contraction a rest period of ten seconds was provided, whilst being rocked to relax their lumbar extensors.

The second day of testing occurred with at least 72 h of rest following the first test day. Prior to testing, participants were required to complete the ODI and mark the VAS. Participants then followed the same protocol for the MedX that was conducted during the familiarisation session.

2.5. Data Analysis

Results from the testing were analysed using the Statistical Package for the Social Sciences 22.0 software (IBM, Portsmouth, Hampshire, UK), with an alpha level of 0.05 set as the level of statistical significance. The Shapiro-Wilk test was used to examine assumptions of normality of distribution as research has shown it to be the most powerful test for all types of distributions and sample sizes [53]. Following the Shapiro-Wilk test, demographic data was examined for between group difference using an independent *t*-test for normally distributed data and a Mann-Whitney U for data which was not normally distributed. Since the data were found to be normally distributed, a Pearson's correlation was calculated to analyse whether there was an association between ILEX and TEX for both the combined sample and the asymptomatic and chronic LBP groups individually. Correlations were also run with additional sub-grouping for sex however results did not differ from the pooled sex analyses and so only the pooled results are reported. Correlation coefficients were interpreted as low (r = 0.30 to 0.50), moderate (r = 0.50 to 0.70) or high (r > 0.70) [54]. TEX endurance is reported as Biering-Sorensen hold time (BSHT) and ILEX as a strength index (SI) which was calculated as the area under the strength curve by the MedX software using the trapezoidal method, incorporating isometric strength at all tested angles.

3. Results

3.1. Participants

Participant demographics are shown in Table 1. An independent *t*-test was conducted on the normally distributed data, which revealed no significant differences between the groups for any of the variables (stature, mass and blood pressure). Age, BMI and ROM were not normally distributed and so a Mann Whitney U test was carried out on these variables. This test also revealed no significant differences between the two groups. The results from the ODI classified the CLBP participants as having only moderate disability, which may explain the lack of difference in lumbar ROM.

Table 1. Participant demographics and descriptive statistics.

Characteristic	Chronic LBP (n = 19)	Asymptomatic (n = 38)	p-Values
Age (year)	28 ± 12	31 ± 12	0.218
Stature (cm)	173.00 ± 0.10	174.00 ± 0.10	0.642
Mass (kg)	75.03 ± 13.15	75.4 ± 12.60	0.918
BMI (kg/m^2)	25.00 ± 3.17	24.82 ± 3.54	0.785
SBP (mmHg)	133.32 ± 13.97	134.47 ± 13.47	0.764
DBP (mmHg)	75.37 ± 10.25	73.90 ± 9.69	0.597
Lumbar ROM (°)	68.05 ± 6.33	68.26 ± 5.25	0.940
VAS (mm)	34.84 ± 24.45	NA	NA
ODI (%)	23.37 ± 12.33	NA	NA

Results are mean ± SD. BMI: Body Mass Index; VAS: Visual Analogue Scale; ODI: Oswestry Disability Index; NA: Not applicable.

3.2. Correlations between BSHT and SI

Pearson's correlation revealed a non-significant very weak positive correlation between ILEX strength and TEX endurance in the combined group (r = 0.035, p = 0.793), and the chronic LBP group

($r = 0.120$, $p = 0.623$). A non-significant very weak negative correlation was found between ILEX strength and TEX endurance in the asymptomatic group ($r = -0.060$, $p = 0.720$). Figures 3–5 present scatter plots of data for ILEX strength (SI) and TEX endurance (BSHT).

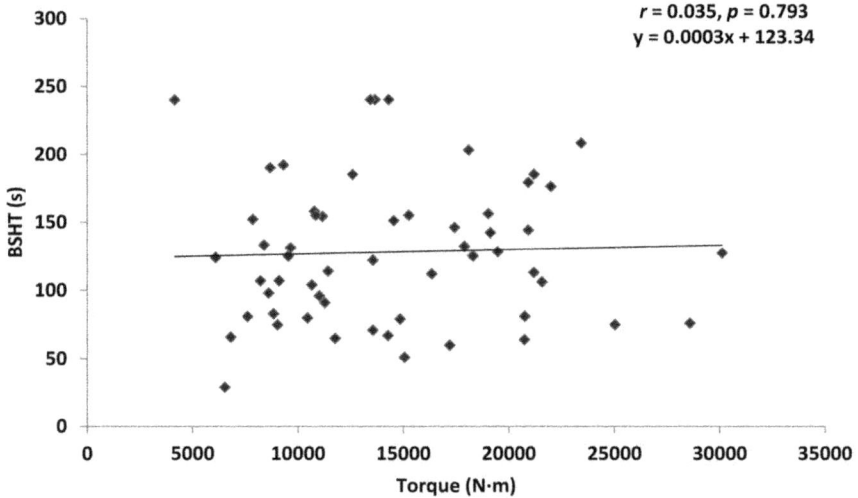

Figure 3. Scatter plot of combined group data for isolated lumbar extension (ILEX) strength index (SI) and trunk extension (TEX) endurance (Biering-Sorensen hold time (BSHT)).

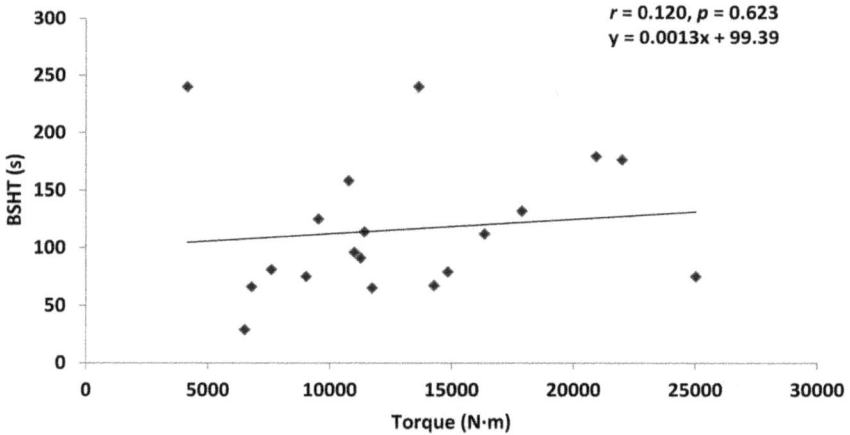

Figure 4. Scatter plot of chronic lower back pain (CLBP) data for ILEX strength (SI) and TEX endurance (BSHT).

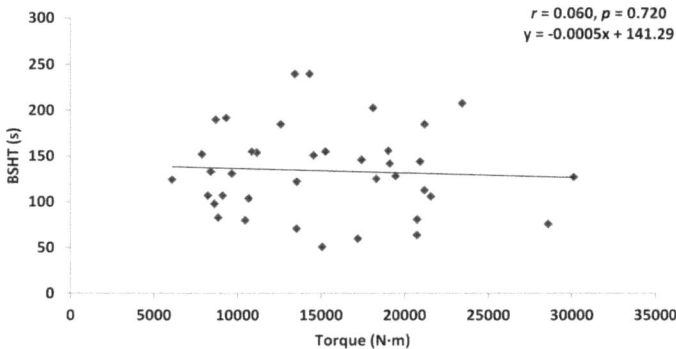

Figure 5. Scatter plot of asymptomatic data for ILEX strength (SI) and TEX endurance (BSHT).

4. Discussion

The aim of this study was to investigate whether there is a relationship between ILEX strength and TEX endurance in chronic LBP and asymptomatic participants. Statistical analysis revealed that there was no significant correlation between the two methods of testing in either the combined group ($r = 0.035$, $p = 0.793$), chronic LBP group ($r = 0.120$, $p = 0.623$) or asymptomatic group ($r = -0.060$, $p = 0.720$). This suggests that TEX endurance is a poor indicator of ILEX strength, thus supporting previous research which suggests that the pelvis must be adequately restrained and stabilised for the purpose of testing ILEX strength [31].

TEX utilises both the paraspinal muscle group and hip extensors in order to extend through a range of motion of approximately 180 degrees [30]. The hip extensors have a larger cross-sectional area and longer moment arms compared to the small lumbar extensors [55]. Further, there is a de-recruitment of the lumbar extensors and a further increase in hip extensor muscle activity during the Biering-Sorensen test [56]. Thus, the torque contributed to TEX by the hip extensors is comparatively greater than the paraspinal musculature [57]. Though, the relative contribution of the hip extensors has produced considerable discourse where some researchers suggest loading activates mostly the lumbar extensors [58,59], whereas others suggest the test indicates more about the endurance of the hip extensors [60,61]. Nonetheless, it is clear that the hip extensor musculature has the potential to influence tests of TEX endurance. Deconditioning in LBP does not appear to be present in the hip extensor musculature [55], which may explain why there is a poor relationship between the two methods of testing in both chronic LBP and asymptomatic participants.

Despite the relationship between strength and absolute endurance [33], the data presented supports previous research suggesting there is a poor relationship between tests of TEX endurance and ILEX strength [62]. As the Biering-Sorensen test utilises both the lumbar extensors and hip extensors, endurance times are not specifically indicative of the lumbar extensors [63]. Therefore, studies implementing an ILEX approach allow a more specific indication of the effects of LBP on the lumbar extensors. This is likely a result of the pelvic stabilisation preventing hip extensor contribution, and isolating the lower spine for ILEX testing [32]. At most, only 3 degrees of pelvic rotation occurs during ILEX, likely as a result of soft tissue compliance. This, in turn, results in greater reliability of results [63].

The present data suggests that ILEX strength testing is required to provide valid information regarding the function of the lumbar extensor musculature specifically. This is particularly important when examining the effects of LBP since atrophy of the lumbar extensors has been well-documented in the literature [55,64,65], potentially resulting in impaired ILEX strength [26,41–43,45,46]. Despite this, consideration of both tests of TEX and ILEX might be valuable when considered together [66]. In combination, the testing might allow for identification of the weak link within the posterior kinetic chain. As a result, an identification of whether differences predominantly lie between the lumbar extensors or hip extensors can be achieved. Therefore, future research examining the relationships between LBP and lumbo-pelvic function should implement a combination of both TEX endurance and ILEX strength tests. Alternatively, it may be that modifications of the Biering-Sorenson test to examine TEX endurance may have greater association with ILEX strength than the one examined here [67].

Limitations

One limitation within this study is the varying group sizes, with a notably smaller sample size for the CLBP group. The sample of subjects may not truly represent the heterogeneity of patients with non-specific CLBP. For instance, results from the ODI classified the CLBP participants as having only moderate disability. As a consequence, this particular sample set may not have been significantly impaired, thus potentially limiting the external validity of the study. Considering this further, the degree to which psychosocial factors, kinesiophobia, or catastraphisation was present in our sample was not investigated and so whether this may have affected the results is unknown.

Intra- and inter-examiner reproducibility tests were not performed prior to the study. Though the reproducibility of TEX and ILEX tests has been previously reported to be moderate to high, this could be considered a potentially limiting factor. Further to this, only ILEX was preceded by a familiarisation with this test. Justifiably, a second session on the MedX was implemented as previous analysis revealed a significant learning effect [31] whereas the Biering-Sorensen test has previously demonstrated no learning effects [68]. However, it may have been appropriate to precede both ILEX and TEX with a familiarisation session. Lastly, for practicality and to represent application in clinical practice, visual inspection was used for the Biering-Sorenson test potentially affecting the validity of the measure in addition to an upper threshold of 240 s. This may have limited the extent to which a relationship was present in those with greater TEX endurance.

5. Conclusions

The present study found that there is a poor relationship between measures of TEX endurance and ILEX strength in both those with and without LBP. Research supports that persons suffering from LBP display atrophy of the lumbar musculature [55,64,65]. Since the lumbar extensors play a significant role in conditions such as LBP [63] it is important that testing mechanisms are able to elucidate which aspects of the musculature are responsible. The poor relationship between TEX endurance and ILEX strength suggests that if information regarding the function of the lumbar extensors is of interest this is best obtained by conducting ILEX testing. Results from TEX tests should only be considered as representing TEX as a compound movement and should not be used to infer results regarding lumbar extensor function specifically. However, a combination of both TEX and ILEX tests offers the greatest and most comprehensive information, by identifying whether differences predominantly lie between the lumbar extensors or hip extensors.

Author Contributions: Rebecca Conway, Jessica Behennah, James Fisher and James Steele conceived and designed the experiments; Rebecca Conway and Jessica Behennah performed the experiments; Rebecca Conway and James Steele analysed the data; Neil Osborne contributed analysis tools; Rebecca Conway drafted the manuscript; Jessica Behennah, James Fisher, Neil Osborne and James Steele reviewed and provided critical feedback regarding the manuscript.

Conflicts of Interest: The authors declare no conflicts of interest.

References

1. Freburger, J.K.; Holmes, G.M.; Agans, R.P.; Jackman, A.M.; Darter, J.D.; Wallace, A.S.; Castel, L.D.; Kalsbeek, W.D.; Carey, T.S. The Rising Prevalence of Chronic Low Back Pain. *Arch. Intern. Med.* **2009**, *169*, 251–258. [CrossRef] [PubMed]
2. Vollin, E. The epidemiology of low back pain in the rest of the world: A review of surveys in low- and middle-income countries. *Spine* **1997**, *22*, 1747–1754. [CrossRef]

3. Hoy, D.; Brooks, P.; Blyth, F.; Buchbinder, R. The epidemiology of low back pain. *Best Pract. Res. Clin. Rheumatol.* **2010**, *24*, 769–781. [CrossRef] [PubMed]

4. Çakmak, A.; Yücel, B.; Özyalçn, S.N.; Bayraktar, B.; Ural, H.I.; Duruöz, M.T.; Genç, A. The frequency and associated factors of low back pain among a younger population in Turkey. *Spine* **2004**, *29*, 1567–1572. [CrossRef] [PubMed]

5. Barrero, L.H.; Hsu, Y.H.; Terwedow, H.; Perry, M.J.; Dennerlein, J.T.; Brain, J.D.; Xu, X. Prevalence and physical determinants of low back pain in a rural Chinese population. *Spine* **2006**, *31*, 2728–2734. [CrossRef] [PubMed]

6. Louw, Q.A.; Morris, L.D.; Grimmer-Somers, K. Prevalence of low back pain in Africa: A systematic Review. *BMC Musculoskelet. Disord.* **2007**. [CrossRef] [PubMed]

7. Ferreira, G.D.; Silva, M.C.; Rombaldi, A.J.; Wrege, E.D.; Siqueira, F.V.; Hallal, P.C. Prevalence and associated factors of back pain in adults from southern Brazil: A population-based study. *Braz. J. Phys. Ther.* **2011**, *15*, 31–36. [CrossRef]

8. Steenstra, I.A.; Verbeek, J.H.; Heymans, M.W.; Bongers, P.M. Prognostic factors for duration of sick leave in patients sick listed with acute low back pain: A systematic review of the literature. *Occup. Environ. Med.* **2005**, *62*, 851–860. [CrossRef] [PubMed]

9. Kent, P.M.; Keating, J.L. The epidemiology of low back pain in primary care. *Chiropr. Osteopat.* **2005**. [CrossRef] [PubMed]

10. Papageorgiou, A.C.; Croft, P.R.; Ferry, S.; Jayson, M.I.; Silman, A.J. Estimating the prevalence of low back pain in the general population: Evidence from the South Manchester Back Pain Survey. *Spine* **1995**, *20*, 1889–1894. [CrossRef] [PubMed]

11. Maniadakis, N.; Gray, A. The economic burden of back pain in the UK. *Pain* **2000**, *84*, 95–103. [CrossRef]

12. Ricci, J.A.; Stewart, W.F.; Chee, E.; Leotta, C.; Foley, K.; Hochberg, M.C. Back pain exacerbations and lost productive time costs in United States workers. *Spine* **2006**, *31*, 3052–3060. [CrossRef] [PubMed]

13. Waddell, G.; Burton, A.K. Occupational health guidelines for the management of low back pain at work: Evidence review. *Occup. Med.* **2001**, *51*, 124–135. [CrossRef]

14. Deyo, R.; Weinstein, J. Low back pain. *N. Engl. J. Med.* **2001**, *344*, 363–370. [CrossRef] [PubMed]

15. Traeger, A.; Henschke, N.; Hübscher, M.; Williams, C.M.; Kamper, S.J.; Maher, C.G.; Moseley, G.L.; McAuley, J.H. Development and validation of a screening tool to predict the risk of chronic low back pain in patients presenting with acute low back pain: A study protocol. *BMJ Open* **2015**, *5*, e007916. [CrossRef] [PubMed]

16. DePalma, M.J.; Ketchum, J.M.; Saullo, T. What is the source of chronic low back pain and does age play a role? *Pain Med.* **2011**, *12*, 224–233. [CrossRef] [PubMed]

17. Bratton, R.L. Assessment and management of acute low back pain. *Am. Fam. Phys.* **1999**, *60*, 2299–2306.

18. Frank, A. Low back pain. *Br. Med. J.* **1993**, *306*, 901–909. [CrossRef]

19. Paasuke, M.; Johanson, E.; Proosa, M.; Ereline, J.; Gapeyeva, H. Back extensor fatigability in chronic low back pain patients and controls: Relationship between electromyogram power spectrum changes and body mass index. *J. Back Musculoskelet. Rehabil.* **2002**, *16*, 17–24. [CrossRef] [PubMed]

20. Cooper, R.G.; Forbes, W.S.; Jayson, M.I. Radiographic demonstration of paraspinal muscle wasting in patients with chronic low back pain. *Rheumatology* **1992**, *31*, 389–394. [CrossRef]

21. Verbunt, J.A.; Seelen, H.A.; Vlaeyen, J.W.; Heijden, G.J.; Heuts, P.H.; Pons, K.; Knottnerus, J.A. Disuse and deconditioning in chronic low back pain: Concepts and hypotheses on contributing mechanisms. *Eur. J. Pain* **2003**, *7*, 9–21. [CrossRef]

22. Wittink, H.; Hoskins, M.T.; Wagner, A.; Sukiennik, A.; Rogers, W. Deconditioning in patients with chronic low back pain: Fact of fiction? *Spine* **2000**, *25*, 2221–2228. [CrossRef] [PubMed]

23. Bousema, E.J.; Verbunt, J.A.; Seelen, H.A.; Vlaeyen, J.W.; Knottnerus, J.A. Disuse and physical deconditioning in the first year after the onset of back pain. *Pain* **2007**, *130*, 279–286. [CrossRef] [PubMed]

24. Smeets, R.J.; Wittink, H. The deconditioning paradigm for chronic low back pain unmasked? *Pain* **2007**, *130*, 201–202. [CrossRef] [PubMed]

25. Roy, S.H.; De Luca, C.J.; Emley, M.; Buijs, R.J. Spectral electromyographic assessment of back muscles in patients with low back pain undergoing rehabilitation. *Spine* **1995**, *20*, 38–48. [CrossRef] [PubMed]

26. Nelson, B.W.; Miller, M.; Hogan, M.; Wegner, J.A.; Kelly, C. The clinical effects of intensive, specific exercise on chronic low back pain: A controlled study of 895 consecutive patients with 1-year follow up. *Orthopedics* **1995**, *18*, 971–981. [PubMed]

27. Danneels, L.A.; Vanderstraeten, G.G.; Cambier, D.C.; Witvrouw, E.E.; De Cuyper, H.J.; Danneels, L. CT imaging of trunk muscles in chronic low back pain patients and healthy control subjects. *Eur. Spine J.* **2000**, *9*, 266–272. [CrossRef] [PubMed]

28. Akuthota, V.; Nadler, S.F. Core Strengthening. *Arch. Phys. Med. Rehabil.* **2004**, *85*, 86–92. [CrossRef]

29. Danneels, L.A.; Vanderstraeten, G.G.; Cambier, D.C.; Witvrouw, E.E.; Bourgois, J.D.; Dankaerts, W.; De Cuyper, H.J. Effects of three different training modalities on the cross sectional area of the lumbar multifidus muscles in patients with chronic low back pain. *Br. J. Sports Med.* **2001**, *35*, 186–191. [CrossRef] [PubMed]

30. Graves, J.E.; Webb, D.C.; Pollock, M.L.; Matkozich, J.; Leggett, S.H.; Carpenter, D.M.; Foster, D.N.; Cirulli, J. Pelvic Stabilization during resistance training: Its effect on the development of lumbar extension strength. *Arch. Phys. Med. Rehabil.* **1994**, *75*, 210–215. [PubMed]

31. Graves, J.E.; Pollock, M.L.; Carpenter, D.M.; Leggett, S.H.; Jones, A.; Macmillan, M.I.; Fulton, M. Quantitative assessment of full range-of-motion isometric lumbar extension strength. *Spine* **1990**, *15*, 288–294. [CrossRef]

32. Pollock, M.L.; Leggett, S.H.; Graves, J.E.; Jones, A.; Fulton, M.; Cirulli, J. Effect of resistance training on lumbar extension strength. *Am. J. Sports Med.* **1989**, *17*, 624–629. [CrossRef] [PubMed]

33. Fisher, J.; Steele, J.; Bruce-Low, S.; Smith, D. Evidence based resistance training recommendations. *Med. Sport.* **2011**, *15*, 147–162. [CrossRef]

34. Luoto, S.; Heliövaara, M.; Hurri, H.; Alaranta, H. Static back endurance and the risk of low-back pain. *Clin. Biomech.* **1995**, *10*, 323–324. [CrossRef]

35. Nicolaisen, T.; Jørgensen, K. Trunk muscle strength, back muscle endurance and low back trouble. *Scand. J. Rehabil. Med.* **1985**, *17*, 121–128. [PubMed]

36. Holmström, E.; Moritz, U.; Andersson, M. Trunk muscle strength and back muscle endurance in construction workers with and without low back disorders. *Scand. J. Rehabil. Med.* **1992**, *24*, 3–10. [PubMed]

37. Salminen, J.J.; Maki, P.; Oksanen, A.; Pentti, J. Spinal mobility and trunk muscle strength in 15 year old school children with and without low back pain. *Spine* **1992**, *17*, 405–411. [CrossRef] [PubMed]

38. Hultman, G.; Nordin, M.; Saraste, H.; Ohlsèn, H. Body composition, endurance, strength, cross-sectional area, and density of MM erector spinae in men and women with and without low back pain. *J. Disord.* **1993**, *6*, 114–123.

39. Crossman, K.; Mahon, M.; Watson, P.J.; Oldham, J.A.; Cooper, R.G. Chronic low back pain-associated paraspinal muscle dysfunction is not the result of a constitutionally "adverse" fibre-type composition. *Spine* **2004**, *29*, 628–634. [CrossRef] [PubMed]

40. Suuden, E.; Ereline, J.; Gapeyeva, H.; Paasuke, M. Low back muscle fatigue during Sorensen endurance test in patients with chronic low back pain: Relationship between electromyographic spectral compression and anthropometric characteristics. *Electromyogr. Clin. Neurophysiol.* **2008**, *48*, 185–192. [PubMed]

41. Mooney, V.; Kron, M.; Rummerfield, P.; Holmes, B. The effects of workplace based strengthening on low back injury rates: A case study in the strip mining industry. *J. Occup. Rehabil.* **1995**, *5*, 157–167. [CrossRef] [PubMed]

42. Boyce, R.O.; Boone, E.; Stallings, J.; Wilde, C. A multidisciplinary approach to a time efficient low back exercise intervention in a small manufacturing plant: A case study. *J. Exerc. Physiol.* **2008**, *11*, 12–24.

43. Cassisi, J.E.; Robinson, M.E.; O'Conner, P.; MacMillan, M. Trunk strength and lumbar paraspinal muscle activity during isometric exercise in chronic low-back pain patients and controls. *Spine* **1993**, *18*, 245–251. [CrossRef] [PubMed]

44. Moreau, C.E.; Green, B.N.; Johnson, C.D.; Moreau, S.R. Isometric back extension endurance tests: A review of the literature. *J. Manip. Physiol. Ther.* **2001**, *24*, 110–122. [CrossRef] [PubMed]

45. Leggett, B.H.; Nichols, V.M.; Hoeyberghs, S.N. Comparison of female geriatric lumbar extension strength: Asymptomatic versus chronic low back pain patients and their response to active rehabilitation. *J. Spinal Disord.* **1996**, *9*, 17–22.

46. Robinson, M.E.; Cassisi, J.E.; O'Connor, P.D.; MacMillan, M. Lumbar iEMG during isotonic exercise: Chronic low back pain patients vs. controls. *J. Spinal Disord.* **1992**, *5*, 8–15. [CrossRef] [PubMed]

47. Larivière, C.; Da Silva, R.A.; Arsenault, A.B.; Nadeau, S.Y.; Plamondon, A.N.; Vadeboncoeur, R.O. Specificity of a back muscle exercise machine in healthy and low back pain subjects. *Med. Sci. Sports Exerc.* **2010**, *42*, 592–599. [CrossRef] [PubMed]

48. Steele, J.; Bruce-Low, S.; Smith, D.; Jessop, D.; Osborne, N. A Randomized controlled trial of limited range of motion lumbar extension exercise in chronic low back pain. *Spine* **2013**, *38*, 1245–1252. [CrossRef] [PubMed]

49. Robinson, M.E.; Greene, A.F.; O'Connor, P.; Graves, J.E.; Mac Millan, M. Reliability of lumbar isometric torque in patients with chronic low back pain. *Phys. Ther.* **1992**, *72*, 186–190. [PubMed]

50. Latimer, J.; Maher, C.G.; Refshauge, K.; Colaco, I. The reliability and validity of the Biering-Sorensen test in asymptomatic subjects and subjects reporting current or previous nonspecific low back pain. *Spine* **1999**, *24*, 2085–2090. [CrossRef] [PubMed]

51. Fairbank, J.C.; Pynsent, P.B. The oswestry disability index. *Spine* **2000**, *25*, 2940–2953. [CrossRef] [PubMed]

52. Ogon, M.; Krismer, M.; Söllner, W.; Kantner-Rumplmair, W.; Lampe, A. Chronic low back pain measurement with visual analogue scales in different settings. *Pain* **1996**, *64*, 425–428. [CrossRef]

53. Razali, N.M.; Wah, Y.B. Power comparisons of Shapiro-Wilk, Kolmogorov-Smirnov, Lilliefors and Anderson-Darling tests. *J. Stat. Model. Anal.* **2011**, *2*, 21–33.

54. Hinkle, D.E.; Wiersma, W.; Jurs, S.G. *Applied Statistics for the Behavioural Sciences*, 5th ed.; Houghton Mifflin Harcourt: Boston, MA, USA, 2003.

55. Kamaz, M.; Kiresi, D.; Oguz, H.; Emlik, D.; Levendoglu, F. CT measurement of trunk muscle areas in patients with chronic low back pain. *Diagn. Interv. Radiol.* **2007**, *13*, 144–148. [PubMed]

56. Clark, B.C.; Manini, T.M.; Ploutz-Snyder, L.L. Derecruitment of the lumbar musculature with fatiguing trunk extension exercise. *Spine* **2003**, *28*, 282–287. [CrossRef] [PubMed]

57. Farfan, H. Muscular mechanism of the lumbar spine and the position of power and efficiency. *Orthop. Clin. N. Am.* **1975**, *6*, 135–144.

58. Sparto, P.J.; Parnianpour, M.; Reinsel, T.E.; Simon, S. Spectral and temporal responses of trunk extensor electromyography to an isometric endurance test. *Spine* **1997**, *22*, 418–426. [CrossRef] [PubMed]

59. Arokoski, J.P.; Kankaanpää, M.; Valta, T.; Juvonen, I.; Partanen, J.; Taimela, S.; Lindgren, K.A.; Airaksinen, O. Back and hip extensor muscle function during therapeutic exercises. *Arch. Phys. Med. Rehabil.* **1999**, *80*, 842–850. [CrossRef]

60. Kankaanpää, M.; Laaksonen, D.; Taimela, S.; Kokko, S.M.; Airaksinen, O.; Hänninen, O. Age, sex, and body mass index as determinants of back and hip extensor fatigue in the isometric Sorensen back endurance test. *Arch. Phys. Med. Rehabil.* **1998**, *79*, 1069–1075. [CrossRef]

61. Moffroid, M.; Reid, S.; Henry, S.M.; Haugh, L.D.; Ricamato, A. Some endurance measures in persons with chronic low back pain. *J. Orthop. Sports Phys. Ther.* **1994**, *20*, 81–87. [CrossRef] [PubMed]

62. Pérez, L.T.; Peiró, O.B.; Díes, T.P.; Navas, R.M.; Ballarini, P.G.; Vives, M.B. Fuerza lumbar en jugadores de hockey hierba. *Apunts Med. L'Esport* **2007**, *155*, 138–144. (In Spanish) [CrossRef]

63. Steele, J.; Bruce-Low, S.; Smith, D. A reappraisal of the deconditioning hypothesis in low back pain: Review of evidence from a triumvirate of research methods on specific lumbar extensor deconditioning. *Curr. Med. Res. Opin.* **2014**, *30*, 865–911. [CrossRef] [PubMed]

64. Barker, K.L.; Shamley, D.R.; Jackson, D. Changes in cross-sectional area of multifidus and psoas in patients with unilateral back pain: The relationship to pain and disability. *Spine* **2004**, *29*, 515–524. [CrossRef]

65. Mooney, V.; Gulick, J.; Perlman, M.; Levy, D.; Pozos, R.; Leggett, S.; Resnick, D. Relationships between myoelectric activity, strength and MRI of lumbar extensor muscles in back pain patients and normal subjects. *J. Spinal Disord.* **1997**, *10*, 348–356. [CrossRef] [PubMed]

66. Smidt, G.; Herring, T.; Amundsen, L.; Rogers, M.; Russell, A.; Lehmann, T. Assessment of abdominal and back extensor function. *Spine* **1983**, *8*, 211–219. [CrossRef] [PubMed]

67. Demoulin, C.; Vanderthommen, M.; Duysens, C.; Crielaard, J.M. Spinal muscle evaluation using the Soresen test: A critical appraisal of the literature. *Jt. Bone Spine* **2006**, *73*, 43–50. [CrossRef] [PubMed]

68. Gruther, W.; Wick, F.; Paul, B.; Leitner, C.; Posch, M.; Matzner, M.; Crevenna, R.; Ebenbichler, G. Diagnostic accuracy and reliability of muscle strength and endurance measurements in patients with chronic low back pain. *J. Rehabil. Med.* **2009**, *41*, 613–619. [CrossRef] [PubMed]

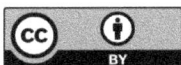

healthcare

MDPI

Review

Revisiting the Corticomotor Plasticity in Low Back Pain: Challenges and Perspectives

Hugo Massé-Alarie [1,*,†] and Cyril Schneider [1,2]

1   Clinical neuroscience and neurostimulation laboratory, Neuroscience Division,
    Research Center of CHU de Québec, Université Laval, Quebec City, QC G1V 4G2, Canada
2   Department of Rehabilitation, Faculty of Medicine, Université Laval, Quebec City, QC G1V 4G2, Canada;
    cyril.schneider@rea.ulaval.ca
*   Correspondence: h.massealarie@uq.edu.au
†   Current address: NHMRC Centre of Clinical Research Excellence in Spinal Pain, Injury & Health,
    School of Health & Rehabilitation Sciences, University of Queensland, Brisbane, QLD 4072, Australia

Academic Editor: Robert J. Gatchel
Received: 24 June 2016; Accepted: 2 September 2016; Published: 8 September 2016

Abstract: Chronic low back pain (CLBP) is a recurrent debilitating condition that costs billions to society. Refractoriness to conventional treatment, lack of improvement, and associated movement disorders could be related to the extensive brain plasticity present in this condition, especially in the sensorimotor cortices. This narrative review on corticomotor plasticity in CLBP will try to delineate how interventions such as training and neuromodulation can improve the condition. The review recommends subgrouping classification in CLBP owing to brain plasticity markers with a view of better understanding and treating this complex condition.

Keywords: chronic low back pain; brain; plasticity; motor cortex; subgrouping; motor control exercise; neuromodulation; transcranial magnetic stimulation; repetitive peripheral magnetic stimulation; spine

1. Lower Back Pain: A Growing Burden for Society

The important burden of lower back pain (LBP) on healthcare systems can be explained by an extremely high annual prevalence worldwide, i.e., up to 36% of the population [1], which still continues to grow [2]. The Global Burden of Disease mega-study classified LBP as the most debilitating condition among more than 300 diseases for both rich and poor countries [3], and the economic burden increased between 1990 and 2010 [4]. Healthcare costs are among the most expensive in many countries, reaching billions for treating and/or alleviating LBP [5]. Although LBP can decrease after acute episodes, its complete resolution is rare [1,6–9], and transition to chronic LBP (CLBP) has been reported in up to 12% of people with LBP [10]. Generic administration of conventional treatments (pharmacology, surgery, and physical therapy) has shown no or minimal improvement of pain and disability [11,12]. The pathophysiological mechanisms of CLBP must therefore be better understood in order to identify which therapy is most efficient per individual and thus overcome refractoriness to treatment. Especially, the plasticity of the central nervous system in response to pain (CNS adaptation to pain) represents one of the most important phenomena that could highlight why people with CLBP are poorly responsive to conventional therapies. For instance, transcranial magnetic stimulation (TMS, see Box 1 and Figure 1, [13]) is a widely used technology that permits the investigation of the excitability, functional organization and integrity of the primary motor cortex (M1) that is largely involved in pain processing and motor control. The present narrative review had three main objectives: (i) to report the current knowledge on the changes of M1 and other cortical motor areas in people with CLBP, (ii) to recommend that the research fields of CLBP subgrouping (to reduce heterogeneity of samples studied) and M1 plasticity (biomarkers of brain adaptation to pain) shall be combined to identify new optimal treatment for each patient, and (iii) to present how current interventions such as motor training and neurostimulation techniques impact pain and M1 plasticity [14–17].

Box 1. Transcranial magnetic stimulation (TMS).

TMS represents a painless and non-invasive technique to investigate the function and integrity of the primary motor cortex (M1) and corticospinal pathway. In 1985, Barker et al. published a game-changer paper in the field of clinical neurophysiology, reporting that the induction of a magnetic field over M1 by a coil (where a transient and large electrical current transits from a capacitor system) could depolarize the corticospinal cells. At a sufficient level of intensity, the stimulus produces a muscle response, referred to as motor evoked potential (MEP) recorded by electromyography (EMG) electrodes [18]. MEP latency and amplitude are considered the primary outcomes studied to probe the corticospinal function. Overall, the integrity of corticospinal, intracortical, interregional and interhemispheric connections can now be assessed by the means of different TMS paradigms that are briefly reviewed below.

Single Pulse TMS

This paradigm provides at least four outcomes used to test the corticospinal excitability and the functional organization of M1.

The motor threshold (MT) reflects the cortico-cortical excitability of M1 axons, their excitatory contact with the corticospinal neurons, and its initial axon segment [19]. It represents the lowest intensity of stimulation producing an MEP in 50% of TMS trials [20].

The MEP amplitude at supra-threshold intensity (e.g., 110%–120% of motor threshold) represents the excitability of the corticospinal tract. This outcome can be influenced by any change of activity at the cortical or spinal level. The use of pharmacological drugs revealed that the MEP amplitude is regulated by the intertwined activation of excitatory (glutamatergic) and inhibitory (GABAergic) interneurons of M1 [19].

The silent period (SP) is tested in preactivated conditions. SP represents the post-MEP shut-off of EMG activity and its duration over 50–75 ms (0–50 ms = motoneurons after-hyperpolarisaton) probes, most likely the activity of $GABA_B$ inhibitory mechanisms of M1 [21].

The M1 mapping is a method to test the functional organization of a muscle representation in M1 and the related corticospinal excitability. TMS at suprathreshold stimulus is applied at multiple sites over M1 and the mean MEP amplitude at each site allows to visually representing the M1 area of the target muscle [22].

Paired-Pulse TMS

Two TMS stimuli are elicited over M1 at a given time-interval through the same coil to probe the excitability of M1 inhibition and facilitation circuits.

The paradigm of short-interval intracortical inhibition (SICI) probes the excitability of $GABA_A$ inhibitory interneurons surrounding M1 corticospinal cells [19]. A subthreshold conditioning TMS elicited 1–5 ms before a suprathreshhold (test) TMS [23] decreases the amplitude of the conditioned MEP (elicited by the paired-pulse TMS) compared to the amplitude of the test MEP (elicited by the test TMS only).

The paradigm of short-interval intracortical inhibiton (SICF) probes the excitability of a chain of glutamatergic excitatory interneurons connecting M1 corticospinal cells. Two near-threshold TMS stimuli are elicited [24] or a suprathreshold TMS is elicited 1.1–1.5,2.3–2.9 and 4.1–4.4 ms before a near-threshold conditioning TMS [25]. The amplitude of the conditioned MEP is higher than the amplitude of the test MEP. More details can be found elsewhere [19].

Box 1. *Cont.*

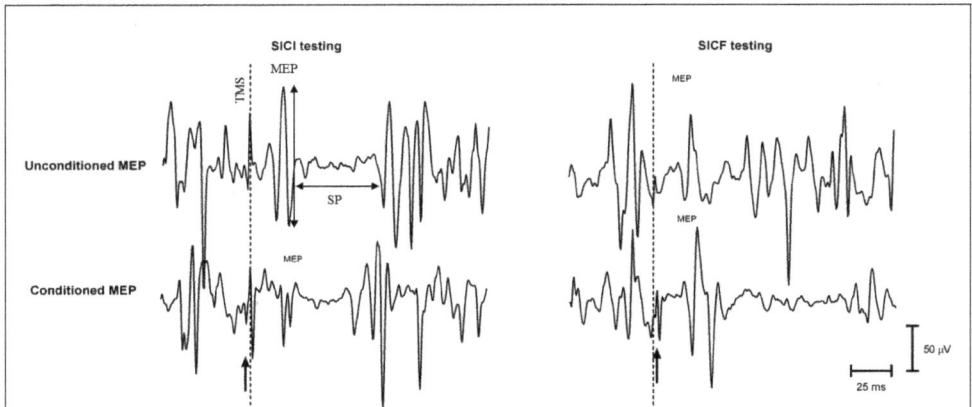

Figure 1. TMS: transcranial magnetic stimulation; SICI: short-interval intracortical inhibition; SICF: short-interval intracortical facilitation; MEP: motor evoked potentials; SP: silent period; small arrow (lower panel): conditioned pulse; dotted line: test pulse.

Double-Coil TMS

This paradigm uses two coils to test the nature (inhibition, facilitation) of other regions' connectivity with M1 areas. The conditioning TMS coil is positioned, for example, over a premotor or cerebellar area and the test TMS coil over the M1 area of a target muscle. Many studies focused on inter-regional connectivity for the control of hand muscles [26]. This functional connectivity has never been studied for the control of postural muscles (e.g., trunk muscles) in pain-free individuals or in people with LBP.

2. Plasticity in M1 and Motor-Related Cerebral Areas

2.1. Can M1 Plasticity Explain Motor Impairment in People with CLBP?

Motor control is an important issue in CLBP given that impairment of spine control (and more precisely of trunk abdominal and paravertebral muscles) is deemed to contribute to pain persistence over time [27]. Disorder of spine control in CLBP is the main rationale behind motor control exercises and manual therapy, i.e., interventions used by healthcare professionals to restore an optimal control and mobility of the spine [28–31]. That is, a large amount of studies have reported that people with CLBP differently plan movement [32,33] and differently react to a postural perturbation [34] as compared to pain-free counterparts. Especially, they present with a later activation of trunk muscle contraction during rapid limb movement, i.e., a delay of the anticipatory postural adjustment (APA) [30], and also less ability to volitionally and specifically contract trunk muscle, abdominal or paravertebral, without recruitment of adjacent muscles [35]. Given the involvement of many cortical structures (M1, supplementary motor area (SMA), cerebellum, basal ganglia, etc.) in APA planning and execution [36], and given that trunk muscles are likely partly controlled by corticospinal pathways [37–40], it was legitimate to anticipate a link between motor impairment and some (plastic) changes in M1 and other cortical motor areas [41]. This assumption was fostered by a first TMS study that unraveled in LBP a direct relation between M1 functional reorganization (changes of M1 maps) and the delay of trunk muscle activation to control for postural perturbation during focal limb movement [42]. Other TMS studies in CLBP then reported a decrease of M1 excitability [43], changes of M1 area localization for the control of trunk muscles [42,44,45] and a lack of intracortical motor inhibition within M1 circuits [46,47], i.e., the loss of an inherent mechanism of motor preparation [48] and planning [49].

M1 integrates information from adjacent sensorimotor areas (e.g., premotor dorsal and ventral cortices, SMA, cerebellum, basal ganglia, primary sensory cortex (S1), etc.) before launching the motor command towards the spinal motoneurons [50]. Thus, beyond the sole M1 plasticity in CLBP, it is important to understand that many structures can be involved in pain and motor disorders in CLBP. In line with this, studies using neuroimaging techniques (electroencephalography (EEG), functional magnetic resonance imaging (fMRI), etc.) did report changes of grey matter density in various brain structures and impairment of connectivity between these structures [17,51–53].

Especially, S1 might be a pivotal stone in the relation between pain and impaired motor control of movement given its substantial role in both the sensory coding of movement and the sensory-discriminative aspects of pain [54,55]. The reciprocal connectivity between S1 and M1 [56] may explain why peripheral inputs (nociceptive, somatosensory) can influence in parallel the plasticity of S1 and of M1 [57,58]. Precisely, in CLBP, S1 grey matter density is different from pain-free couterparts [59], S1 areas receiving information from the trunk are shifted, and connectivity with M1 is impaired [60]. All of these changes likely contribute to the distortion of body image and tactile dysfunction [61,62] but also to the lesser performance in spine motor control by people with CLBP [61]. In addition, abnormal neural processing and connectivity of SMA [52,63] and altered connectivity and change in white matter density of cerebellum [52,64] have been reported in CLBP. These structures are known to be involved in postural control of external perturbations [63] and in APA [36] via transcortical and cerebello-cortical connections with M1 areas. The modifications of cerebellum have been observed in parallel with a slower performance at the sit-to-stand task and an altered proprioceptive integration [52,64].

Interestingly, from a psychological perspective, morphology and connectivity of the brain have also been reported for structures involved in the perception and evaluation of fear, such as amygdala and insula [65,66], these changes having recently been identified as neural correlates of the fear of movement (kinesiophobia) in CLBP [67]. These psychological aspects can alter motor control in CLBP given the correlations found between scores of kinesiophobia or fear-avoidance belief and activation of trunk muscles [47,68–70], trunk stiffness [71], and the increased stress on spine structures (spine loading) [72].

However, the causal relations in CLBP between pain persistence, motor control and brain plasticity have not been appropriately addressed in the literature with most studies being cross-sectional. However, a few longitudinal studies pointed out that the strength of the connection between mesolimbic and prefrontal area could be an important predictor of pain chronicity [51,73]. Future longitudinal studies in CLBP should thus more thoroughly test the role of M1 and other motor control-related cerebral plasticity in the persistence of LBP. For instance, the integrity of M1 functional interregional connectivity with SMA and cerebellum and the remote inhibitory and excitatory influence of these structures on M1 excitability could be assessed by means of TMS paradigms using two coils (see Figure 2). These paradigms might help unravel the mechanisms underlying the impaired corticomotor control of trunk muscles in people with CLBP and the transition from acute to chronic pain.

2.2. Discrepancies between TMS Studies in CLBP: How to Reconcile the Controversial Results?

A closer look at the studies that pointed out differences of M1 maps, excitability and function between people with CLBP and pain-free subjects [42–45,47,74,75] reveals important discrepancies between the results. For instance, Strutton et al. reported that people with CLBP presented with a lower M1 excitability (measured by motor threshold—MT) and a decreased GABA (γ-aminobutyric acid) inhibition (measured by the silent period duration, see Box 1) [34]. However, these findings have not been yet reproduced [46,47,76]. In addition, our recent TMS studies in CLBP did not detect any difference of MT or SP duration but rather a reduction of $GABA_A$ short-interval intracortical inhibition (SICI) in the M1 area of internal oblique/transversus abdominis muscles [47] and superficial multifidus [46]. Our more recent works even conversely showed that a subgroup of people with right-sided CLBP presented with a higher M1 excitability (lower MT) compared to pain-free counterparts (Massé-Alarie et al., *in revisions* [77]). In the same vein, Hodges' group studies in CLBP showed the impaired organization of trunk muscles M1 areas (for erector spinae [44] and transversus abdominis muscles [42]), M1 plasticity being more important in a subgroup of people with severe CLBP (>5 on numerical rating scale) than moderate and mild CLBP [45] and upper CLBP relating to smaller map volumes, thus likely a decrease of corticospinal excitability [45].

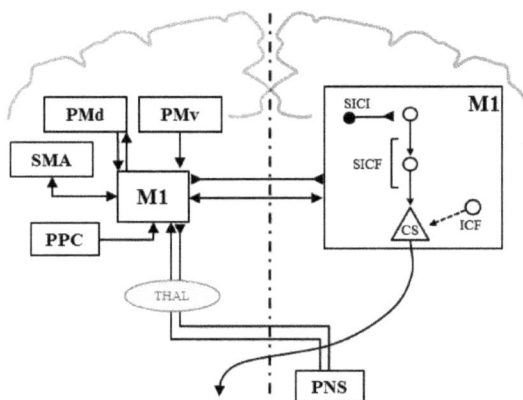

Figure 2. The nature of interregional and interhemispheric connectivity with M1 (left brain) and intracortical connections in M1 (right brain) for hand muscles. M1: primary motor cortex; PMd/v: dorsal/ventral premotor cortex; SMA: supplementary motor area; PPC: parietal posterior cortex; THAL: thalamus; PNS: peripheral nervous system: SICI: short-interval intracortical inhibition; SICF: short-interval intracortical facilitation; arrow: excitatory influence; inverted triangle: inhibitory influence. Adapted with permission from Reis et al. [49].

Therefore, even though most of these studies reported changes in one or more TMS outcomes, no one has been replicated yet. In line with Schabrun et al. (2015) [36] and our unpublished data [77], it is proposed that the heterogeneity of the nonspecific CLBP population tested has hindered specific differences of M1 function in literature, some subgroups presenting with M1 plasticity and others not. The next section briefly reviews some classification known in LBP and how this could be useful in TMS and neuroimaging studies to detect changes specific to subgrouping.

3. Subgrouping of CLBP in Neuroplasticity Studies

The inherent heterogeneity of CLBP population affects the understanding of plastic phenomena and thus hinders the knowledge of the actual clinical impact of novel and conventional therapies. Despite the validation of several models of classification in the last two decades [78,79], only a few neuroimaging or TMS studies have used subgrouping of people with CLBP. A better delineation of the link between characteristics of CLBP (subgrouping) and components of brain plasticity, and a better understanding of the significance of this plasticity in pain processing and disability, are, therefore, current challenges to better managing CLBP and guiding rehabilitation.

3.1. Subgroups Based on the Nature of CLBP

Smart et al. (2010) proposed classifying people with CLBP into three subgroups relative to the nature of pain, i.e., nociceptive pain (peripheral structure injury, 55% of CLBP population), neuropathic (nerve lesion, 22%) or "central sensitization" (characterized by a diffuse disproportioned pain and exaggerated response of CNS to sensory inputs, 23%, see Box 2 [80–82]). Brain plasticity has, however, never been tested as a function of the nature of CLBP. Interestingly, TMS studies on other pain conditions showed that changes of M1 function and excitability were more important in people with neuropathic pain (radiculopathy [83]) or "central sensitization" (fibromyalgia or complex regional pain syndrome (CRPS) [84–86]) than in people suffering from specific nociceptive pain (finger osteoarthrosis) [87]. For instance, people suffering from CRPS, fibromyalgia and people with neuropathic pain were all tested with a reduction of the level of inhibition (measured by SICI, see Box 1) [84–86,88]. Thus, testing nonspecific CLBP, i.e., a heterogeneous population, may explain the inconsistent, even controversial, findings on M1 excitability and function across studies. Future studies should indeed enroll subgroups of patients with CLBP in order to better tackle the link of nociceptive, neuropathic or centrally sensitized CLBP with the plasticity of M1 circuits that likely contributes to pain and motor impairment. If brain plasticity, as tested by TMS of M1, is different between subgroups of CLBP, then TMS will be a useful tool to identify, for example, the sensorimotor mechanisms impaired in people with "central sensitization", and thus will help to manage each person with the most appropriate treatment (e.g., with neuromodulation technique, see Section 4). Some challenges have to be overcome, however, in order to utilize TMS for that purpose. First, normative values of the M1 control of trunk muscles, for example, have to be determined in order to assess any M1 dysfunction in CLBP. This will be challenging given the important variability in TMS outcomes. In addition, TMS markers of M1 function, such as M1 inhibition and facilitation (SICI, ICF), are changed in various pathological conditions (e.g., psychiatric or neurological diseases [89,90], likely because of the multiple cerebral and peripheral influences onto M1 circuits [26] (Figure 2). Thus, and as already mentioned, future longitudinal studies should use double-coil TMS paradigms or TMS tools combined with neuroimaging techniques to unravel the faulty mechanisms (structures, connectivity) in specific subgroups of CLBP.

Box 2. Central sensitization

"Central sensitization" is defined as "an amplification of neural signaling within the CNS that elicits pain hypersensitivity" [91]. The term was introduced to describe changes found at the spinal cord level ([92]), i.e., a post-injury amplification of the peripheral nociceptive signal by CNS hyperexcitability. "Central sensitization" implies that innocuous inputs from the periphery might be perceived as painful if the "pain pathway" is facilitated either at the spinal or cerebral level. By extension, the hyperalgesia documented in subgroups of people with CLBP [93], in addition to the alteration of brain connectivity and morphology (e.g., dorsolateral prefrontal cortex [14–17], periaqueductal grey matter), could be interpreted as "central sensitization" because it likely reflects the alteration of pain modulation by descending pathways that might favour pain persistence.

The term "central sensitization" is used in clinical practice to describe a subgroup of people with specific clinical characteristics [80]. In CLBP, this corresponds to three criteria: (i) disproportionate pain, (ii) neuroanatomically illogical pain pattern, and (iii) hypersensitivity of senses unrelated to the musculoskeletal system [80]. These criteria can delineate people with "central sensitization" patterns from people with nociceptive and neuropathic pain.

Nociceptive pain refers to pain coming from the activation of nociceptors of non-neural tissue in response to noxious chemical, mechanical or thermal stimuli [80,81] (e.g., the activation of the nociceptors in lumbar ligaments, thoraco-lumbar fascia or zygapophyseal joints). Neuropathic pain refers to pain secondary to a disease or a lesion of the somatosensory nervous system [80] (e.g., LBP associated with lumbar radiculopathy).

In recent studies, people with CLBP are classified in three different subgroups owing to the nature of pain: nociceptive, neuropathic or "central sensitization" [80–82,94–98]. Please refer to the clinical guideline proposed by Nijs et al. (2015) for additional details about this classification [80].

3.2. Subgroups Based on the Nociceptive Somatosensory Processing: Mechanical vs. Non-Mechanical CLBP

The O'Sullivan's group published a series of studies lately that insisted further on the need to monitor heterogeneity of samples in CLBP research [93,99,100]. Precisely, nociceptive and somatosensory processing appeared to be significantly different in people with a mechanical CLBP (i.e., pain increased by a specific movement, posture or activity) as compared to people with a non-mechanical CLBP (i.e., spontaneous pain not related to a specific movement, posture or activity). Only people with non-mechanical CLBP presented with a decrease in cold pain threshold as compared to pain-free subjects [99]. In addition, differences of somatosensory nociceptive processing were detected in a large CLBP cohort where three subgroups were differentiated, but only two of them behaved differently than the pain-free subjects [93]. This mechanical vs. non-mechanical CLBP classification could also help to discriminate plastic changes in the brain. Indeed, given tight functional connections between S1 and M1 areas [101], it is likely that subgroups presenting with impaired somatosensory nociceptive processing and S1 plasticity will also undergo plasticity of M1 areas.

3.3. Subgroups Bbased on Movement Disorders

Many classifications based on the type of movement disorders and on movements generating pain in LBP have been validated in the last years [78]. For instance, people with CLBP predominantly triggered during lumbar extension did present with an increase of paravertebral muscles activity in sitting [102] and during forward bending [103] as compared to pain-free participants, whereas people with CLBP triggered primarily during flexion did not. These differences were masked when the two CLBP subgroups were considered as one CLBP group [103]. Such classification should be tested to detect whether M1 plasticity is specific to movement disorders in CLBP. This will help to identify biomarkers of brain function and excitability that will be useful in the management of the clinical outcomes specific to each subgroup. The next section will present how different types of interventions such as motor training and neuromodulation technologies might impact pain and the brain.

4. Interventions Targeting M1 Plasticity

4.1. Learning-Dependent Plasticity in CLBP: How Motor Training Impacts M1?

Studies revealing the extensive brain plasticity in CLBP contribute to a better understanding of the physiopathology mechanisms present in pain pathologies. This ought to guide the development of therapies that will better cope with brain adaptation. In other words, the induction of plasticity that promotes the function and reduces pain (positive plasticity) should become the rule in pain rehabilitation. For instance, training the tactile acuity normalized S1 maps and in parallel improved sensory integration in CLBP [104,105]. The same is true for motor training in CLBP since the practice of isometric activation of the trunk muscles normalized M1 maps [106] and influenced the intracortical inhibition required for planning the action [47] and the corticospinal excitability [107]. In fact, the induction of a positive plasticity (favoring functional recovery) requires a task-oriented practice, i.e., the repetition of a specific task, whose complexity is increased with improvement of performance over the sessions and attention/motivation of the trainee [108]. Usually, the improvement of a motor skill is accompanied by changes of M1 protein synthesis (for instance, tyrosine kinase), synaptogenesis and reorganization of S1 and M1 maps [108]. In addition, a local release from GABAergic inhibition in M1 areas recruited by task-specific training and an increase of corticospinal excitability related to the muscles engaged in the task are usually observed in the minutes following motor learning [109–112]. These plastic mechanisms of motor learning belong to the LTP-like phenomenon that strengthens the synapses efficacy and includes the activation of post-synaptic NMDA (N-methyl-D-aspartate) receptors and the increase of AMPA (α-amino-3-hydroxy-5-methyl-4-isoxazolepropionic acid) receptor density [110,111]. However, the question remains whether these learning-related mechanisms of plasticity do properly work in the presence of pain.

Motor training influences brain plasticity and this contributes to motor learning. For example, motor control exercise (MCE) is used in CLBP physical therapy to restore the proper balance of activation between trunk muscles (usually increasing deep muscle activation and reducing superficial) and, eventually, to transfer this re-learned muscle coordination in functional tasks [30]. In line with this, it was shown that MCE could normalize M1 maps in people with LBP [106], downregulate the exaggerated corticospinal excitability related to superficial paravertebral muscles and upregulate the missing intracortical inhibition needed for motor planning [107]. This influence of MCE on corticomotor plasticity is thought to promote the postural function of the trunk muscles (e.g., APA) in CLBP, thus normalizing the postural control of the spine [106]. However, despite these intertwined cerebral and functional changes, meta-analyses and systematic reviews underlined that exercise therapy and motor control training worked poorly on pain and disability in CLBP [11,113,114], and no therapy seems more effective than another [114]. In addition to subgrouping (focus on specific subgroups of CLBP) and/or patient-oriented training (personalized care), as discussed above, an increasing number of studies investigated whether new techniques of modulation of CNS excitability could further influence pain intensity, brain plasticity, and motor disorders in CLBP beyond the gains already reached by conventional therapies alone.

4.2. Noninvasive and Painless Neuromodulation in CLBP

Noninvasive and painless neuromodulation in CLBP is a new area of research to influence CNS plasticity directly by stimulation of brain circuits (central stimulation: top-down mechanisms involved) or indirectly by stimulation of the lower back (peripheral stimulation: bottom-up). This influence on CNS plasticity ought to help decrease pain, improve sensory integration, and normalize the sensorimotor control of posture and movement (all being intertwined in the management of CLBP). Neuromodulation techniques that are known to increase the corticospinal excitability (e.g., high-frequency repetitive transcranial magnetic stimulation (rTMS), intermittent theta-burst stimulation (iTBS) or anodal transcranial direct current stimulation (tDCS)) share similar mechanisms of neuroplasticity with motor learning, i.e., LTP-like phenomenon with changes of M1 GABAergic inhibition and NMDA-dependent facilitation (for an extensive review on plastic mechanisms following noninvasive neurostimulation, see [19]). Thus, these mechanisms influenced by neuromodulation could prime the brain before beginning a conventional therapy, and this may increase gains beyond those reached by each intervention alone. The next sections present the literature on central and peripheral neurostimulation and their combination with therapy in CLBP to decrease pain and promote the function.

4.3. Central Stimulation

The mechanisms' underlying pain decrease following M1 stimulation could rely on the activation of thalamus by cortico-thalamic projections [115], on the inhibition of spinal cord circuits (likely at the dorsal horn) by corticospinal modulatory projections, and on the activation of μ-opioid receptors [116]. Central neurostimulation has been used in research for chronic pain conditions like CRPS, neuropathic pain and fibromyalgia [116,117]. However, only a few studies used rTMS and tDCS in people with CLBP, and evidence of effectiveness is lacking. For example, one study showed that one session of rTMS over M1 improved CLBP intensity and the cold/heat pain threshold [118], but no study has ever tested longer-lasting after-effects following multiple sessions of rTMS [116]. In addition, two recent randomized double-blind designed studies reported that multiple sessions of tDCS over M1 did not improve CLBP [119,120], and one experimental study did not report immediate impact on pain threshold [121]. Thus, due to scarce data published on that topic, there is no clear evidence that central stimulation impacts pain or disability in CLBP.

4.4. Peripheral Stimulation

Repetitive magnetic stimulation over muscles, nerves or spinal roots (RPMS) is used in exploratory research to improve motor impairments in brain-injured people [122,123]. The rationale for using RPMS is based on the production of contractions that send massive flows of ascending movement-related proprioceptive information to the brain and influence M1 excitability via thalamo-cortical (lemniscal) and spino-cerebellar pathways [124]. It has been shown that this synchronizes the activity of the fronto-parietal networks involved in motor planning [125]. RPMS is a novel, not yet evidence-based, but promising experimental approach in people living with chronic pain and presenting with motor disability. One study showed that a single session of RPMS applied over the lumbar spine in people with CLBP could decrease pain and the after-effects persisted for least four days [126]. In addition, RPMS applied over the deep abdominal muscles not only reduced CLBP and improved postural control

(APA becoming earlier) but also reactivated proper mechanisms of M1 intracortical inhibition [127], which was shown to be missing or lower in people with CLBP [47]. Altogether, these findings emphasize the potential of this novel approach to act on brain plasticity for decreasing pain and improving motor control. Further investigations are warranted to better understand the link between RPMS and brain adaptation and to determine whether RPMS activates the different components of the endogenous pain modulation system.

4.5. Combination of Interventions

The combination of two interventions that influence brain plasticity could impact pain intensity more than each intervention used separately. This was tested in CLBP by tDCS of M1 combined with peripheral electrical stimulation over paravertebral muscles [121]. The authors showed a reduction of pain that was accompanied by M1 reorganization and by improvements of forward bending, pressure pain threshold, and two-point discrimination. However, these after-effects did not last after the end of stimulation [128]. Short-lasting effects could be related to the fact that, in the absence of a lesion, brain circuits can adapt rapidly to any change of activation and could re-balance the synaptic excitability back to physiological ranges of homeostasis: this phenomenon is referred to as metaplasticity [129]. Metaplasticity implies that all increases or decreases of excitability will eventually return to baseline unless repeated over multiple sessions or combined with other therapies, such as motor training that favors similar mechanisms of synaptic plasticity [130]. Changes of M1 excitability following neurostimulation could indeed open a "therapeutic" window during which a task-oriented practice is easier, and, in turn, makes plastic changes more persistent, thus facilitating learning and retention [130], therefore improving motor control and pain over a longer period of time. This was tested by two original studies that combined RPMS with motor control training in people with CLBP in a single session for deep abdominal muscles [127] and over one week for the paravertebral multifides muscles (Massé-Alarie et al., *in revisions* [131]). It was shown that the combination decreased pain more than training alone and that one-week of training induced the normalization of superficial multifides activation in parallel with up regulation of M1 facilitation mechanisms (Massé-Alarie et al., *in revisions* [131]).

Combining neurostimulation with motor training could act at the spinal, brainstem and cerebral levels of the endogenous pain modulation system to re-balance the activity of cerebral networks and areas that do not work properly in CLBP. This may provide gains in pain and disability beyond those already reached by conventional treatments. Therefore, priming the brain with neuromodulation techniques to enlarge the after-effects of conventional therapy [132] represents a research field that ought to be pursued in CLBP.

5. How Can Neuroplasticity Studies Better Reduce Pain and Disability in CLBP?

5.1. Identifying Brain Biomarkers in CLBP

5.1.1. "Central Sensitization" or Non-Mechanical CLBP

Neuroimaging and TMS studies on neuroplasticity in CLBP can help determine biomarkers that will contrast between people with "central sensitization" (see Box 2) and people with nociceptive pain. These biomarkers may inform on unsuspected impaired function, thus easing the adaptation of the therapeutic approach. For example, "central sensitization" and non-mechanical CLBP that share a common definition (pain not related to a specific spine movement, posture and activity) may be less responsive to conventional motor control exercises, stabilization or passive mobility (e.g., manual therapy or stretching) because of somatosensory nociceptive processing impairments [99] and extensive changes of M1 maps and excitability [84–86]. That said, it was shown that the neural connections between medial PFC (mPFC) and NAc were stronger in people with persistent LBP (less than 20% improvement at one year after the first LBP episode) [51]. These people with central sensitization reported higher scores for affective dimension of CLBP (i.e., the pain was considered more threatening), and this is in line with the fact that stronger mPFC-NAc connections could induce negative pain conditioning with aversive or fear-related behavior [51]. In order to influence such behaviors related to pain-related plasticity, novel approaches targeting psychological factors were proposed, such as pain conditioning extinction [133], pain neuroscience education [134], motor control exercise [94] and cognitive-based intervention [135]. These approaches tended to address the psychosocial risk factors associated with CLBP (especially for people with "central sensitization") [6,80] and took into account that the activation of sensory-discriminative brain areas in subacute pain was switched to the activation of emotional areas during the transition to chronic pain [136]. As a matter of fact, people identified with specific biomarkers of brain plasticity (for instance, a stronger connection between mPFC and NAc) could be subclassified according to their clinical characteristics related to plasticity (for instance, a high score for affective dimension of pain at the McGill Pain Questionnaire) and might be better responders to cognitive-related therapy targeting psychosocial factors than to motor control exercises or to neuromodulation of mPFC to downregulate the facilitation of NAc. Future investigations are warranted to test whether such specific approaches dedicated to people with strong mPFC-NAc (or high affective dimension of pain) better impacts pain persistence. It is also questioned whether neuromodulation of DLPFC could be an interesting adjuvant to cognitive-related therapies in people with important psychosocial factors and central sensitization. Indeed, DLPFC is often targeted with rTMS in chronic pain condition [116], it is implied in endogenous pain system [137,138] and its function is altered in CLBP [15]). Of note, given that M1 (opiate system) and DLPFC (non-opiate system) [116] can have a different influence on CLBP, the choice of stimulating one or the other in combination with a therapy may depend on the patient's characteristics and biomarkers of neuroplasticity and underlying mechanisms have still to be studied.

5.1.2. Nociceptive or Mechanical CLBP

People who present nociceptive or mechanical CLBP can be divided into subgroups according to movement disorders and thus be treated accordingly. For instance, it was shown that people with a treatment adapted to their clinical profile (according to the Classification Based Cognitive Functional Therapy (CB-CFT) [139]) had larger decrease of pain than people treated with conventional exercise therapy combined with manual therapy [140]. The same results were reproduced in subacute LBP (CB-CFT was more effective than "general exercise"), but with the exclusion of people with high psychosocial risk factors (fear-avoidance, kinesiophobia, depression) and with poor scores on the Motor Control Abilities Questionnaire (MCAQ, which identifies people unable to learn motor control exercise) [88]. The authors suggested that the improvement in the CB-CFT group in their study was actually due to the exclusion of people with poor MCAQ scores. In fact, a lower capacity of motor learning has already been associated with a polymorphism of brain-derived neurotrophic factor (BDNF) [141]. More precisely, these authors showed that the increase of M1 excitability following training, thus usually favoring learning, was reduced in healthy subjects with BDNF polymorphism compared to healthy subjects without. Thus, people with CLBP could also be classified owing to their BDNF polymorphism (blood sampling) or, more conveniently, owing to their responsiveness to a complex motor learning task (increase or not of M1 excitability as tested by TMS), in order to detect rapidly those who might better respond to motor training. In support, we showed that training at isometric activation of the multifides muscles could influence the corticospinal excitability and the intracortical inhibition of M1 (SICI) related to these muscles [107]. Future studies should test whether such changes after one training session (biomarkers of learning-related plasticity) are correlated with MCAQ scores and thus could be useful predictors to identify people who might be responsive to motor control training (i.e., significant increase of M1 excitability, high MCAQ scores) or not (i.e., small or no change of M1 excitability, low MCAQ scores). In addition, peripheral neurostimulation could be an efficient adjuvant in people with CLBP to influence brain plasticity and improve motor learning and pain beyond gains already reached by more conventional therapies (Massé-Alarie et al. *in revisions* [131]). This work denoted that larger improvements were obtained after one week of training in people who presented with lower M1 excitability at baseline. It will thus be important to understand the clinical significance of a low vs. a high M1 excitability in CLBP at enrollment for better identifying people who will be responsive, for example, to peripheral neurostimulation and motor training.

6. Conclusions: Avoiding *One Size Fits All* Treatments to M1 Plasticity in CLBP

The extensive brain plasticity in chronic pain has been depicted in the last years with a view of tackling the cortical processes under the clinical characteristics and making recommendations of more efficient interventions [135,142]. Thus, a better understanding of the neurophysiology of pain, and, more precisely, the physiopathology of CLBP (in the absence of any peripheral lesion) did revolutionize the way chronic pain was understood and people with CLBP were managed (integration of the psychological, environmental and social factors, in addition to conventional therapies). However, careful examination of neuroplasticity studies revealed that some CLBP subgroups did not present changes of M1 function, maps or excitability [45] and that literature discrepancies hinder the comprehension, e.g., of whether grey matter density is increased or decreased in target structures [15]. In addition, larger plastic changes of M1 areas were detected for people with "central sensitization" and in relation to psychosocial factors, but this subgroup represents 23% of people with CLBP. Thus, the sole cognitive-based intervention may not be efficient for most patients and motor control disorders have to be considered. Avoiding amalgam for treating CLBP is necessary to better understand and treat this condition appropriately in each individual in consideration of M1 plasticity, motor impairments (posture, movement), psychological issues and social characteristics. Thus, a thorough evaluation of the initial condition of the patients will help personalize treatment owing to clinical characteristics, although it remains challenging to get a clear difference between subgroups (since all pain is in the brain, nociceptive pain likely embedded a certain component of "central sensitization" [80]). Future studies in CLBP will have to consider the recruitment of subgroups of patients in order to identify specific biomarkers of brain plasticity and motor disorders, thus markers of responsiveness to approaches based on individuals' clinical profile, including peripheral or central neurostimulation as adjuvants to more conventional treatments. The development of such new guidelines, along with the one published in Nijs et al. [80], and integrating the diversity of people with CLBP in relation to clinical features, biomarkers of neuroplasticity, and motor disorders is warranted for the researchers to better test new interventions and for the clinicians to better cope with this condition and decrease the societal burden of CLBP.

Acknowledgments: The authors acknowledge financial support from the Canadian Foundation for Innovation (Cyril Schneider's laboratory infrastructure), the Fonds de Recherche du Québec-Santé and the Canadian Institutes for Health Research (Hugo Massé-Alarie's studentships).

Author Contributions: Hugo Massé-Alarie wrote the draft of the manuscript and Cyril Schneider and Hugo Massé-Alarie reviewed the version submitted together.

Conflicts of Interest: The authors declare no conflict of interest.

References

1. Hoy, D.; Brooks, P.; Blyth, F.; Buchbinder, R. The epidemiology of low back pain. *Best Pract. Res. Clin. Rheumatol.* **2010**, *24*, 769–781. [CrossRef] [PubMed]
2. Freburger, J.K.; Holmes, G.M.; Agans, R.P.; Jackman, A.M.; Darter, J.D.; Wallace, A.S.; Castel, L.D.; Kalsbeek, W.D.; Carey, T.S. The rising prevalence of chronic low back pain. *Arch. Intern. Med.* **2009**, *169*, 251–258. [CrossRef] [PubMed]
3. Buchbinder, R.; Blyth, F.M.; March, L.M.; Brooks, P.; Woolf, A.D.; Hoy, D.G. Placing the global burden of low back pain in context. *Best Pract. Res. Clin. Rheumatol.* **2013**, *27*, 575–589. [CrossRef] [PubMed]
4. Hoy, D.; March, L.; Brooks, P.; Blyth, F.; Woolf, A.; Bain, C.; Williams, G.; Smith, E.; Vos, T.; Barendregt, J.; et al. The global burden of low back pain: Estimates from the global burden of disease 2010 study. *Ann. Rheum. Dis.* **2014**, *73*, 968–974. [CrossRef] [PubMed]

5. Dagenais, S.; Caro, J.; Haldeman, S. A systematic review of low back pain cost of illness studies in the united states and internationally. *Spine J.* **2008**, *8*, 8–20. [CrossRef] [PubMed]
6. Dunn, K.M.; Hestbaek, L.; Cassidy, J.D. Low back pain across the life course. *Best Pract. Res. Clin. Rheumatol.* **2013**, *27*, 591–600. [CrossRef] [PubMed]
7. Lemeunier, N.; Leboeuf-Yde, C.; Gagey, O. The natural course of low back pain: A systematic critical literature review. *Chiropr. Man. therap.* **2012**. [CrossRef] [PubMed]
8. Macedo, L.G.; Maher, C.G.; Latimer, J.; McAuley, J.H.; Hodges, P.W.; Rogers, W.T. Nature and determinants of the course of chronic low back pain over a 12-month period: A cluster analysis. *Phys. Ther.* **2014**, *94*, 210–221. [CrossRef] [PubMed]
9. Vasseljen, O.; Woodhouse, A.; Bjorngaard, J.H.; Leivseth, L. Natural course of acute neck and low back pain in the general population: The hunt study. *Pain* **2013**, *154*, 1237–1244. [CrossRef] [PubMed]
10. Krismer, M.; van Tulder, M. Strategies for prevention and management of musculoskeletal conditions. Low back pain (non-specific). *Best Pract. Res. Clin. Rheumatol.* **2007**, *21*, 77–91. [CrossRef] [PubMed]
11. Hayden, J.; van Tulder, M.W.; Malmivaara, A.; Koes, B.W. Exercise therapy for treatment of non-specific low back pain. *Cochrane Database Syst. Rev.* **2005**. [CrossRef]
12. Rubinstein, S.M.; van Middelkoop, M.; Assendelft, W.J.; de Boer, M.R.; van Tulder, M.W. Spinal manipulative therapy for chronic low-back pain. *Cochrane Database Syst. Rev.* **2011**. [CrossRef]
13. Kobayashi, M.; Pascual-Leone, A. Transcranial magnetic stimulation in neurology. *Lancet Neurol.* **2003**, *2*, 145–156. [CrossRef]
14. Apkarian, A.V.; Sosa, Y.; Sonty, S.; Levy, R.M.; Harden, R.N.; Parrish, T.B.; Gitelman, D.R. Chronic back pain is associated with decreased prefrontal and thalamic gray matter density. *J. Neurosci.* **2004**, *24*, 10410–10415. [CrossRef] [PubMed]
15. Kregel, J.; Meeus, M.; Malfliet, A.; Dolphens, M.; Danneels, L.; Nijs, J.; Cagnie, B. Structural and functional brain abnormalities in chronic low back pain: A systematic review. *Semin. Arthritis. Rheum.* **2015**, *45*, 229–237. [CrossRef] [PubMed]
16. Schmidt-Wilcke, T.; Leinisch, E.; Ganssbauer, S.; Draganski, B.; Bogdahn, U.; Altmeppen, J.; May, A. Affective components and intensity of pain correlate with structural differences in gray matter in chronic back pain patients. *Pain* **2006**, *125*, 89–97. [CrossRef] [PubMed]
17. Ceko, M.; Shir, Y.; Ouellet, J.A.; Ware, M.A.; Stone, L.S.; Seminowicz, D.A. Partial recovery of abnormal insula and dorsolateral prefrontal connectivity to cognitive networks in chronic low back pain after treatment. *Hum. Brain Mapp.* **2015**, *36*, 2075–2092. [CrossRef] [PubMed]
18. Hodges, P.W.; Ferreira, H.F.; Ferreira, M.L. Lumbar spine: Treatment of instability and disorders of movement control. In *Pathology and Intervention in Musculoskeletal Rehabilitation*; Magee, D.J., Zachazewski, J.E., Quillen, W.S., Eds.; Saunders Elsevier: St. Louis, MO, USA, 2009; pp. 389–425.
19. Lee, D.G. *The Pelvic Girdle: An Integration of Clinical Expertise and Research*; Elsevier Health Sciences: New York, NY, USA, 2011.
20. McGill, S.M. *Low Back Disorders: Evidence-Based Prevention and Rehabilitation*, 2nd ed.; Human Kinetics: Champaign, IL, USA, 2007; p. 328.
21. Richardson, C.A.; Paul, H.; Hides, J.A. *Therapeutic Exercise for Lumbopelvic Stabilization: A Motor Control Approach for the Treatment and Prevention of Low Back Pain*, 2nd ed.; Churchill Livingston: London, UK, 2004; p. 271.
22. Sahrmann, S. *Diagnosis and Treatment of Movement Impairment Syndromes*, 1st ed.; Mosby: St. Louis, MO, USA, 2002; p. 380.
23. Hodges, P.W.; Richardson, C.A. Inefficient muscular stabilization of the lumbar spine associated with low back pain: A motor control evaluation of transversus abdominis. *Spine* **1996**, *21*, 2640–2650. [CrossRef] [PubMed]
24. Smith, J.A.; Kulig, K. Altered multifidus recruitment during walking in young asymptomatic individuals with a history of low back pain. *J. Orthop. Sports Phys. Ther.* **2016**, *46*, 365–374. [CrossRef] [PubMed]
25. Radebold, A.; Cholewicki, J.; Polzhofer, G.K.; Greene, H.S. Impaired postural control of the lumbar spine is associated with delayed muscle response times in patients with chronic idiopathic low back pain. *Spine* **2001**, *26*, 724–730. [CrossRef] [PubMed]

26. Hides, J.; Stanton, W.; Mendis, M.D.; Sexton, M. The relationship of transversus abdominis and lumbar multifidus clinical muscle tests in patients with chronic low back pain. *Man. Ther.* **2011**, *16*, 573–577. [CrossRef] [PubMed]

27. Massion, J. Movement, posture and equilibrium: Interaction and coordination. *Prog. Neurobiol.* **1992**, *38*, 35–56. [CrossRef]

28. Ferbert, A.; Caramia, D.; Priori, A.; Bertolasi, L.; Rothwell, J.C. Cortical projection to erector spinae muscles in man as assessed by focal transcranial magnetic stimulation. *Electroencephalogr. Clin. Neurophysiol.* **1992**, *85*, 382–387. [CrossRef]

29. Strutton, P.H.; Beith, I.D.; Theodorou, S.; Catley, M.; McGregor, A.H.; Davey, N.J. Corticospinal activation of internal oblique muscles has a strong ipsilateral component and can be lateralised in man. *Exp. Brain Res.* **2004**, *158*, 474–479. [CrossRef] [PubMed]

30. Tsao, H.; Danneels, L.; Hodges, P.W. Individual fascicles of the paraspinal muscles are activated by discrete cortical networks in humans. *Clin. Neurophysiol.* **2011**, *122*, 1580–1587. [CrossRef] [PubMed]

31. Tsao, H.; Galea, M.P.; Hodges, P.W. Concurrent excitation of the opposite motor cortex during transcranial magnetic stimulation to activate the abdominal muscles. *J. Neurosci. Methods* **2008**, *171*, 132–139. [CrossRef] [PubMed]

32. Hodges, P.W. Changes in motor planning of feedforward postural responses of the trunk muscles in low back pain. *Exp. Brain Res.* **2001**, *141*, 261–266. [CrossRef] [PubMed]

33. Tsao, H.; Galea, M.P.; Hodges, P.W. Reorganization of the motor cortex is associated with postural control deficits in recurrent low back pain. *Brain* **2008**, *131*, 2161–2171. [CrossRef] [PubMed]

34. Strutton, P.H.; Theodorou, S.; Catley, M.; McGregor, A.H.; Davey, N.J. Corticospinal excitability in patients with chronic low back pain. *J. Spinal Disord. Tech.* **2005**, *18*, 420–424. [CrossRef] [PubMed]

35. Tsao, H.; Danneels, L.A.; Hodges, P.W. Issls prize winner: Smudging the motor brain in young adults with recurrent low back pain. *Spine* **2011**, *36*, 1721–1727. [CrossRef] [PubMed]

36. Schabrun, S.M.; Elgueta-Cancino, E.L.; Hodges, P.W. Smudging of the motor cortex is related to the severity of low back pain. *Spine* **2015**. [CrossRef] [PubMed]

37. Massé-Alarie, H.; Beaulieu, L.D.; Preuss, R.; Schneider, C. Corticomotor control of lumbar multifidus muscles is impaired in chronic low back pain: Concurrent evidence from ultrasound imaging and double-pulse transcranial magnetic stimulation. *Exp. Brain Res.* **2016**, *234*, 1033–1045. [CrossRef] [PubMed]

38. Massé-Alarie, H.; Flamand, V.H.; Moffet, H.; Schneider, C. Corticomotor control of deep abdominal muscles in chronic low back pain and anticipatory postural adjustments. *Exp. Brain Res.* **2012**, *218*, 99–109. [CrossRef] [PubMed]

39. Duque, J.; Ivry, R.B. Role of corticospinal suppression during motor preparation. *Cereb. Cortex.* **2009**, *19*, 2013–2024. [CrossRef] [PubMed]

40. Stinear, C.M.; Byblow, W.D. Role of intracortical inhibition in selective hand muscle activation. *J. Neurophysiol.* **2003**, *89*, 2014–2020. [CrossRef] [PubMed]

41. Barker, A.; Jalinous, R.; Freeston, I. Non-invasive magnetic stimulation of human motor cortex. *Lancet* **1985**, *1*, 1106–1107. [CrossRef]

42. Ziemann, U.; Reis, J.; Schwenkreis, P.; Rosanova, M.; Strafella, A.; Badawy, R.; Muller-Dahlhaus, F. TMS and drugs revisited 2014. *Clin. Neurophysiol.* **2014**, *126*, 1847–1868. [CrossRef] [PubMed]

43. Rossini, P.M.; Burke, D.; Chen, R.; Cohen, L.G.; Daskalakis, Z.; Di Iorio, R.; Di Lazzaro, V.; Ferreri, F.; Fitzgerald, P.B.; George, M.S.; et al. Non-invasive electrical and magnetic stimulation of the brain, spinal cord, roots and peripheral nerves: Basic principles and procedures for routine clinical and research application. An updated report from an i.F.C.N. Committee. *Clin. Neurophysiol.* **2015**, *126*, 1071–1107. [CrossRef] [PubMed]

44. Inghilleri, M.; Berardelli, A.; Cruccu, G.; Manfredi, M. Silent period evoked by transcranial stimulation of the human cortex and cervicomedullary junction. *J. Physiol.* **1993**, *466*, 521–534. [PubMed]

45. Wassermann, E.M.; McShane, L.M.; Hallett, M.; Cohen, L.G. Noninvasive mapping of muscle representations in human motor cortex. *Electroencephalogr. Clin. Neurophysiol.* **1992**, *85*, 1–8. [CrossRef]

46. Kujirai, T.; Caramia, M.D.; Rothwell, J.C.; Day, B.L.; Thompson, P.D.; Ferbert, A.; Wroe, S.; Asselman, P.; Marsden, C.D. Corticocortical inhibition in human motor cortex. *J. Physiol.* **1993**, *471*, 501–519. [CrossRef] [PubMed]

47. Tokimura, H.; Ridding, M.C.; Tokimura, Y.; Amassian, V.E.; Rothwell, J.C. Short latency facilitation between pairs of threshold magnetic stimuli applied to human motor cortex. *Electroencephalogr. Clin. Neurophysiol.* **1996**, *101*, 263–272. [CrossRef]

48. Ziemann, U.; Tergau, F.; Wassermann, E.M.; Wischer, S.; Hildebrandt, J.; Paulus, W. Demonstration of facilitatory I wave interaction in the human motor cortex by paired transcranial magnetic stimulation. *J. Physiol.* **1998**, *511*, 181–190. [CrossRef] [PubMed]

49. Reis, J.; Swayne, O.B.; Vandermeeren, Y.; Camus, M.; Dimyan, M.A.; Harris-Love, M.; Perez, M.A.; Ragert, P.; Rothwell, J.C.; Cohen, L.G. Contribution of transcranial magnetic stimulation to the understanding of cortical mechanisms involved in motor control. *J. Physiol.* **2008**, *586*, 325–351. [CrossRef] [PubMed]

50. Lemon, R.N. Descending pathways in motor control. *Annu. Rev. Neurosci.* **2008**, *31*, 195–218. [CrossRef] [PubMed]

51. Baliki, M.N.; Petre, B.; Torbey, S.; Herrmann, K.M.; Huang, L.; Schnitzer, T.J.; Fields, H.L.; Apkarian, A.V. Corticostriatal functional connectivity predicts transition to chronic back pain. *Nat. Neurosci.* **2012**, *15*, 1117–1119. [CrossRef] [PubMed]

52. Pijnenburg, M.; Brumagne, S.; Caeyenberghs, K.; Janssens, L.; Goossens, N.; Marinazzo, D.; Swinnen, S.P.; Claeys, K.; Siugzdaite, R. Resting-state functional connectivity of the sensorimotor network in individuals with nonspecific low back pain and the association with the sit-to-stand-to-sit task. *Brain Connect.* **2015**, *5*, 303–311. [CrossRef] [PubMed]

53. Seminowicz, D.A.; Wideman, T.H.; Naso, L.; Hatami-Khoroushahi, Z.; Fallatah, S.; Ware, M.A.; Jarzem, P.; Bushnell, M.C.; Shir, Y.; Ouellet, J.A.; et al. Effective treatment of chronic low back pain in humans reverses abnormal brain anatomy and function. *J. Neurosci.* **2011**, *31*, 7540–7550. [CrossRef] [PubMed]

54. Bingel, U.; Lorenz, J.; Glauche, V.; Knab, R.; Gläscher, J.; Weiller, C.; Büchel, C. Somatotopic organization of human somatosensory cortices for pain: A single trial fmri study. *Neuroimage* **2004**, *23*, 224–232. [CrossRef] [PubMed]

55. Mazzola, L.; Isnard, J.; Mauguiere, F. Somatosensory and pain responses to stimulation of the second somatosensory area (SII) in humans. A comparison with si and insular responses. *Cerebral. Cortex.* **2006**, *16*, 960–968. [CrossRef] [PubMed]

56. Karhu, J.; Tesche, C.D. Simultaneous early processing of sensory input in human primary (SI) and secondary (SII) somatosensory cortices. *J. Neurophysiol.* **1999**, *81*, 2017–2025. [PubMed]

57. Schabrun, S.M.; Jones, E.; Kloster, J.; Hodges, P.W. Temporal association between changes in primary sensory cortex and corticomotor output during muscle pain. *Neuroscience* **2013**, *235*, 159–164. [CrossRef] [PubMed]

58. Schabrun, S.M.; Ridding, M.C.; Galea, M.P.; Hodges, P.W.; Chipchase, L.S. Primary sensory and motor cortex excitability are co-modulated in response to peripheral electrical nerve stimulation. *PLoS ONE* **2012**, *7*, e51298. [CrossRef] [PubMed]

59. Kong, J.; Spaeth, R.B.; Wey, H.Y.; Cheetham, A.; Cook, A.H.; Jensen, K.; Tan, Y.; Liu, H.; Wang, D.; Loggia, M.L.; et al. S1 is associated with chronic low back pain: A functional and structural mri study. *Mol. Pain* **2013**. [CrossRef] [PubMed]

60. Flor, H.; Braun, C.; Elbert, T.; Birbaumer, N. Extensive reorganization of primary somatosensory cortex in chronic back pain patients. *Neurosci. Lett.* **1997**, *224*, 5–8. [CrossRef]

61. Luomajoki, H.; Moseley, G.L. Tactile acuity and lumbopelvic motor control in patients with back pain and healthy controls. *Br. J. Sports Med.* **2011**, *45*, 437–440. [CrossRef] [PubMed]

62. Moseley, G.L. I can't find it! Distorted body image and tactile dysfunction in patients with chronic back pain. *Pain* **2008**, *140*, 239–243. [CrossRef] [PubMed]

63. Jacobs, J.V.; Henry, S.M.; Nagle, K.J. People with chronic low back pain exhibit decreased variability in the timing of their anticipatory postural adjustments. *Behav. Neurosci.* **2009**, *123*, 455–458. [CrossRef] [PubMed]

64. Pijnenburg, M.; Caeyenberghs, K.; Janssens, L.; Goossens, N.; Swinnen, S.P.; Sunaert, S.; Brumagne, S. Microstructural integrity of the superior cerebellar peduncle is associated with an impaired proprioceptive weighting capacity in individuals with non-specific low back pain. *PLoS ONE* **2014**, *9*, e100666. [CrossRef] [PubMed]

65. Baliki, M.N.; Schnitzer, T.J.; Bauer, W.R.; Apkarian, A.V. Brain morphological signatures for chronic pain. *PLoS ONE* **2011**, *6*, e26010. [CrossRef] [PubMed]

66. Mao, C.P.; Yang, H.J. Smaller amygdala volumes in patients with chronic low back pain compared with healthy control individuals. *J. Pain* **2015**, *16*, 1366–1376. [CrossRef] [PubMed]

67. Meier, M.L.; Stampfli, P.; Vrana, A.; Humphreys, B.K.; Seifritz, E.; Hotz-Boendermaker, S. Neural correlates of fear of movement in patients with chronic low back pain vs. Pain-free individuals. *Front. Hum. Neurosci.* **2016**. [CrossRef] [PubMed]

68. Alschuler, K.N.; Neblett, R.; Wiggert, E.; Haig, A.J.; Geisser, M.E. Flexion-relaxation and clinical features associated with chronic low back pain: A comparison of different methods of quantifying flexion-relaxation. *Clin. J. Pain* **2009**, *25*, 760–766. [CrossRef] [PubMed]

69. Geisser, M.E.; Haig, A.J.; Wallbom, A.S.; Wiggert, E.A. Pain-related fear, lumbar flexion, and dynamic emg among persons with chronic musculoskeletal low back pain. *Clin. J. Pain* **2004**, *20*, 61–69. [CrossRef] [PubMed]

70. Watson, P.J.; Booker, C.K.; Main, C.J. Evidence for the role of psychological factors in abnormal paraspinal activity in patients with chronic low back pain. *J. Musculoskelatal Pain* **1997**, *5*, 41–56. [CrossRef]

71. Karayannis, N.V.; Smeets, R.J.; van den Hoorn, W.; Hodges, P.W. Fear of movement is related to trunk stiffness in low back pain. *PLoS ONE* **2013**, *8*, e67779. [CrossRef] [PubMed]

72. Marras, W.S.; Davis, K.G.; Heaney, C.A.; Maronitis, A.B.; Allread, W.G. The influence of psychosocial stress, gender, and personality on mechanical loading of the lumbar spine. *Spine* **2000**, *25*, 3045–3054. [CrossRef] [PubMed]

73. Mansour, A.R.; Baliki, M.N.; Huang, L.; Torbey, S.; Herrmann, K.M.; Schnitzer, T.J.; Apkarian, A.V. Brain white matter structural properties predict transition to chronic pain. *Pain* **2013**, *154*, 2160–2168. [CrossRef] [PubMed]

74. Chiou, S.Y.; Shih, Y.F.; Chou, L.W.; McGregor, A.H.; Strutton, P.H. Impaired neural drive in patients with low back pain. *Eur. J. Pain* **2014**, *18*, 794–802. [CrossRef] [PubMed]

75. Massé-Alarie, H.; Beaulieu, L.D.; Preuss, R.; Schneider, C. Impairment of Corticomotor Control of Lumbar Multifidus in Chronic Low Back Pain. In Proceedings of the 35th Annual Scientific Meeting of the Canadian Pain Society, Quebec City, QC, Canada, 20–23 May 2014.

76. Chiou, S.Y.; Jeevathol, A.; Odedra, A.; Strutton, P.H. Voluntary activation of trunk extensors appears normal in young adults who have recovered from low back pain. *Eur. J. Pain* **2015**, *19*, 1506–1515. [CrossRef] [PubMed]

77. Massé-Alarie, H.; Beaulieu, L.D.; Preuss, R.; Schneider, C. The side of chronic low back pain matters: Evidence from the primary motor cortex excitability and the postural adjustments of multifidi muscles, experimental brain research. *Exp. Brain Res.* Unpublished work, **2016**.

78. Karayannis, N.V.; Jull, G.A.; Hodges, P.W. Physiotherapy movement based classification approaches to low back pain: Comparison of subgroups through review and developer/expert survey. *BMC Musculoskelet. Disord.* **2012**. [CrossRef] [PubMed]

79. Foster, N.E.; Hill, J.C.; O'Sullivan, P.; Hancock, M. Stratified models of care. *Best Pract. Res. Clin. Rheumatol.* **2013**, *27*, 649–661. [CrossRef] [PubMed]

80. Nijs, J.; Apeldoorn, A.; Hallegraeff, H.; Clark, J.; Smeets, R.; Malfliet, A.; Girbes, E.L.; De Kooning, M.; Ickmans, K. Low back pain: Guidelines for the clinical classification of predominant neuropathic, nociceptive, or central sensitization pain. *Pain Physician.* **2015**, *18*, E333–E346. [PubMed]

81. Smart, K.M.; Blake, C.; Staines, A.; Doody, C. Clinical indicators of "nociceptive", "peripheral neuropathic" and "central" mechanisms of musculoskeletal pain. A Delphi survey of expert clinicians. *Man. Ther.* **2010**, *15*, 80–87. [CrossRef] [PubMed]

82. Smart, K.M.; Blake, C.; Staines, A.; Doody, C. The discriminative validity of "nociceptive", "peripheral neuropathic", and "central sensitization" as mechanisms-based classifications of musculoskeletal pain. *Clin. J. Pain* **2011**, *27*, 655–663. [CrossRef] [PubMed]

83. Strutton, P.H.; Catley, M.; McGregor, A.H.; Davey, N.J. Corticospinal excitability in patients with unilateral sciatica. *Neurosci. Lett.* **2003**, *353*, 33–36. [CrossRef] [PubMed]

84. Eisenberg, E.; Chistyakov, A.V.; Yudashkin, M.; Kaplan, B.; Hafner, H.; Feinsod, M. Evidence for cortical hyperexcitability of the affected limb representation area in crps: A psychophysical and transcranial magnetic stimulation study. *Pain* **2005**, *113*, 99–105. [CrossRef] [PubMed]

85. Schwenkreis, P.; Janssen, F.; Rommel, O.; Pleger, B.; Volker, B.; Hosbach, I.; Dertwinkel, R.; Maier, C.; Tegenthoff, M. Bilateral motor cortex disinhibition in complex regional pain syndrome (crps) type I of the hand. *Neurology* **2003**, *61*, 515–519. [CrossRef] [PubMed]

86. Mhalla, A.; de Andrade, D.C.; Baudic, S.; Perrot, S.; Bouhassira, D. Alteration of cortical excitability in patients with fibromyalgia. *Pain* **2010**, *149*, 495–500. [CrossRef] [PubMed]

87. Schwenkreis, P.; Scherens, A.; Ronnau, A.K.; Hoffken, O.; Tegenthoff, M.; Maier, C. Cortical disinhibition occurs in chronic neuropathic, but not in chronic nociceptive pain. *BMC Neurosci* **2010**. [CrossRef] [PubMed]

88. Lehtola, V.; Luomajoki, H.; Leinonen, V.; Gibbons, S.; Airaksinen, O. Sub-classification based specific movement control exercises are superior to general exercise in sub-acute low back pain when both are combined with manual therapy: A randomized controlled trial. *BMC Musculoskelet. Disord.* **2016**. [CrossRef] [PubMed]

89. Bareš, M.; Kaňovský, P.; Klajblová, H.; Rektor, I. Intracortical inhibition and facilitation are impaired in patients with early parkinson's disease: A paired tms study. *Eur. J. Neurol.* **2003**, *10*, 385–389. [CrossRef] [PubMed]

90. Di Lazzaro, V.; Oliviero, A.; Pilato, F.; Saturno, E.; Dileone, M.; Marra, C.; Daniele, A.; Ghirlanda, S.; Gainotti, G.; Tonali, P. Motor cortex hyperexcitability to transcranial magnetic stimulation in alzheimer's disease. *J. Neurol. Neurosurg. Psychiatry* **2004**, *75*, 555–559. [CrossRef] [PubMed]

91. Woolf, C.J. Central sensitization: Implications for the diagnosis and treatment of pain. *Pain* **2011**, *152*, S2–S15. [CrossRef] [PubMed]

92. Woolf, C.J. Evidence for a central component of post-injury pain hypersensitivity. *Nature* **1983**, *306*, 686–688. [CrossRef] [PubMed]

93. Rabey, M.; Slater, H.; O'Sullivan, P.; Beales, D.; Smith, A. Somatosensory nociceptive characteristics differentiate subgroups in people with chronic low back pain: A cluster analysis. *Pain* **2015**, *156*, 1874–1884. [CrossRef] [PubMed]

94. Nijs, J.; Meeus, M.; Cagnie, B.; Roussel, N.A.; Dolphens, M.; Van Oosterwijck, J.; Danneels, L. A modern neuroscience approach to chronic spinal pain: Combining pain neuroscience education with cognition-targeted motor control training. *Phys. Ther.* **2014**, *94*, 730–738. [CrossRef] [PubMed]

95. Smart, K.M.; Blake, C.; Staines, A.; Doody, C. Self-reported pain severity, quality of life, disability, anxiety and depression in patients classified with "nociceptive", "peripheral neuropathic" and "central sensitisation" pain. The discriminant validity of mechanisms-based classifications of low back (+/−leg) pain. *Man. Ther.* **2012**, *17*, 119–125. [PubMed]

96. Smart, K.M.; Blake, C.; Staines, A.; Thacker, M.; Doody, C. Mechanisms-based classifications of musculoskeletal pain: Part 1 of 3: Symptoms and signs of central sensitisation in patients with low back (+/−leg) pain. *Man. Ther.* **2012**, *17*, 336–344. [CrossRef] [PubMed]

97. Smart, K.M.; Blake, C.; Staines, A.; Thacker, M.; Doody, C. Mechanisms-based classifications of musculoskeletal pain: Part 2 of 3: Symptoms and signs of peripheral neuropathic pain in patients with low back (+/−leg) pain. *Man. Ther.* **2012**, *17*, 345–351. [CrossRef] [PubMed]

98. Smart, K.M.; Blake, C.; Staines, A.; Thacker, M.; Doody, C. Mechanisms-based classifications of musculoskeletal pain: Part 3 of 3: Symptoms and signs of nociceptive pain in patients with low back (+/−leg) pain. *Man. Ther.* **2012**, *17*, 352–357. [CrossRef] [PubMed]

99. O'Sullivan, P.; Waller, R.; Wright, A.; Gardner, J.; Johnston, R.; Payne, C.; Shannon, A.; Ware, B.; Smith, A. Sensory characteristics of chronic non-specific low back pain: A subgroup investigation. *Man. Ther.* **2014**, *19*, 311–318. [CrossRef] [PubMed]

100. Rabey, M.; Beales, D.; Slater, H.; O'Sullivan, P. Multidimensional pain profiles in four cases of chronic non-specific axial low back pain: An examination of the limitations of contemporary classification systems. *Man. Ther.* **2015**, *20*, 138–147. [CrossRef] [PubMed]

101. Erpelding, N.; Moayedi, M.; Davis, K.D. Cortical thickness correlates of pain and temperature sensitivity. *Pain* **2012**, *153*, 1602–1609. [CrossRef] [PubMed]

102. Dankaerts, W.; O'Sullivan, P.; Burnett, A.; Straker, L. Altered patterns of superficial trunk muscle activation during sitting in nonspecific chronic low back pain patients: Importance of subclassification. *Spine* **2006**, *31*, 2017–2023. [CrossRef] [PubMed]

103. Dankaerts, W.; O'Sullivan, P.; Burnett, A.; Straker, L.; Davey, P.; Gupta, R. Discriminating healthy controls and two clinical subgroups of nonspecific chronic low back pain patients using trunk muscle activation and lumbosacral kinematics of postures and movements: A statistical classification model. *Spine* **2009**, *34*, 1610–1618. [CrossRef] [PubMed]

104. Gutknecht, M.; Mannig, A.; Waldvogel, A.; Wand, B.M.; Luomajoki, H. The effect of motor control and tactile acuity training on patients with non-specific low back pain and movement control impairment. *J. Bodyw. Mov. Ther.* **2015**, *19*, 722–731. [CrossRef] [PubMed]

105. Morone, G.; Iosa, M.; Paolucci, T.; Fusco, A.; Alcuri, R.; Spadini, E.; Saraceni, V.M.; Paolucci, S. Efficacy of perceptive rehabilitation in the treatment of chronic nonspecific low back pain through a new tool: A randomized clinical study. *Clin. Rehabil.* **2012**, *26*, 339–350. [CrossRef] [PubMed]

106. Tsao, H.; Galea, M.P.; Hodges, P.W. Driving plasticity in the motor cortex in recurrent low back pain. *Eur. J. Pain.* **2010**, *14*, 832–839. [CrossRef] [PubMed]

107. Massé-Alarie, H.; Beaulieu, L.D.; Preuss, R.; Schneider, C. Influence of paravertebral muscles training on brain plasticity and postural control in chronic low back pain. *Scand. J. Pain.* **2016**, *12*, 74–83. [CrossRef]

108. Adkins, D.L.; Boychuk, J.; Remple, M.S.; Kleim, J.A. Motor training induces experience-specific patterns of plasticity across motor cortex and spinal cord. *J. Appl. Physiol.* **2006**, *101*, 1776–1782. [CrossRef] [PubMed]

109. Liepert, J.; Classen, J.; Cohen, L.G.; Hallett, M. Task-dependent changes of intracortical inhibition. *Exp. Brain Res.* **1998**, *118*, 421–426. [CrossRef] [PubMed]

110. Pascual-Leone, A.; Grafman, J.; Hallett, M. Modulation of cortical motor output maps during development of implicit and explicit knowledge. *Science* **1994**, *263*, 1287–1289. [CrossRef] [PubMed]

111. Pascual-Leone, A.; Nguyet, D.; Cohen, L.; Brasil-Neto, J.; Cammarota, A.; Hallett, M. Modulation of muscle responses evoked by transcranial magnetic stimulation during the acquisition of new fine motor skills. *J. Neurophysiol.* **1995**, *74*, 1037–1045. [PubMed]

112. Ziemann, U.; Ilic, T.V.; Pauli, C.; Meintzschel, F.; Ruge, D. Learning modifies subsequent induction of long-term potentiation-like and long-term depression-like plasticity in human motor cortex. *J. Neurosci.* **2004**, *24*, 1666–1672. [CrossRef] [PubMed]

113. Bystrom, M.G.; Rasmussen-Barr, E.; Grooten, W.J. Motor control exercises reduces pain and disability in chronic and recurrent low back pain: A meta-analysis. *Spine* **2013**, *38*, E350–E358. [CrossRef] [PubMed]

114. Saragiotto, B.T.; Maher, C.G.; Yamato, T.P.; Costa, L.O.; Menezes Costa, L.C.; Ostelo, R.W.; Macedo, L.G. Motor control exercise for chronic non-specific low-back pain. *Cochrane Database Syst. Rev.* **2016**. [CrossRef]

115. Garcia-Larrea, L.; Peyron, R.; Mertens, P.; Gregoire, M.C.; Lavenne, F.; Le Bars, D.; Convers, P.; Mauguiere, F.; Sindou, M.; Laurent, B. Electrical stimulation of motor cortex for pain control: A combined pet-scan and electrophysiological study. *Pain* **1999**, *83*, 259–273. [CrossRef]

116. Galhardoni, R.; Correia, G.S.; Araujo, H.; Yeng, L.T.; Fernandes, D.T.; Kaziyama, H.H.; Marcolin, M.A.; Bouhassira, D.; Teixeira, M.J.; de Andrade, D.C. Repetitive transcranial magnetic stimulation in chronic pain: A review of the literature. *Arch. Phys. Med. Rehabil.* **2015**, *96*, S156–S172. [CrossRef] [PubMed]

117. Lefaucheur, J.P.; Andre-Obadia, N.; Antal, A.; Ayache, S.S.; Baeken, C.; Benninger, D.H.; Cantello, R.M.; Cincotta, M.; de Carvalho, M.; De Ridder, D.; et al. Evidence-based guidelines on the therapeutic use of repetitive transcranial magnetic stimulation (rtms). *Clin. Neurophysiol.* **2014**, *125*, 2150–2206. [CrossRef] [PubMed]

118. Johnson, S.; Summers, J.; Pridmore, S. Changes to somatosensory detection and pain thresholds following high frequency repetitive tms of the motor cortex in individuals suffering from chronic pain. *Pain* **2006**, *123*, 187–192. [CrossRef] [PubMed]

119. Luedtke, K.; Rushton, A.; Wright, C.; Jurgens, T.; Polzer, A.; Mueller, G.; May, A. Effectiveness of transcranial direct current stimulation preceding cognitive behavioural management for chronic low back pain: Sham controlled double blinded randomised controlled trial. *BMJ* **2015**. [CrossRef] [PubMed]

120. O'Connell, N.E.; Cossar, J.; Marston, L.; Wand, B.M.; Bunce, D.; De Souza, L.H.; Maskill, D.W.; Sharp, A.; Moseley, G.L. Transcranial direct current stimulation of the motor cortex in the treatment of chronic nonspecific low back pain: A randomized, double-blind exploratory study. *Clin. J. Pain* **2013**, *29*, 26–34. [CrossRef] [PubMed]

121. Schabrun, S.M.; Jones, E.; Elgueta Cancino, E.L.; Hodges, P.W. Targeting chronic recurrent low back pain from the top-down and the bottom-up: A combined transcranial direct current stimulation and peripheral electrical stimulation intervention. *Brain Stimul.* **2014**, *7*, 451–459. [CrossRef] [PubMed]

122. Struppler, A.; Angerer, B.; Havel, P. Modulation of sensorimotor performances and cognition abilities induced by rpms: Clinical and experimental investigations. *Suppl. Clin. Neurophysiol.* **2003**, *56*, 358–367. [PubMed]

123. Struppler, A.; Havel, P.; Müller-Barna, P. Facilitation of skilled finger movements by repetitive peripheral magnetic stimulation (RPMS)—A new approach in central paresis. *NeuroRehabilitation* **2003**, *18*, 69–82. [PubMed]

124. Krause, P.; Straube, A. Peripheral repetitive magnetic stimulation induces intracortical inhibition in healthy subjects. *Neurol. Res.* **2008**, *30*, 690–694. [CrossRef] [PubMed]

125. Struppler, A.; Binkofski, F.; Angerer, B.; Bernhardt, M.; Spiegel, S.; Drzezga, A.; Bartenstein, P. A fronto-parietal network is mediating improvement of motor function related to repetitive peripheral magnetic stimulation: A PET-H2O15 study. *Neuroimage* **2007**, *36*, T174–T186. [CrossRef] [PubMed]

126. Lo, Y.L.; Fook-Chong, S.; Huerto, A.P.; George, J.M. A randomized, placebo-controlled trial of repetitive spinal magnetic stimulation in lumbosacral spondylotic pain. *Pain Med.* **2011**, *12*, 1041–1045. [CrossRef] [PubMed]

127. Massé-Alarie, H.; Flamand, V.H.; Moffet, H.; Schneider, C. Peripheral neurostimulation and specific motor training of deep abdominal muscles improve posturomotor control in chronic low back pain. *Clin. J. Pain* **2013**, *29*, 814–823. [CrossRef] [PubMed]

128. Maeda, F.; Keenan, J.; Tormos, J.; Topka, H.; Pascual-Leone, A. Interindividual variability of the modulatory effects of repetitive transcranial magnetic stimulation on cortical excitability. *Exp. Brain Res.* **2000**, *133*, 425–430. [CrossRef] [PubMed]

129. Ziemann, U.; Siebner, H.R. Modifying motor learning through gating and homeostatic metaplasticity. *Brain Stimul.* **2008**, *1*, 60–66. [CrossRef] [PubMed]

130. Massé-Alarie, H.; Schneider, C. Cerebral reorganization in chronic low back pain and neurostimulation to improve motor control. *Neurophysiol. Clin.* **2011**, *41*, 51–60. [CrossRef] [PubMed]

131. Massé-Alarie, H.; Beaulieu, L.D.; Preuss, R.; Schneider, C. Peripheral magnetic neurostimulation of multifidus muscles combined with motor training influenced spine motor control and chronic low back pain. *Clin. Neurophysiol.* Unpublished work, **2016**.

132. Schabrun, S.M.; Chipchase, L.S. Priming the brain to learn: The future of therapy? *Man. Ther.* **2012**, *17*, 184–186. [CrossRef] [PubMed]

133. Moseley, G.L.; Vlaeyen, J.W. Beyond nociception: The imprecision hypothesis of chronic pain. *Pain* **2015**, *156*, 35–38. [CrossRef] [PubMed]

134. Butler, D.S.; Moseley, G.L. *Explain Pain*, 2nd ed.; NOI group: Adelaide, Austrlia, 2013.

135. Pelletier, R.; Higgins, J.; Bourbonnais, D. Addressing neuroplastic changes in distributed areas of the nervous system associated with chronic musculoskeletal disorders. *Phys. Ther.* **2015**, *95*, 1582–1591. [CrossRef] [PubMed]

136. Hashmi, J.A.; Baliki, M.N.; Huang, L.; Baria, A.T.; Torbey, S.; Hermann, K.M.; Schnitzer, T.J.; Apkarian, A.V. Shape shifting pain: Chronification of back pain shifts brain representation from nociceptive to emotional circuits. *Brain* **2013**, *136*, 2751–2768. [CrossRef] [PubMed]

137. Krummenacher, P.; Candia, V.; Folkers, G.; Schedlowski, M.; Schonbachler, G. Prefrontal cortex modulates placebo analgesia. *Pain* **2010**, *148*, 368–374. [CrossRef] [PubMed]

138. Tracey, I.; Mantyh, P.W. The cerebral signature for pain perception and its modulation. *Neuron* **2007**, *55*, 377–391. [CrossRef] [PubMed]

139. O'Sullivan, P. Diagnosis and classification of chronic low back pain disorders: Maladaptive movement and motor control impairments as underlying mechanism. *Man. Ther.* **2005**, *10*, 242–255. [CrossRef] [PubMed]

140. Vibe Fersum, K.; O'Sullivan, P.; Skouen, J.S.; Smith, A.; Kvale, A. Efficacy of classification-based cognitive functional therapy in patients with non-specific chronic low back pain: A randomized controlled trial. *Eur. J. Pain* **2013**, *17*, 916–928. [CrossRef] [PubMed]

141. Kleim, J.A.; Chan, S.; Pringle, E.; Schallert, K.; Procaccio, V.; Jimenez, R.; Cramer, S.C. BDNF val66met polymorphism is associated with modified experience-dependent plasticity in human motor cortex. *Nat. Neurosci.* **2006**, *9*, 735–737. [CrossRef] [PubMed]

142. Moseley, G.L.; Flor, H. Targeting cortical representations in the treatment of chronic pain: A review. *Neurorehabil. Neural. Repair.* **2012**, *26*, 646–652. [CrossRef] [PubMed]

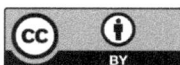

Review

Core Outcome Sets and Multidimensional Assessment Tools for Harmonizing Outcome Measure in Chronic Pain and Back Pain

Ulrike Kaiser [1,*], **Katrin Neustadt** [1], **Christian Kopkow** [2], **Jochen Schmitt** [2] and **Rainer Sabatowski** [1,3]

[1]   Comprehensive Pain Center, University Hospital "Carl Gustav Carus", Technical University Dresden, Dresden 01307, Germany; katrin.neustadt@uniklinikum-dresden.de (K.N.); rainer.sabatowski@uniklinikum-dresden.de (R.S.)

[2]   Center for Evidence-Based Healthcare, Medical Faculty, Technical University Dresden, Dresden 01307, Germany; christian.kopkow@uniklinikum-dresden.de (C.K.); jochen.schmitt@uniklinikum-dresden.de (J.S.)

[3]   Department of Anesthesiology and Intensive Care, University Hospital "Carl Gustav Carus", Technical University Dresden, Dresden 01307, Germany

*   Correspondence: ulrike.kaiser.usc-tkl@uniklinikum-dresden.de; Tel.: +49-0351-458-4547; Fax: +49-0351-458-6391

Academic Editor: Robert J. Gatchel
Received: 6 May 2016; Accepted: 17 August 2016; Published: 29 August 2016

Abstract: Core Outcome Sets (COSs) are a set of domains and measurement instruments recommended for application in any clinical trial to ensure comparable outcome assessment (both domains and instruments). COSs are not exclusively recommended for clinical trials, but also for daily record keeping in routine care. There are several COS recommendations considering clinical trials as well as multidimensional assessment tools to support daily record keeping in low back pain. In this article, relevant initiatives will be described, and implications for research in COS development in chronic pain and back pain will be discussed.

Keywords: core outcome set; effectiveness; efficacy; pain management; chronic pain; back pain; daily record keeping; clinical trials

1. Introduction

Chronic pain, especially non-specific chronic low back pain (NLBP), is a frequently encountered phenomenon with considerable psychosocial and overall socio-economic consequences. In recent decades, clinical and health care service research has provided substantial international contribution to several approaches in pain management. Particularly in relation to NLBP and interdisciplinary multidisciplinary pain therapy (IMPT), numerous studies formed the basis for a large number of systematic reviews and meta-analyses (e.g., [1–4]). However, there are still unsolved problems in analyzing IMPT such as the heterogeneity of outcome assessment in clinical trials and interventional studies which hamper drawing conclusions out of those studies and/or systematic reviews. e.g., for multidisciplinary pain therapy systematic reviews express the need for a standardized use of outcome parameters for measuring treatment success in those programs, and for a consideration of reliability and validity of measuring instruments. This leads to significant limitations in the interpretability of results. The problems observed in integrating results on a meta-perspective are exemplarily for most of the systematic reviews and meta-analyses at the moment [5–7].

2. Developing COS for Clinical Trials-Introduction to Method and Development

Establishing Core Outcome Sets is recommended to overcome such limitations and to enable researchers to integrate data in systematic reviews and meta-analyses. A Core Outcome Set (COS) is defined as a minimum set of outcome domains, which are recommended to be applied in each clinical trial and to be extended by other domains according to the specific study design [6]. Some authors extend the definition of COS including further relevant, reliable and valid measurement instruments as well [8]. The development of a COS has once been pioneered by OMERACT (Outcome Measures in Rheumatology; [5]). First guidance in developing COS has been presented by HOME (Harmonizing Outcome Measures in Eczema; [8]) and COMET (Core Outcome Measures in Effectiveness Trials; [6]). According to Schmitt et al. [8] developing COSs consists of several different steps, frequently beginning with a systematic review of all outcomes reported in clinical trials and a subsequent consensus process to vote for relevant outcome domains which should be assessed in clinical trials. Of high importance are relevant and important stakeholders joining the expert panel, including patient representatives who are expected to best decide about relevant outcomes [9]. Online surveys are common for achieving consensus, but still the methodology of COS development is various and heterogeneous [10]. Alongside the discussion of COS domain development, psychometric properties of measurement instruments to measure COS domains have been questioned and guidelines have been developed by COSMIN (COnsensus-based Standards for the selection of health Measurement Instruments; [11–14]). Further, outcome measures of COS should adequately meet the criteria of truth (i.e., validity; measure what they intend to measure), discrimination (i.e., reliability and sensitivity to change; discriminate between situations), and feasibility (i.e., be applied and interpreted easily) in order to be meaningful and relevant [15]. According to the notion that studies are only as credible as their outcome measures [15] measures have to be validated on target population [13]. This is always an important issue especially when considering comprehensive therapy approaches and/or heterogeneous patient populations.

Naturally standardization in developing COS consisting of relevant domains and valid and reliable measurement instruments is work in progress. Updates will become necessary due to advances in research, therapy provision, quality of conceptual definitions and measurement instruments.

3. Core Outcome Sets for Low Back Pain in Clinical Trials

Based on the described obstacles in practicing evidence-based medicine, some outcome initiatives with special focus on chronic pain in general [16,17] and non-specific low back pain [18–23] have been established. The main objective of these initiatives is to recommend a consensus on COS of outcome domains and measures that should be used in each clinical trial to enable comparison estimates of the benefits of different pain interventions (e.g., medication, surgery). An overview of the different recommendations is provided in Table 1.

The IMMPACT initiative (Initiative on Methods, Measurement, and Pain Assessment in Clinical Trials) recommended 6 outcome domains to be included in any clinical trial of therapy approaches in chronic pain in general, including NLBP: pain, physical functioning, emotional functioning, participant's ratings of global improvement, symptoms and adverse events, and participant's disposition (including adherence to the treatment regimen and reasons for premature withdrawal from the trial) [16]. Additional domains were recommended to be assessed optionally according to study question and aim (role functioning, interpersonal functioning, pharmacoeconomic measures and health care utilization, biological markers, coping, clinician or surrogate ratings of global improvement, neuropsychological assessments of cognitive and motor function, and suffering and other end of life issues). Panel members of IMMPACT consisted of different professions (see Table 1). However, patient representatives had not been included [16]. A survey performed with patients suffering from chronic pain indicated other outcome domains as compared to the first recommendations [16,24]. Patients rated the domains sleep, sexual activities, ability to fulfill role function, work ability, several forms of activities (physical, homework, work, and social activities), emotional wellbeing, weakness and fatigue, and cognitive impairment to be obligatory in assessing therapy effectiveness [24]. The patient relevant outcome domains are in accordance with the additional recommendations of IMMPACT [16], but not with the main recommendation (see Table 1).

Alongside these recommendations for chronic pain in general, there are others which are more disease specific. Especially for non-specific low back pain a long history of attempts to standardize outcome exists [18–23]. Quite recently, an update of a former recommendation by Deyo [23] for NLBP (consisting of pain symptoms, function, well-being, disability (physical and social roles) and satisfaction with care) was published by Chiarotto et al. [18]. A group of 280 researchers of different professions and backgrounds, patients and health care providers guided by a steering committee was led through a complex Delphi process with clearly specified definition of consensus. Starting with 41 outcome domains derived from systematic reviews in 3 Delphi rounds (response rates 45%–52%) finally 3 domains were recommended to be COS relevant: physical functioning, pain intensity and health related quality of life, whereby health related quality of life was not supported by the patient group. The steering committee decided to include an additional domain "number of deaths" (as recommended by OMERACT [15]) into the COS even though they stated occurring death in clinical trials in NLBP to be a rare event. The COS is assumed to serve for all clinical trials in NLBP. All domains were accompanied by a consented definition. Defining measurement instruments is now work in progress and will complete the recommendation [18]. Other initiatives for NLBP recommended further overlapping or distinct outcome domains by different kinds of decision making processes [21,22]. They mainly included clinicians and researchers to identify relevant outcome domains.

A setting specific approach for vocational rehabilitation of NLBP and musculoskeletal pain patients in the Netherlands is pursued by Reneman et al. [20] who developed a COS integrating ICF (International Classification of Function) for low back pain [19] and IMMPACT [16] recommendations, resulting in 18 outcome domains assessed by 12 measurement instruments. Reneman et al. kept the ICF framework and extended it by primary and supplemental outcome domains as recommended by IMMPACT. Patient participation in the process of defining COS was not considered and the panel consisted mainly of physicians specialized in rehabilitation medicine. Psychometric properties of measurement instruments were discussed as satisfactory [20]. Recommended domains are provided in Table 1.

Since the therapy of chronic pain can pursue different aims the question emerged to what extent a more unspecific recommendation, e.g., IMMPACT recommendation, can be applied to a specific therapy approach in chronic pain. The VAPAIN initiative (Validation and Application of patient reported outcome domains to assess in multimodal pain therapy) targets to assessing effectiveness of an interdisciplinary multimodal therapy (IMPT) of chronic pain [17]. The project is a comprehensive and multi-method approach consisting of several steps of systematic reviews (domains [25], instruments (in preparation)), a multistep consensus process on domains and instruments accomplished by validation studies investigating psychometric properties of potential instruments. According to previous recommendations [9] panelists experienced in IMPT or COS development and with international and multi-professional background (consisting of patient representatives, physicians specialized in pain medicine, physiotherapists, psychotherapists and methodological experts) were invited. The challenge of VAPAIN is the biopsychosocial model of chronic pain as a fundamental basis of the chosen therapy approach, leading to a complex intervention. This means that all future included outcome domains shall cover biological, psychological and social aspects affected by chronic pain.

Table 1. Recommendations for core outcome sets for clinical trial and/or effectiveness studies in chronic pain and back pain (table modified and adapted from Deckert et al. [25]).

Name of Initiative/Author	(a) Condition (b) Intervention (c) Scope of application (d) Location	Core Outcome Set -Domains-	Core Outcome Set -Measurement Instruments-	Stakeholders	Additional Comments
ICF Core sets for low back pain Cieza et al. 2004 [19]	(a) Low back pain (b) Not reported (c) Not reported (d) International	**4 outcome domains** body functions body structures activities and participation environmental factors Different number of second level categories for a *comprehensive set* and *a brief set*	ICF category system	Panel consisted of 18 experts (3 occupational therapists, 1 physical therapists, 14 physicians with various sub-specializations)	Formal decision-making and consensus process with systematic review, Delphi exercise and empirical data collection The both sets were recommended for validation only
ICF/IMMPACT for vocational rehabilitation Reneman et al. 2013 [20]	Musculoskeletal pain (subacut and chronic) Vocational rehabilitation Clinical research and clinical practice Regional (The Netherlands)	**18 outcome domains** (based on IMMPACT and ICF), e.g., Quality of life Physical functioning Pain intensity Emotional functioning Coping	12 measurement instruments such as: EuroQuol-5D Pain Disability Index (PDI); RAND 36-Item Health Survey Numerical Rating Scale (NRS) Work Reintegration Questionnaire (Distress sub-scale) Work Reintegration Questionnaire (Distress Avoidance and Persistence Sub-scale)	Preliminary core set was presented to 3 groups: Dutch Vocational rehabilitation center (n = 13; user, clinicians, management) Dutch pain rehabilitation development centers (n = 4; pain rehabilitation experts) Members of the consensus group (vocational rehabilitation) (n = 23; vocational rehabilitation experts)	Elaborate procedure to identify relevant outcome domains and measurement instruments: 1. Domains were identified according to ICF and IMMPACT recommendations 2. Domains were classified and judged by panel and authors (also according to the use in economic evaluation) 3. Instruments were identified for the included domains according to specific requirements of psychometric property

Table 1. *Cont.*

Name of Initiative/Author	(a) Condition (b) Intervention (c) Scope of application (d) Location	Core Outcome Set -Domains-	Core Outcome Set -Measurement Instruments-	Stakeholders	Additional Comments
IMMPACT Turk et al. 2003 [16] Dworkin et al. 2005 [26]	Chronic pain No specific Clinical trials International	**6 outcome domains** (1) Pain (2) Physical functioning (3) Emotional functioning (4) Participant's ratings of global improvement (5) Symptoms and adverse events, and (6) Participant's disposition **additional domains** according to study aim: - role functioning— interpersonal functioning— pharmacoeconomic measures and health care utilization, - biological markers, - coping, - clinician or surrogate ratings of global improvement— neuropsychological assessments of cognitive and motor function, and—suffering and other end of life issues	(1) 11 point (0–10) numerical rating scale of pain intensity (NRS) Usage of rescue analgesics Categorical rating of pain intensity (none, mild, moderate, severe) in circumstances in which numerical ratings may be problematic (2) Multidimensional Pain Inventory Interference Scale or Brief Pain Inventory Interference Items (3) Beck Depression Inventory (BDI) or Profile of Mood States (PMS) (4) Patient global assessment of change (PGIC) (5) Passive capture of spontaneously reported adverse events and symptoms and use of open-ended prompts (6) Detailed information regarding participant recruitment and progress through the trial, including all information specified in the CONSORT guidelines No measurement recommendations for the additional outcome domains	Domains [16] 27 participants with backgrounds in anesthesiology, biostatistics, clinical pharmacology, epidemiology, geriatrics, internal medicine, neurology, nursing, oncology, pediatric pain, physical medicine and rehabilitation, psychology, and rheumatology, all with research, clinical, or administrative expertise relevant to evaluating chronic pain treatment outcomes additionally representatives from the pharmaceutical industry and an attorney for specific expertise Measurement instruments [26] 35 participants from academia, governmental agencies, a self-help organization, and the pharmaceutical industry	Consensus process consisting of presence meeting and preselected clinical trials to identify relevant outcome domains Other issues have been published for assessing effectiveness in chronic pain, e.g.,: - Analyzing multiple endpoints [27] - Interpreting the clinical importance of group differences [28] - Interpreting the clinical importance of treatment outcomes [29] - Developing patient reported outcome measures [30] - COS for pediatric acute pain in clinical trials [31] #

Table 1. *Cont.*

Name of Initiative/Author	(a) Condition (b) Intervention (c) Scope of application (d) Location	Core Outcome Set -Domains-	Core Outcome Set -Measurement Instruments-	Stakeholders	Additional Comments
IMMPACT Survey with patient representatives Turk et al. 2008 [24]	Chronic pain No specific Clinical trials International	**19 outcome domains e.g.,:** - sleep, - sexual activities, - ability to fulfill role function, - work ability, - several forms of activities (physical, homework, work, and social activities), - emotional wellbeing, weakness and fatigue, - cognitive impairment (e.g., concentrating and remembering)	Not reported	Patient representatives Preparing focus groups $n = 31$ Web survey $n = 959$	Preparing of relevant outcome domains via focus groups Validating via web survey
Low back pain Deyo et al. 1998 [23]	Low back pain No specific Clinical trials and other kinds of research (also routine care) International	**6 outcome domains** (1) Pain symptoms (2) (Physical) function (3) Well being (4) Disability (5) Disability (social role) (6) Satisfaction with care	**For routine clinical use, quality improvement and as a component of formal research** All domains form a set of six questions (six items), adapted from several instruments such as Short- Form 36 Questionnaire (SF-36(SF36), Roland and Morris disability scale (RMDS), EuroQuol and others **For researchers** (1) Bothersomeness or severity and frequency of low back pain and leg pain (2) Roland and Morris Disability scale (RMDS) or Oswestry Disability Questionnaire (ODQ) (3) Short- Form 12 Health Survey (SF-12) or EuroQuol (4) not mentioned (5) Days of work absenteeism, cut down activities, bed rest (6) single question on overall satisfaction (optional)	A multinational group of investigators	Consensus process not reported

Table 1. *Cont.*

Name of Initiative/Author	(a) Condition (b) Intervention (c) Scope of application Setting (d) Location	Core Outcome Set -Domains-	Core Outcome Set -Measurement Instruments-	Stakeholders	Additional Comments
Low back pain Bombardier 2000 [21]	Low back pain No specific Clinical and health policy setting International	**5 outcome domains** (1) Back specific function (2) Generic health status (3) Pain (4) Work disability (5) Patient satisfaction	(1) Oswestry Disability Questionnaire (ODQ) or Roland Morris Disability Questionnaire (RMDQ) (2) Short Form 36 (SF-36) (3) Bodily pain Scale (SF-36), optional Chronic pain grade (CPG) (4) Work status; #days off work and day of cut down work, # of day return to work (5) Patient satisfaction scale (PSS) and Satisfaction with treatment (one item)	Clinicians (physicians, psychologists, researchers experienced in pain medicine, outcome research and development of questionnaires)	non-formal consensus process not further described
Low back pain Chiarotto et al. 2015 [18]	Non-specific low back pain No specific Clinical trials International	**4 outcome domains** Physical functioning Pain intensity Health related quality of life * Number of deaths ** (for * and ** please refer to *additional comments*)	In preparation	Steering group consisting of members from four continents, including researchers, health care providers and patient representatives Panel was identified by systematic review about number of publications as an indicator for expertise, including representatives from health care researchers, health care providers, professionals working both as researchers and providers and patients with non-specific low back pain; *n* = 280	Three stage online Delphi and consensus exercise As an update of the former recommendation by Deyo et al. [23] * health related quality of life was not supported by the patient group. **Based on OMERACT 2.0 Filter framework [15]

Table 1. *Cont.*

Name of Initiative/Author	(a) Condition (b) (c) Intervention Scope of application (d) Location	Core Outcome Set -Domains-	Core Outcome Set -Measurement Instruments-	Stakeholders	Additional Comments
VAPAIN Kaiser et al. 2015 [17]	Chronic pain Interdisciplinary multimodal pain therapy Effectiveness studies and daily record keeping International	In preparation	In preparation	Panel consists of 25 participants, 5 of each patient representatives, physicians, psychotherapists, physiotherapists with experience in interdisciplinary multimodal pain therapy and researches with methodological expertise in COS development and development of questionnaires	The VAPAIN process targets also towards the development and/or validation of measurement instruments for effectiveness studies and daily record keeping in MPT Multi-methodic consensus process with online exercises, structured consensus process and moderated face to face meeting Based on PROMIS framework [32]
WHO back pain initiative Ehrlich 2003 [22]	Low back pain No specific In all studies international (to all cultures)	Not specified	(1) Appropriate history and physical examination (2) Modified Schober Test of spinal mobility (3) Measurement of pain via visual analogue scale (4) Oswestry disability questionnaire (ODQ) (5) Modified Zung Questionnaire (6) Modified somatic perception questionnaire	Not reported	Consensus process not reported

IMMPACT: Initiative on Methods, Measurement, and Pain Assessment in Clinical Trials; ICF: International Classification of Functioning, Disability, and Health; VAPAIN: Validation and Application of a patient relevant core outcome set to assess effectiveness of multimodal pain therapy; # Recommended outcome domains for children and adolescents consist of Pain intensity, Global judgment of satisfaction with treatment, Symptoms and adverse events, Physical recovery, Emotional response, Economic factors.

4. COS Measurement Instruments to Be Applied in Chronic Pain

Application of COS requires associated measurement instruments. For the purpose of assessment in pain therapy there is a broad variety of measurement instruments, covering many aspects of a biopsychosocial model of chronic pain. Deckert et al. identified more than 140 outcome domains in the setting of IMPT [33], but even more applied instruments limiting comparisons between studies and meta-analyses. e.g., pain intensity was measured in 56 out of 70 included studies, the variety of the different instruments and their presentation was considerable (e.g., time period, interval of Likert-scales, specific categories of pain levels etc.) [33]. Currently the psychometric properties of measurement instruments for pain intensity are critically reflected [34–36].

IMMPACT proposed measurement instruments for their primary outcome recommendation [26]. The authors reported that psychometric property particularly of the psychological scales (e.g., Beck Depression Inventory, Profile of Mood States) was lacking or insufficient. Despite of this problem and due to the absence of alternatives between one and three measurement instruments for each domain were recommended (Table 1).

In a recently published overview representatives of IMMPACT and OMERACT discussed existing measurement instruments for physical function and participation [37]. The authors reported a considerable variety of such instruments but still open questions for example according to the discrepancies between patient reported outcome (PRO) instruments and objective measures of physical function and influencing psychosocial factors. The need for PROs and inclusion of patient representatives into developmental processes for PROs assessing physical function and participation was repeatedly emphasized [37].

The functional barometer [38] has been developed as a measurement tool to assess ICF criteria in patients with long term pain accompanied by pain related problems with function, activity and quality of life. It consists of items for patient reporting and correspondingly a classification form for professionals to assess patients' problems from the clinicians' perspective. Norrefalk reported a significantly underestimation of the patients' perceived problems followed by a large variability between the different observers, and assumed that integrating the patients' perception of pain related problems should be regarded as to be of high value within the assessment in clinical trials [38]. A review by Jelsma [39] demonstrated that ICF was broadly applied, but main critic refers to complication in coding pain and the lack of codes for personal factors (such as satisfaction with specific aspects, personal experience or emotional states).

Ashburn et al. [40] highlights that lacking data may put the specialty of pain medicine at risk and calls researchers to redouble the efforts "to demonstrate that what we do, in fact, matters- and that the care we provide improves the lives of those we serve as well as society as a whole" [40]. One way to do so is to clear up the situation of heterogeneous and therefore incomparable outcome domains and measurement tools to enhance meta-analyses. This also includes a careful work on psychometric properties of measurement instruments in pain therapy, consequently considering the characteristics and specialties of its very heterogeneous population. It is necessary to acknowledge the requirements of the process of investigating instruments as well as the amount of resources and effort to ensure high validity and reliability of concepts and instruments in pain therapy.

5. Core Outcome Sets for Daily Record Keeping in Routine Care for Patients with Back Pain

Several initiatives have worked on recommendation and standardization on outcome assessment in daily record keeping (DRK; [41–46], see Table 2). The German Pain Questionnaire [41,42] is provided to all specialized pain centers throughout Germany and supports quality management of the diagnostic and therapeutic process. Via an electronic platform benchmarking for each institution is possible. To fulfill requirements of diagnosis and therapy in different settings (outpatients, inpatients, specific approaches in pain therapy) the included variables are comprehensive comprising sociodemographic data, pain variables (e.g., pain sites, temporal characteristics, duration, intensity), pain associated symptoms, affective and sensory qualities of pain, pain relieving and intensifying factors, previous treatment procedures, pain related impairment, and psychosocial factors (see Table 2). For users the authors provide normative data and cut-off points for several scales.

For multidisciplinary outpatient treatment the Treatment Outcome of Pain Survey (TOPS) has been developed and completed by norms for initial values and treatment related improvements [43,44]. A short form has been published recently [45]. Basing on the SF-36 the original TOPS-version was generated by incorporating specific additional variables following a scientific model of disablement [47], consisting of pain symptoms, functional limitations, perceived family/social disability, objective family/social disability, and objective work disability (see Table 2). To complete the biopsychosocial perspective other items concerning life control, passive coping, solicitous responses, fear avoidance, upper body functional limitations, satisfaction with care and outcomes, and work limitation have been included as well. The authors reported sufficient psychometric properties (reliability and validity). As the authors concluded, the TOPS distinguishes from other pain and quality-of–life instruments, e.g., it bases on a treatment model, it comprises both treatment and context factors and it tracks individual change as well as documents the outcomes of groups of patients [44]. Rogers furthermore recommended the time line of providing the TOPS to patients and for a fast and efficient administration process in routine clinical care [44].

Since the original TOPS consisted of 14 subscales and 8 subscales of the SF-36 a previous initiative has tried to come up with a reduced version to improve feasibility [45]. A multi-methodic approach has been conducted including judgment of experienced clinicians as well as criteria of psychometric property and patients were asked about the acceptable amount of items. Finally, seven subscales, including 4 out of 6 IMMPACT domains, were recommended (physical function lower body, physical function upper body, pain symptom, role-emotional disability, family and social disability, patient satisfaction with outcomes, patient satisfaction with care) accomplished by the SF-12 subscales replacing the former SF-36 subscales [45]. To complete the recommended set of scales Haroutiunian et al. suggested two more scales—performance/work disability scale and sleep scale [45]. The authors recommended these instruments for patient reported outcome assessment for monitoring chronic pain treatment by individual change and reported sufficient psychometric properties (reliability, validity, and sensitivity to change), emphasizing that the inclusion of IMMPACT recommendations should enhance the process of translation from research into immediate clinical practice.

A patient centered approach was presented by Casarett et al. [46], where patients were asked by qualitative interviewing and quantitative assessment about the most relevant outcome domains for medication treatment. Patients indicated 20 outcome domains, e.g., decrease pain, decrease opioid dose, decrease frequency of scheduled dose, increased ability to function, decrease frequency of breakthrough dose and improve sleep. The authors concluded, that the opinion of patients' needs to be valued when designing studies and defining relevant outcome. The Patient Centered Outcome Questionnaire (PCOQ, [48]) targets 4 outcome domains such as pain, fatigue, emotional distress, and interference with daily activities. The origin of the chosen outcome domains unfortunately remains unclear. Notable is the focus of judging the outcome domains by the patients in 3 levels: usual level, desired level, and level of success [48]. This way therapy success is clearly defined by patients' expectations and differs from clinicians' definition of treatment success in chronic back pain [46].

For Germany an initiative provides another tool to picture effectiveness in daily routine care of IMPT institutions [49]. The authors selected items and scales from the German Pain Questionnaire [41,42] such as average pain intensity (NRS, 0–10), Pain Disability Index (PDI), German version of the Center of Epidemiologic Studies Depression Scale (CES-D) and the SF-36. The authors suggested a combined criterion consisting of the presented instruments and the criteria that 4 out of 5 scales should have changed at least 0.5 standard deviations to indicate a successful change. The tool was reported to be useful to identify more than 50% of patients to have recovered in at least 4 of the 5 recommended criteria [49]. The preference of the patients about the different success criteria and their cut-off had not been considered. Including the perspective of patients might have led to completely different criteria and their combination.

Table 2. Recommendations for core outcome sets for daily record keeping in chronic pain and back pain.

Name of Initiative/Authors		(a) Condition (b) Intervention (c) Scope of application (d) Location	Core Outcome Set -Domains-	Core Outcome Set -Measurement Instruments-	Stakeholders	Additional Comments
German Pain Questionnaire (DSF) Casser et al. 2012 [42]		(a) Chronic pain (b) Specialized pain management, (c) Daily practice (d) Germany	several domains consisting of: (1) Patient's demographic data of patient (2) Biographic data (3) Description of pain - Pain drawing and verbal description - Pain duration, frequency, course - Qualitative pain description - Pain intensity - Pain related disability - Causal- and control attribution (4) Psychological wellbeing - General wellbeing - Screening of anxiety, depression, and stress (5) Comorbidity (6) History of medical pretreatment - Physicians and interventions - medication	(1) self-report items (2) self-report items (3) self-report items, adaptation of the Brief Pain Inventory (BPI), Numerical Rating Scale for pain intensity (NRS.), Pain perception scale (SES), Chronic pain grade questionnaire (CPG) (4) Marburg Questionnaire of habitual wellbeing (MFHW), Depression-Anxiety-Stress-Scale (DASS) (5) self-report items (6) self-report items	Panel consisted of physicians specialized in pain medicine, psychotherapists, and researcher experienced in public health	Several updates Completed validation of the questionnaire Implementation in Germany via an electronical platform Benchmarking and observational studies by the German Pain Questionnaire supported Questionnaire supports diagnostic and therapeutic process
Treatment Outcomes in Pain Survey (TOPS) Rogers et al. 2000 [43] Rogers et al. 2000 [44]		(a) Chronic pain (b) Interdisciplinary pain management (c) Daily clinical care (d) International	**14 outcome domains** (1) Pain symptom (2) Perceived family/social disability (3) Objective family/social disability (4) Work limitations (5) Objective work disability (6) Lower body functional limitations (7) Upper body functional limitations (8) Fear avoidance (9) Passive coping (10) Life control (11) Solicitous responses (12) Patient satisfaction with care (13) Patient satisfaction with outcome (14) Total pain experience	A 120-item questionnaire constructed according to the identified domains for administration For follow-up were 61 items were provided	Not applicable	The tool was statistically derived from Short Form 36 (SF-36), Multidimensional Pain Inventory (MPI), Oswestry Disability Questionnaire (ODQ and), Brief pain Inventory (BPI) accomplished by several items to role-functioning, coping and pain (MOS)

156

Table 2. *Cont.*

Name of Initiative/Authors		Condition (a) Intervention (b) Scope of application (c) Location (d)	Core Outcome Set -Domains-	Core Outcome Set -Measurement Instruments-	Stakeholders	Additional Comments
Treatment Outcomes in Pain Survey short version (S-TOPS) Haroutiunian et al. 2012 [45]	(a) (b) (c) (d)	chronic pain interdisciplinary pain management daily clinical care/individual patient monitoring international	**7 outcome domains** * (1) physical function lower body (2) physical function upper body (3) pain symptom (4) role-emotional disability (5) family and social disability (6) patient satisfaction with outcomes (7) patient satisfaction with care (for * please refer to *additional comments*)	Reanalyzes from original TOPS via factor analyzes Reducing the health related quality scale by replacing the original SF 36 by the shorter SF 12	Panel consisted of 11 clinicians (medical $n = 4$, physical therapy $n = 3$, behavioral medicine $n = 2$, pharmacotherapy $n = 2$) experienced in pain medicine Patients were asked about the acceptable length of the questionnaire	A multi-methodic approach has been conducted including judgement of experienced clinicians, defined criteria of psychometric property, inclusion of IMMPACT recommended domains (4/6), factor analyzes, and patients were asked about the acceptable amount of items for individual patient Aim of the tool is monitoring in multidisciplinary chronic pain treatment * To complete the recommended set of scales Haroutiunian et al. [34] suggested including two more scales performance/work disability scale and sleep scale
Patient Centered Outcome Questionnaire (PCOQ) Robinson et al. 2005 [48]	(a) (b) (c) (d)	Chronic pain No specific No specific International	**4 outcome domains** Considering usual level, desired level and level of success for: (1) Pain (2) Fatigue (3) Emotional distress (4) Interference with daily activities	Single item assessment of (1) NRS pain (0–10) (2) NRS fatigue (0–10) (3) NRS emotional distress (0–10) (4) NRS interference with daily activities (0–10) For three levels: - usual level - desired level - level of success	Not reported	The identification of the domains and development of the scales was not clearly described Patient expectation were assessed for low back pain and fibromyalgia [50]
Patient reported outcome criterion for operationalizing success in multi-modal pain therapy Donath et al. 2015 [49]	(a) (b) (c) (d)	Chronic pain Interdisciplinary multimodal pain therapy Daily practice Germany	**5 outcome domains** (1) Pain severity (2) Disability due to pain (3) Depressiveness (4) Physical health related quality of life (5) Mental health related quality of life	(1) Average pain severity (NRS 0–10) (2) Pain disability Index (PDI) (3) German version of the CESD (4) S-36,Short Form 26 (SF36), physical composite score (5) S-36,Short Form 26 (SF36), mental composite score	Not applicable	The tool was statistically derived from scales and items of the German Pain Questionnaire

Regarding these different approaches it becomes obvious that each approach has focused on a specific aspect or function. Some want to support diagnostic and therapeutic process; others want to ensure high quality of array of treatment. Several issues have been picked up, such as success criteria or the distinction between individual or group change. All of these initiatives have brought up important, yet until today unsolved parts of therapy quality assessment. An overarching work would help to set the frame of definition and requirements of COS in DRK.

6. Issues for Further Consideration in the Discussion of COS for Chronic Pain

6.1. General Issues

Considering core outcome domains there is an overlap in recommended outcome domains or areas of the different initiatives on chronic pain comprising pain (intensity), physical function, and psychological factors (distress, emotional wellbeing, emotional functioning). Nevertheless there are still significant gaps between these different recommendations. Primarily, the scope of the domains varies significantly, for instance focusing on emotional functioning [16] or emotional wellbeing [24]. Even though the area of the domains is the same (psychological) the underlying concepts might be wide apart. A definition of theoretical constructs of domains was not always provided. Many of the presented initiatives have included biological and emotional areas and domains but still lack social components [16,18,22] (see Table 1). Some initiatives have tried to connect with other initiatives [20,34]. This has led to a greater overlap between the different recommendations and seems to be a promising way to close the existing gaps. For daily record keeping the recommendations are even more heterogeneous, both in recommended domains and number of domains (see Table 2). The recommendations vary according to national or international focus as well as to the setting they consider (e.g., individual patient monitoring [36] or support of therapy and diagnostic approach [38]). Different outcome measurement instruments might be a consequence and still hamper standardized outcome measurement in effectiveness studies in chronic pain as described on the example of the domain of pain intensity. From the current point of view it needs to be stated that there is still a considerable lack of valid and reliable measurement instruments or unclear evidence of psychometric properties of existing instruments. Previous reports about measurement instruments and their properties for pain intensity vary significantly, from no evidence of psychometric property for pain intensity [30], unclear evidence because of low report quality [29] to good results in psychometric property for patient reported outcome questionnaires for people with pain in any spine region while mainly fair methodological quality [51]. Lacking methodological quality is a well-known problem in the field of measurement instruments and affects most of the instruments in pain research [26]. The work of the COSMIN group is therefore promising and gratifying [11,12,14]. The basis of methodological standards need to be reinforced by thoroughly designed validation studies, starting with content validity and taking into account patients' perspectives while designing scales [13]. Existing scales should be careful investigated according to their psychometric properties in the sample of patients with chronic pain [13]. Other aspects of applying scales and interpreting their results affect the context of assessment. Relevance and sensitivity of outcome measurement instruments might interact with acquainted active components of therapy approaches. It seems considerable that domains might be more useful when linked to an attribute targeted by therapy. For instance, depression will only consistently and consequently change according to an intervention when it is specifically aimed for. Further the requirement of patient reported outcomes (outcomes picturing domains relevant to patients) necessitates the consideration of patient aims, which depend also on the applied intervention. Further concerning DRK measurement instruments should be sensitive to individual's change as well as to group effects. The translation of clinical results into practice as being part of treatment research needs to consider both, requirements for DRK as well as for clinical trials/effectiveness studies, which have not been discussed until today but are necessary to further establish COS in specific settings.

6.2. Implementing and Updating COS

Implementation of a COS as part of the complete process has been highlighted by Schmitt et al. [8]. There are at least two important issues to be considered for this step: Feasibility and content validity of a COS will certainly influence implementation. In addition to the domains which are part of a specific COS, other outcome domains can be of relevance for specific study objectives. Therefore the reasonably limited number of required COS domains shall enable researchers to add other domains and still keep the set of questionnaires feasible to use. Another important issue is the existence of competing COS recommendations as observed in chronic pain. Naturally competing COS will not solve the existent situation of incomparable studies. An initiative to bring together the different COS recommendations with focus of clinical trials to find consensus on recommended overlap and further indicators for a specific COS application might help researchers to decide which COS is appropriate for a designed clinical trial.

The application of such COS's should not be restricted to clinical trials only. The attempt to translate the knowledge about efficacy from clinical, standardized investigation of a therapy approach into effectiveness of daily routine care needs at least an overlap of relevant domains. Therefore, a COS is also relevant within routine care [52]. None of existing initiatives focused on therapy effects of interventions for chronic pain for both effectiveness studies and daily recordkeeping in particular. Yet, for DRK an international recommendation for one COS seems to be illusory at the moment considering the different national requirements of structural and procedural characteristics of health care delivery, health care politics and grown landscape of therapy approaches.

Developing COS is work in progress. Concepts of therapy or methodological approaches change as well as the perspective of clinicians, researchers and patients. A COS will need to be updated considering advances in all those areas in a manageable time period.

7. Conclusions

Core Outcome Initiatives in chronic pain target on harmonizing outcome assessment in clinical trials, but frequently focus on different aspects, such as specific conditions, therapy approaches or clinical settings. Implementing COS, as proposed to be part of an extended process of COS development [8], depends on distinct indicators when to apply a specific COS, especially when competing COS exist. Implementation also requires the application of valid and reliable measurement instruments. At the moment the psychometric property of several instruments is either unknown or insufficient. The careful identification of stake holders, patient representatives and scope of a COS will strongly influence its acceptance and its implementation. Only accomplished by reliable, valid and feasible instruments a COS serves well for meta analyses in evidence based medicine.

Acknowledgments: VAPAIN is funded by the German Federal Ministry of Education and Research (BMBF 01GY1326).

Author Contributions: Ulrike Kaiser prepared the draft of the paper. All other authors contributed to this work by discussion as well as correction and adjustment of the article.

Conflicts of Interest: Ulrike Kaiser, Katrin Neustadt and Christian Kopkow are team members of VAPAIN and receive funding from BMBF. Ulrike Kaiser is principal investigator of the project. Rainer Sabatowski and Jochen Schmitt declare that they have no competing interests.

References

1. Kamper, S.J.; Apeldoorn, A.T.; Chiarotto, A.; Smeets, R.J.E.M.; Ostelo, R.W.J.G.; Guzman, J.; van Tulder, M.W. Multidisciplinary biopsychosocial rehabilitation for chronic low back pain: Cochrane systematic review and meta-analysis. *BMJ* **2015**, *350*. [CrossRef] [PubMed]
2. Waterschoot, F.P.; Dijkstra, P.U.; Hollak, N.; de Vries, H.J.; Geertzen, J.H.; Reneman, M.F. Dose or content? Effectiveness of pain rehabilitation programs for patients with chronic low back pain: A systematic review. *Pain* **2014**, *155*, 179–189. [CrossRef] [PubMed]

3.   Norlund, A.; Ropponen, A.; Alexanderson, K. Multidisciplinary interventions: Review of studies of return to work after rehabilitation for low back pain. *J. Rehabil. Med.* **2009**, *41*, 115–121. [CrossRef] [PubMed]

4.   Guzmán, J.; Esmail, R.; Karjalainen, K.; Malmivaara, A.; Irvin, E.; Bombardier, C. Multidisciplinary rehabilitation for chronic low back pain: Systematic review. *BMJ* **2001**, *322*, 1511–1516. [CrossRef] [PubMed]

5.   Tugwell, P.; Bombardier, C. A methodologic framework for developing and selecting endpoints in clinical trials. *J. Rheumatol.* **1982**, *9*, 758–762. [PubMed]

6.   Williamson, P.R.; Altman, D.G.; Blazeby, J.M.; Clarke, M.; Devane, D.; Gargon, E.; Tugwell, P. Developing core outcome sets for clinical trials: Issues to consider. *Trials* **2012**, *13*. [CrossRef] [PubMed]

7.   Schmitt, J.; Langan, S.; Stamm, T.; Williams, H.C.; Harmonizing Outcome Measurements in Eczema (HOME) Delphi panel. Core outcome domains for controlled trials and clinical recordkeeping in eczema: International multiperspective Delphi consensus process. *J. Investig. Dermatol.* **2011**, *131*, 623–630. [CrossRef] [PubMed]

8.   Schmitt, J.; Apfelbacher, C.; Spuls, P.I.; Thomas, K.S.; Simpson, E.L.; Furue, M.; Chalmers, J.; Williams, H.C. The Harmonizing Outcome Measures for Eczema (HOME) roadmap: A methodological framework to develop core sets of outcome measurements in dermatology. *J. Investig. Dermatol.* **2015**, *135*, 24–30. [CrossRef] [PubMed]

9.   Sanderson, T.; Morris, M.; Calnan, M.; Richards, P.; Hewlett, S. Patient perspective of measuring treatment efficacy: The rheumatoid arthritis patient priorities for pharmacologic interventions outcomes. *Arthritis Care Res.* **2010**, *62*, 647–656. [CrossRef] [PubMed]

10.   Gargon, E.; Gurung, B.; Medley, N.; Altman, D.G.; Blazeby, J.M.; Clarke, M.; Williamson, P.R. Choosing important health outcomes for comparative effectiveness research: A systematic review. *PLoS ONE* **2014**, *9*, e99111. [CrossRef] [PubMed]

11.   Mokkink, L.B.; Terwee, C.B.; Patrick, D.L.; Alonso, J.; Stratford, P.W.; Knol, D.L.; Bouter, L.M.; de Vet, H.C. The COSMIN study reached international consensus on taxonomy, terminology, and definitions of measurement properties for health-related patient-reported outcomes. *J. Clin. Epidemiol.* **2010**, *63*, 737–745. [CrossRef] [PubMed]

12.   Mokkink, L.B.; Terwee, C.B.; Knol, D.L.; Stratford, P.W.; Alonso, J.; Patrick, D.L.; Bouter, L.M.; De Vet, H.C. The COSMIN checklist for assessing the methodological quality of studies on measurement properties of health status measurement instruments: An international Delphi study. *Qual. Life Res.* **2010**, *19*, 539–549. [CrossRef] [PubMed]

13.   De Vet, H.C.; Terwee, C.B.; Mokkink, L.B.; Knol, D.L. *Measurement in Medicine: A Practical Guide*; Cambridge University Press: New York, NY, USA, 2011.

14.   Terwee, C.B.; Mokkink, L.B.; Knol, D.L.; Ostelo, R.W.; Bouter, L.M.; de Vet, H.C. Rating the methodological quality in systematic reviews of studies on measurement properties: A scoring system for the COSMIN checklist. *Qual. Life Res.* **2012**, *21*, 651–657. [CrossRef] [PubMed]

15.   Boers, M.; Kirwan, J.R.; Wells, G.; Beaton, D.; Gossec, L.; d'Agostino, M.A.; Conaghan, P.G.; Bingham, C.O., III; Brooks, P.; Landew, R.; et al. Developing core outcome measurement sets for clinical trials: OMERACT filter 2.0. *J. Clin. Epidemiol.* **2014**, *67*, 745–753. [CrossRef] [PubMed]

16.   Turk, D.C.; Dworkin, R.H.; Allen, R.R.; Bellamy, N.; Brandenburg, N.; Carr, D.B.; Cleeland, C.; Dionne, R.; Farrar, J.T.; Galer, B.S.; et al. Core outcome domains for chronic pain clinical trials: IMMPACT recommendations. *Pain* **2003**, *106*, 337–345. [CrossRef] [PubMed]

17.   Kaiser, U.; Kopkow, C.; Deckert, S.; Sabatowski, R.; Schmitt, J. Validation and application of a core set of patient-relevant outcome domains to assess the effectiveness of multimodal pain therapy (VAPAIN): A study protocol. *BMJ Open* **2015**, *5*, e008146. [CrossRef] [PubMed]

18.   Chiarotto, A.; Deyo, R.A.; Terwee, C.B.; Boers, M.; Buchbinder, R.; Corbin, T.P.; Costa, L.O.P.; Foster, N.E.; Grotle, M.; Koes, B.W.; et al. Core outcome domains for clinical trials in non-specific low back pain. *Eur. Spine J.* **2015**, *24*, 1127–1142. [CrossRef] [PubMed]

19.   Cieza, A.; Stucki, G.; Weigl, M.; Disler, P.; Jackel, W.; van der Linden, S.; Kostenjsek, N.; de Bie, R. ICF Core Sets for low back pain. *J. Rehabil. Med.* **2004**, *36*, 69–74. [CrossRef] [PubMed]

20.   Reneman, M.F.; Beemster, T.T.; Edelaar, M.J.A.; van Velzen, J.M.; van Bennekom, C.; Escorpizo, R. Towards an ICF-and IMMPACT-based pain vocational rehabilitation core set in The Netherlands. *J. Occup. Rehabil.* **2013**, *23*, 576–584. [CrossRef] [PubMed]

21.   Bombardier, C. Outcome assessments in the evaluation of treatment of spinal disorders: Summary and general recommendations. *Spine* **2000**, *25*, 3100–3103. [CrossRef] [PubMed]

22. Ehrlich, G.E. Back pain. *J. Rheumatol.* **2003**, *67*, 26–31.
23. Deyo, R.A.; Battie, M.; Beurskens, A.J.; Bombardier, C.; Croft, P.; Koes, B.; Malmivaara, A.; Roland, M.; Von Korff, M.; Waddell, G. Outcome measures for low back pain research: A proposal for standardized use. *Spine* **1998**, *23*, 2003–2013. [CrossRef] [PubMed]
24. Turk, D.C.; Dworkin, R.H.; Revicki, D.; Harding, G.; Burke, L.B.; Cella, D.; Cleeland, C.S.; Cowan, P.; Farrar, J.T.; Hertz, S.; et al. Identifying important outcome domains for chronic pain clinical trials: An IMMPACT survey of people with pain. *Pain* **2008**, *137*, 276–285. [CrossRef] [PubMed]
25. Deckert, S.; Sabatowski, R.; Schmitt, J.; Kaiser, U. Clinical studies on multimodal pain therapy—Standardized measurement of therapy outcomes with a core outcome set. *Schmerz* **2016**. [CrossRef]
26. Dworkin, R.H.; Turk, D.C.; Farrar, J.T.; Haythornthwaite, J.A.; Jensen, M.P.; Katz, N.P.; Kerns, R.D.; Stucki, G.; Allen, R.R.; Bellamy, N.; et al. Core outcome measures for chronic pain clinical trials: IMMPACT recommendations. *Pain* **2005**, *113*, 9–19. [CrossRef] [PubMed]
27. Turk, D.C.; Dworkin, R.H.; McDermott, M.P.; Bellamy, N.; Burke, L.B.; Chandler, J.M.; Cleeland, C.S.; Cowan, P.; Dimitrova, R.; Farrar, J.T.; et al. Analyzing multiple endpoints in clinical trials of pain treatments: IMMPACT recommendations. *Pain* **2008**, *139*, 485–493. [CrossRef] [PubMed]
28. Dworkin, R.H.; Turk, D.C.; McDermott, M.P.; Peirce-Sandner, S.; Burke, L.B.; Cowan, P.; Farrar, J.T.; Hertz, S.; Raja, S.N.; Rappaport, B.A.; et al. Interpreting the clinical importance of group differences in chronic pain clinical trials: IMMPACT recommendations. *Pain* **2009**, *146*, 238–244. [CrossRef] [PubMed]
29. Dworkin, R.H.; Turk, D.C.; Wyrwich, K.W.; Beaton, D.; Cleeland, C.S.; Farrar, J.T.; Haythornthwaite, J.A.; Jensen, M.P.; Kerns, R.D.; Ader, D.N.; et al. Interpreting the clinical importance of treatment outcomes in chronic pain clinical trials: IMMPACT recommendations. *J. Pain* **2008**, *9*, 105–121. [CrossRef] [PubMed]
30. Turk, D.C.; Dworkin, R.H.; Burke, L.B.; Gershon, R.; Rothman, M.; Scott, J.; Allen, R.R.; Atkinson, J.H.; Chandler, J.; Cleeland, J.; et al. Developing patient-reported outcome measures for pain clinical trials: IMMPACT recommendations. *Pain* **2006**, *125*, 208–215. [CrossRef] [PubMed]
31. McGrath, P.J.; Walco, G.A.; Turk, D.C.; Dworkin, R.H.; Brown, M.T.; Davidson, K.; Eccleston, C.; Finley, G.A.; Goldschneider, K.; Haverkos, L.; et al. Core outcome domains and measures for pediatric acute and chronic/recurrent pain clinical trials: PedIMMPACT recommendations. *J. Pain* **2008**, *9*, 771–783. [CrossRef] [PubMed]
32. Idzerda, L.; Rader, T.; Tugwell, P.; Boers, M. Can we decide which outcomes should be measured in every clinical trial? A scoping review of the existing conceptual frameworks and processes to develop core outcome sets. *J. Rheumatol.* **2014**, *41*, 986–993. [CrossRef] [PubMed]
33. Deckert, S.; Kaiser, U.; Kopkow, C.; Trautmann, F.; Sabatowski, R.; Schmitt, J. A systematic review of the outcomes reported in multimodal pain therapy for chronic pain. *Eur. J. Pain* **2016**, *20*, 51–63. [CrossRef] [PubMed]
34. Smith, S.M.; Hunsinger, M.; McKeown, A.; Parkhurst, M.; Allen, R.; Kopko, S.; Lu, Y.; Wilson, H.D.; Burke, L.B.; Desjardins, P.; et al. Quality of Pain Intensity Assessment Reporting: ACTTION Systematic Review and Recommendations. *J. Pain* **2015**, *16*, 299–305. [CrossRef] [PubMed]
35. Dworkin, R.H.; Burke, L.B.; Gewandter, J.S.; Smith, S.M. Reliability is necessary but far from sufficient: How might the validity of pain ratings be improved? *Clin. J. Pain* **2015**, *31*, 599–602. [CrossRef] [PubMed]
36. Ballantyne, J.C.; Sullivan, M.D. Intensity of Chronic Pain—The Wrong Metric? *N. Engl. J. Med.* **2015**, *373*, 2098–2099. [CrossRef] [PubMed]
37. Taylor, A.M.; Phillips, K.; Patel, K.V.; Turk, D.C.; Dworkin, R.H.; Beaton, D.; Clauw, D.J.; Gignac, M.A.M.; Markman, J.D.; Williams, D.A.; et al. Assessment of physical function and participation in chronic pain clinical trials: IMMPACT/OMERACT recommendations. *Pain* **2016**. [CrossRef] [PubMed]
38. Norrefalk, J.R.; Svensson, E. The functional barometer—A self-report questionnaire in accordance with the international classification of functioning, disability and health for pain related problems; validity and patient-observer comparisons. *BMC Health Serv. Res.* **2014**, *14*. [CrossRef] [PubMed]
39. Jelsma, J. Use of the International Classification of Functioning, Disability and Health: A literature survey. *J. Rehabil. Med.* **2009**, *41*, 1–12. [CrossRef] [PubMed]
40. Ashburn, M.A.; Witkin, L. Integrating outcome data collection into the care of the patient with pain. *Pain* **2012**, *153*, 1549–1550. [CrossRef] [PubMed]
41. Nagel, B.; Gerbershagen, H.U.; Lindena, G.; Pfingsten, M. Development and evaluation of the multidimensional German pain questionnaire. *Schmerz* **2002**, *16*, 263–270. [CrossRef] [PubMed]

42. Casser, H.R.; Hüppe, M.; Kohlmann, T.; Korb, J.; Lindena, G.; Maier, C.; Nagel, B.; Pfingsten, M.; Thoma, R. German pain questionnaire and standardised documentation with the KEDOQ-Schmerz. A way for quality management in pain therapy. *Der Schmerz* **2012**, *26*, 168–175. [CrossRef] [PubMed]

43. Rogers, W.H.; Wittink, H.; Wagner, A.; Cynn, D.; Carr, D.B. Assessing Individual Outcomes during Outpatient Multidisciplinary Chronic Pain Treatment by Means of an Augmented SF-36. *Pain Med.* **2000**, *1*, 44–54. [CrossRef] [PubMed]

44. Rogers, W.H.; Wittink, H.M.; Ashburn, M.A.; Cynn, D.; Carr, D.B. Using the "TOPS" an outcomes instrument for multidisciplinary outpatient pain treatment. *Pain Med.* **2000**, *1*, 55–67. [CrossRef] [PubMed]

45. Haroutiunian, S.; Donaldson, G.; Yu, J.; Lipman, A.G. Development and validation of shortened, restructured Treatment Outcomes in Pain Survey instrument (the S-TOPS) for assessment of individual pain patients' health-related quality of life. *Pain* **2012**, *153*, 1593–1601. [CrossRef] [PubMed]

46. Casarett, D.; Karlawish, J.; Sankar, P.; Hirschman, K.; Asch, D.A. Designing pain research from the patient's perspective: What trial end points are important to patients with chronic pain? *Pain Med.* **2001**, *2*, 309–316. [CrossRef] [PubMed]

47. Nagi, S.Z. Disability concepts revisited: Implications for prevention. In *Disability in America: Toward a National Agenda for Prevention 1991*; The National Academies Press: Washington, DC, USA, 1991; pp. 309–327.

48. Robinson, M.E.; Brown, J.L.; George, S.Z.; Edwards, P.S.; Atchison, J.W.; Hirsh, A.T.; Waxenberg, L.B.; Wittmer, V.; Fillingim, R.B. Multidimensional success criteria and expectations for treatment of chronic pain: The patient perspective. *Pain Med.* **2005**, *6*, 336–345. [CrossRef] [PubMed]

49. Donath, C.; Dorscht, L.; Graessel, E.; Sittl, R.; Schoen, C. Searching for success: Development of a combined patient-reported-outcome ("PRO") criterion for operationalizing success in multi-modal pain therapy. *BMC Health Serv. Res.* **2015**, *15*. [CrossRef] [PubMed]

50. O'Brien, E.M.; Staud, R.M.; Hassinger, A.D.; McCulloch, R.C.; Craggs, J.G.; Atchison, J.W.; Price, D.D.; Robinson, M.E. Patient-Centered Perspective on Treatment Outcomes in Chronic Pain. *Pain Med.* **2010**, *11*, 6–15. [CrossRef] [PubMed]

51. Leahy, E.; Davidson, M.; Benjamin, D.; Wajswelner, H. Patient-Reported Outcome (PRO) questionnaires for people with pain in any spine region. A systematic review. *Man. Ther.* **2016**, *22*, 22–30. [CrossRef] [PubMed]

52. Clarke, M. Standardising outcomes for clinical trials and systematic reviews. *Trials* **2007**, *8*. [CrossRef] [PubMed]

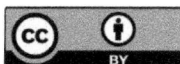

healthcare

MDPI

Article

Relationships between Paraspinal Muscle Activity and Lumbar Inter-Vertebral Range of Motion

Alister du Rose [1,2,*,†] **and Alan Breen** [1,†]

1   Institute for Musculoskeletal Research and Clinical Implementation, Anglo-European College of
     Chiropractic, Parkwood Road, Bournemouth BH5 2DF, UK; imrci.ABreen@aecc.ac.uk
2   Faculty of Science and Technology, Bournemouth University, Fern Barrow, Poole BH12 5B, UK
*   Correspondence: adurose@aecc.ac.uk; Tel.: +44-(0)1202-436-353
†   These authors contributed equally to this work.

Academic Editor: Robert J. Gatchel
Received: 2 December 2015; Accepted: 24 December 2015; Published: 5 January 2016

Abstract: Control of the lumbar spine requires contributions from both the active and passive sub-systems. Identifying interactions between these systems may provide insight into the mechanisms of low back pain. However, as a first step it is important to investigate what is normal. The purpose of this study was to explore the relationships between the lumbar inter-vertebral range of motion and paraspinal muscle activity during weight-bearing flexion in healthy controls using quantitative fluoroscopy (QF) and surface electromyography (sEMG). Contemporaneous lumbar sEMG and QF motion sequences were recorded during controlled active flexion of $60°$ using electrodes placed over Longissimus thoracis pars thoracis (TES), Longissimus thoracis pars lumborum (LES), and Multifidus (LMU). Normalised root mean square (RMS) sEMG amplitude data were averaged over five epochs, and the change in amplitude between epochs was calculated. The sEMG ratios of LMU/LES LMU/TES and LES/TES were also determined. QF was used to measure the maximum inter-vertebral range of motion from L2-S1, and correlation coefficients were calculated between sEMG amplitude variables and these measurements. Intra- and inter-session sEMG amplitude repeatability was also assessed for all three paraspinal muscles. The sEMG amplitude measurements were highly repeatable, and sEMG amplitude changes correlated significantly with L4-5 and L5-S1 IV-RoMmax ($r = -0.47$ to 0.59). The sEMG amplitude ratio of LES/TES also correlated with L4-L5 IV-RoMmax ($r = -0.53$). The relationships found may be important when considering rehabilitation for low back pain.

Keywords: spine kinematics; fluoroscopy; surface electromyography; reliability; agreement

1. Introduction

Optimal control of the spine during voluntary trunk bending requires fine-tuned coordination of numerous trunk muscles [1]. This dynamic control is believed to be modulated by communication between three sub-systems, the passive (vertebrae, discs, and ligaments), the active (muscles and tendons), and the control (central nervous system and nerves) systems [2,3]. Investigating the interplay between sub-systems however is difficult, as the spine is a complex structure; and a hidden kinematic chain. Several different technologies are therefore typically required, each with their own limitations.

In order to directly investigate the passive and active sub-systems of the spine, there have been many efforts to concurrently measure spinal kinematics and muscle activity [4–12]. The majority of these studies have used surface electromyography combined with skin surface kinematic measurement techniques such as Fastrak [8,13], Isotrak [9,11,12], or cameras [4,5,7]. These are limited to the investigation of gross spinal motion. To include segmental data usually requires invasive techniques such as the surgical insertion of intra-osseous pins. In this way Kaigle *et al.* (1998) investigated the reduction in lumbar muscular activity during full flexion (flexion relaxation) and spinal kinematics at an inter-vertebral level [10]. However, typically only single motion segments were considered, and EMG was also only recorded from one level (e.g., lumbar longissimus thoracis) [10].

1.1. Contemporaneous Monitoring of Inter-Vertebral Passive and Motor Control Systems

Study of the integrated function of the joints and muscles of the spine requires contemporaneous multi-level kinematic and electromyographic monitoring throughout the motion. This is necessary to incorporate timing, magnitude, and segmentation in the two systems to characterise control. Multi-level surface electromyography fulfils these requirements for motor control and quantitative fluoroscopy measures a range of continuous inter-vertebral motion variables [14]. Contemporaneous recording of these measures therefore provides an integrated assessment of the passive and active systems of the spine, and it is proposed that this may be useful when assessing patients with low back pain (LBP) [4,15]. This study therefore deployed quantitative fluoroscopy (QF), and surface electromyography (sEMG) of the lumbar spine together for the first time. The study investigated the biomechanics of the lumbar spine in a healthy control population in order to potentially better understand the significance of biomechanical changes in LBP populations.

1.2. Variable Selection

In order to investigate relationships between segmental kinematics and local muscle activity, suitable variables from each must be identified. While responses to perturbation [16], and the flexion relaxation phenomenon (an absence of paraspinal muscle activity during full sagittal flexion (FRP)) have been investigated [17,18], few studies have included sEMG amplitude changes throughout the cycle, be they increases or decreases. This study therefore addressed these parameters. QF measures continuous intervertebral rotation and translation in the coronal and sagittal planes during weight-bearing or recumbent motion and can also extrapolate the instant axis of rotation (IAR) and rotational range attainment rate from this. However, the need to also compare intervertebral range of motion (IV-RoM) with sEMG in the present studies, dictates the need for continuous motion information. Therefore IAR rotation and attainment rate were not likely to be so useful. In addition, the small ranges of translation make this measure unsuitable for numerical comparisons, leaving maximum rotational motion as the preferred measure.

To investigate the relationships between lumbar muscle activity and inter-vertebral restraint during bending requires access to the maximum IV-RoM (IV-RoMmax). Continuous intervertebral rotation data allows both temporal comparisons with other variables and the actual maximum IV-RoM (IV-RoMmax), rather than IV-RoM at the limit of voluntary trunk bending, to be extracted. Recording in the standing orientation allows these comparisons.

1.3. Enhanced Functional Assessment

Sanchez-Zuriaga *et al.* (2015) suggest that there are only subtle differences between various low back patient groups and healthy controls in terms of paraspinal muscle activity and regional lumbar movement [4]. This means that either muscle activity has no effect on the range of motion, or that we are missing the detail of what is happening at individual levels. For example it may be that whereas there is an increase in paraspinal activity in recurrent LBP patients during flexion, but no difference in RoM, the share of RoM may have shifted between levels at different stages in the motion. The primary role of the paraspinal muscle during flexion is to resist inter-vertebral motion [19] and so it may be that the motion is restricted at a specific level, and compensated for elsewhere, be this at other lumbar levels, or in the thoracic spine or pelvis. It is essential therefore, when attempting to understand the relationships between functional impairments and LBP that specific inter-vertebral levels are assessed both in terms of kinematics and associated muscle activity.

1.4. Repeatability

The development of QF techniques has seen its use in LBP research become more common [20–22]. IV-RoM has been the most common QF measure of inter-vertebral motion [22–24], where it has been shown to be accurate and reliable [22,25]. It is known however that sEMG recordings, by contrast, are inherently variable [26,27]. Therefore, a sub-study was conducted to assess the intra and inter-session repeatability (reliability and agreement) of the mean normalised root mean square (RMS) sEMG amplitude recordings from the entire flexion and return cycle.

1.5. Aim of the Study

The purpose of this study was to quantify the relationships between IV-RoMmax during flexion of the lumbar spine with the accompanying paraspinal muscle activity.

1.6. Specific Objectives

To determine the inter- and intra-session reliability and agreement of normalised sEMG amplitudes during weight-bearing sagittal flexion and return.

- To determine whether ratios of inter-level lumbar paraspinal sEMG amplitudes are related to the IV-RoMmax at lumbar inter-vertebral levels.
- To determine whether changes in sEMG amplitudes during different phases of the forward bending cycle are related to IV-RoMmax at lumbar inter-vertebral levels.

2. Experimental Section

2.1. Participants

The eligibility criteria for the study are shown in Table 1. Twenty male participants from the Anglo-European College of Chiropractic (AECC) student population were recruited. National Research Ethics Service (NRES) approval was gained for the study (Bristol 10/H0106/65) and written informed consent was obtained from all participants prior to data collection. The QF and sEMG data collection was conducted concurrently. In order to minimise the potential impact of variations in parameters such as soft tissue thickness (STT) and spinal degeneration (e.g., reduced disc heights), recruitment was restricted to young adult males.

Table 1. Eligibility criteria.

Inclusion	Exclusion
Males aged 20–40 years	Poor understanding of English
Able to understand written information	Having treatment for osteoporosis
Willing to participate and able to give informed consent	Recent abdominal or pelvic surgery
Consent to GP being informed	Previous lumbar spine surgery
BMI < 30	BMI > 30
No history of low back pain that prevented normal activity for at least one day in the previous year	Any medical radiation exposure in the past year or exposure in the past two years with a dose greater than 8mSv
	Current involvement in any other research study

2.2. Kinematic Data Collection and Processing (Quantitative Fluoroscopy)

Lumbar spine fluoroscopic images were collected at 15 Hz using a Siemens Arcadis Avantic VC10A digital fluoroscope (CE0123) and an upright motion frame, which stabilised participants and guided their bending motion. Participants were asked to stand with their right side against the motion frame (Figure 1), and follow a rotating arm rest which guided them through a range of 60° of forward flexion and a return to upright during continuous fluoroscopic imaging over a period of 20 seconds. A range of 60° was selected on the basis that the lumbar spine has an overall range of 80° (Flexion and extension components) [28]. The motion frame apparatus could be fully adjusted in accordance with the participant's stature, and the central ray was positioned at L4 to ensure that all vertebrae (L2-S1) were included in the image field.

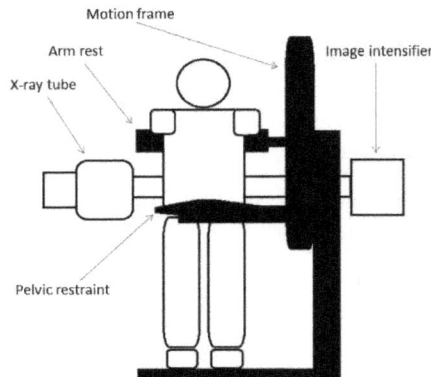

Figure 1. Fluoroscope and motion frame set-up.

Before image acquisition commenced, participants were taken in 20° increments through to the full 60° to ensure that they were able to tolerate the motion. The movement of the motion frame was recorded by electronic feedback from its motor drive and synchronised with the fluoroscopic imaging. To avoid bending at the hip joints, the pelvis was stabilised using a belt secured around the anterior superior iliac spine and secured to a bracing pad placed against the lower sacral segments. A lead apron was worn to shield the gonads.

Flexion and return sequences were then transferred to a desktop computer for analysis using bespoke image processing codes written in Matlab (The Mathworks, Cambridge) [14]. The vertebral outlines from L2-S1 in the first image in each sequence were manually marked with an electronic template using the screen cursor. This process was repeated five times for each sequence and the results averaged to increase precision. In each subsequent image frame the software programme automatically tracked each vertebra, producing a continuous measurement of its movement throughout the bending sequence [14]. Template tracking was checked visually via video playback to ensure the templates maintained the correct alignment throughout the sequence.

The data extracted comprised the continuous inter-vertebral angle in flexion and the IV-RoMmax. IV-RoMmax for each inter-vertebral level (L2-3, L3-4, L4-5 and L5-S1) was calculated as the maximum angular range reached at any point throughout the 60° trunk flexion and return cycle.

2.3. Electromyography

Prior to the commencement of data collection, participants lay prone in order for 12 electrode sites to be marked on their backs with a skin pencil. In preparation for this, the skin over their lower backs was prepared for sEMG electrode application by light abrasion, cleaning with an alcohol swab, and when necessary, shaving of the area. Disposable pre-gelled self-adhesive Ag-AgCl electrodes were then applied over three bilateral muscle groups with a 20 mm centre-to-centre inter-electrode distance as follows: Thoracic erector spinae (TES) (5 cm lateral to the T9 spinous process) [12,29], the lumbar erector spinae (LES), and lumbar multifidus (LMU) (2 cm lateral to the L2 and L5 spinous processes) [18,30] whilst the participant was in slight flexion (Figure 2).

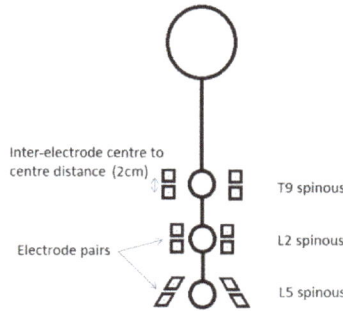

Figure 2. Electrode positioning sites. (Note: T9 spinous refers to the spinous process of the ninth thoracic vertebra, L2 to the second lumbar vertebra and L5 to the fifth lumbar vertebra.)

Although cross talk from multiple muscles will inevitably contribute to the signal recorded at each electrode site, cross-sections of the spine at each electrode site showed that the muscles that will predominate at T9 (TES) and L2 (LES) is longissimus thoracis, and at L5 (LMU) multifidus [31]. Three Biopac wireless transmitters (Bionomadix Dual Channel Wireless EMG) were then placed on the lower back attached by self-adhesive Velcro pads. There was no significant difference between the normalised mean sEMG amplitudes recorded over left and right sides during the flexion and return cycle. Therefore, an average of the mean amplitudes from both sides was used for all analysis [15].

2.4. Electrode Positioning Accuracy

Electrode application accuracy is dependent on the subjective identification of bony anatomical landmarks, and current methods used are therefore limited by human subjectivity and variation in individual anatomy [32–35]. It has been suggested however that accuracy can be improved significantly when techniques are combined [36]. This investigation was integrated into a larger ongoing normative database study, which required recumbent QF imaging before weight-bearing imaging commenced. In order to improve electrode positioning accuracy, an electrode was placed over the spinous process of L3 during the recumbent protocol. This provided an improved anatomical reference point for the application of the electrodes (Figure 3).

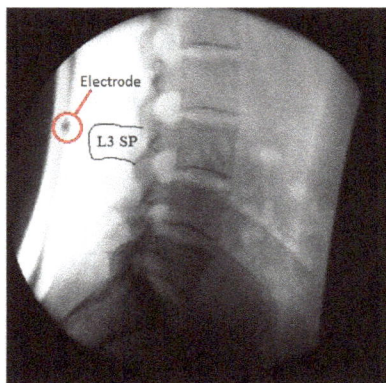

Figure 3. An electrode placed over the spinous process of L3.

2.5. The sEMG Equipment

The sEMG signal data were recorded at a sampling rate of 2000 Hz using a common-mode rejection ratio (CMRR) of 110 dB and an input impedance of 1000 MOhms.

The six signals were band pass filtered at 10–500 Hz and full wave rectified. The root mean square (RMS) amplitude was calculated for individual participant cycles and normalised during post-processing to sub-maximal voluntary contractions expressed as a percentage of the sMVC.

2.6. Reference Contraction

When data collection had been completed, and in order to provide a sub-maximal reference contraction (sMVC) [37], participants were asked to lie prone on a padded bench with their hands behind their head. They were then required to raise their torso off the couch and hold this position for five seconds whilst their legs and pelvis were stabilised. This process was repeated three times and the average sMVC was used as a reference. This technique was selected over a normalisation to a peak, primarily due to the even loading of the investigated muscle groups, but also to avoid the problem of variations in participant's muscle activation patterns in order to produce the same movement.

2.7. Synchronisation

The QF motion frame controller recording and the sEMG data recording were co-ordinated using a trip switch attached to the motion arm of the frame. This registered a data point on the sEMG timeline (Figure 4).

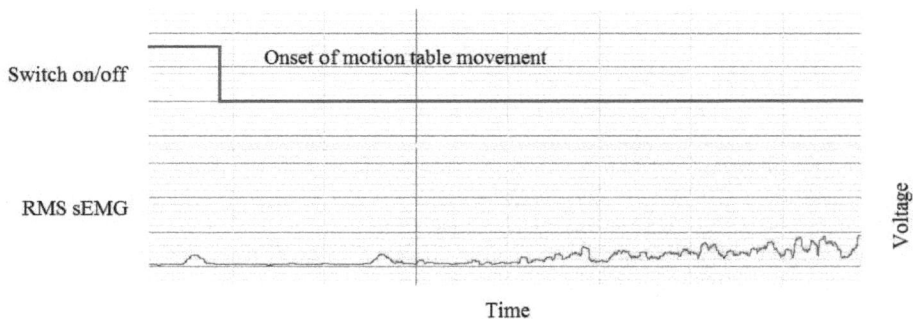

Figure 4. Synchronisation of the motion frame movement and sEMG recordings.

2.8. The sEMG Amplitude Repeatability Study

A separate convenience sample of 10 participants was used for the sEMG amplitude intra- and inter-subject repeatability studies. These studies were done without QF imaging. The acquisition cycle was repeated four times (several minutes apart) at baseline and follow up. Intra-session results compared cycles 1 and 2 (of the four), whereas inter-session results were calculated as an average of the four mean (left and right) normalised amplitudes recorded over the cycle duration. All analysis was conducted by ADR.

2.9. Data Analysis

sEMG ratios [38,39] were calculated from the mean left-right normalised sEMG (RMS) amplitudes during the flexion phase only as follows, LMU/LES, LES/TES and LMU/TES. In order to calculate sEMG changes at different stages of the flexion cycle, the forward bending phase was divided into five epochs for each participant [15]. The change in mean sEMG between epochs was then calculated (e.g., the change during the early stage of flexion was calculated as (epoch 1–2) for each of TES, LES, and LMU). This was repeated to determine changes between all epochs at all levels.

All data were tested for normality using the Shapiro-Wilk test. Relationships between IV-RoMmax and sEMG ratios and changes from normally distributed data were analysed using the Pearson product-moment correlation coefficient, and non-normal data using the Spearman's Rank Correlation. Significant relationships (p values < 0.05) were further analysed using simple linear regression. Intra-subject reliability and agreement of the mean normalised RMS sEMG amplitudes throughout the flexion and return cycle were assessed using intra-class correlations (ICC 3, 1) [40], and the standard error of measurement (SEM) respectively [41]. Statistical analysis was performed using IBM SPSS (version 21).

3. Results and Discussion

3.1. Results

Twenty males with no history of low back pain over the previous year consented to participate. Failed template tracking occurred in two participants' sequences, and their QF and sEMG data were therefore discarded. The mean (SD) age, height, and body mass Index (BMI) were 27.6 years (4.4), 1.8 m (0.06), and 24 (2.2), respectively. Average radiographic exposure factors for the group were recorded as 79.7 kV SD (5.4) and 55.4 mA SD (3.4). The mean effective dose was calculated using ICRP103 conversion software PCXMC (Monte Carlo Simulation Package) [42], and was 0.143 mSv. A complete motion sequence of the lumbar spine therefore requires less radiation than a single traditional radiograph [14]. Mean normalised RMS sEMG during the flexion cycle ranged between 3% and 21% for the TES, 2% and 31% for the LES and 13% and 40% for the LMU.

3.1.1. Reliability and Agreement

Intra- and inter-session reliability and agreement for normalised muscle activity during the bending sequence was high for all muscle levels (Table 2). The highest ICC was for LMU intra-session (ICC = 0.990, 95% CI 0.961–0.998), and the lowest SEM was 0.5% for TES intra-session. The lowest ICC was for LES inter-session (ICC = 0.872, 95% CI 0.508–0.968) and the highest SEM was for LES inter-session (SEM = 3.9%).

Table 2. Intra- and inter-session reliability and agreement for normalised RMS sEMG amplitudes during the weight-bearing sagittal plane QF protocol (n = 10).

	Intra-Session ICC (3, 1) (95% CI)	Inter-Session ICC (3, 1) (95% CI)	Intra-Session SEM (%)	Inter-Session SEM (%)
TES	0.996 (0.986–0.999)	0.895 (0.606–0.974)	0.5	2.7
LES	0.984 (0.939–0.996)	0.872 (0.508–0.968)	1.2	3.9
LMU	0.990 (0.961–0.998)	0.974 (0.902–0.993)	1.4	2.8

3.1.2. Correlations between Muscle Activity Changes and IV-RoMmax

A summary of all correlations between changes in muscle activity and IV-RoMmax is given in (Table 3). Significant correlations were only found with lower lumbar segmental motion (L4-5 and L5-S1). These were consistently of mid-level strength (r-values ranging from −0.48 to 0.59), and include inter-vertebral relationships with all three muscle levels. The results also demonstrate a number of correlations that approach significance; these did include relationships with motion at upper inter-vertebral lumbar levels (L2-3 and L3-4).

All significant correlations were further analysed using simple linear regression. The effects of muscle activity changes on IV-RoMmax are shown in (Table 4). The table shows that r^2 values range from 0.177 to 0.247.

Table 3. Correlations* between muscle activity changes (three groups, five epochs) and IV-RoMmax at all inter-vertebral levels (n = 18).

		Inter-Vertebral level			
Muscle activity change		L2-L3	L3-L4	L4-L5	L5-S1
TES epoch 1-2	r	**0.404**	0.316	−0.164	0.224
	p	**0.097**	0.201	0.516	0.371
TES epoch 2-3	r	0.083	−0.02	0.036	*−0.477*
	p	0.743	0.938	0.888	*0.045*
TES epoch 3-4*	r	−0.059	−0.077	−0.171	−0.434
	p	0.817	0.760	0.496	0.072
TES epoch 4-5	r	−0.124	−0.194	−0.134	−0.103
	p	0.625	0.441	0.596	0.683
LES epoch 1-2*	r	−0.203	0.070	*0.595*	0.391
	p	0.418	0.782	*0.009*	0.108
LES epoch 2-3	r	−0.045	0.257	0.295	*0.497*
	p	0.86	0.303	0.234	*0.036*
LES epoch 3-4	r	−0.117	−0.118	0.211	0.266
	p	0.645	0.642	0.4	0.286
LES epoch 4-5*	r	0.228	0.215	−0.088	−0.055
	p	0.362	0.392	0.729	0.829
LMU epoch 1-2	r	0.14	0.334	0.314	−0.144
	p	0.58	0.176	0.204	0.567
LMU epoch 2-3*	r	0.021	0.062	0.317	0.139
	p	0.935	0.807	0.200	0.581
LMU epoch 3-4	r	−0.039	0.164	**0.455**	0.273
	p	0.877	0.517	**0.058**	0.272
LMU epoch 4-5	r	−0.159	0.067	**0.429**	*0.461*
	p	0.53	0.793	**0.076**	*0.027*

Significant correlations are highlighted in bold italic. Correlations that approach significance are highlighted in bold. * Indicates a row that includes non-parametric data and therefore a Spearman's Rank Correlation was used. All other normally distributed data were analysed using the Pearson product-moment correlation coefficient. r = correlation co-efficient, p = p-value.

Table 4. Simple linear regression analysis: significant correlations.

Variable	Inter-Vertebral Level	r	p	r^2
LMU Epoch 4-5	L5-S1	0.461	0.027	0.212
LES Epoch 2-3	L5-S1	0.497	0.036	0.247
TES Epoch 2-3	L5-S1	−0.477	0.045	0.227
LES Epoch 1-2*	L4-5	0.595	0.009	0.177

* Indicates a row that includes non-parametric data and therefore a Spearman's Rank Correlation was used. All other normally distributed data was analysed using the Pearson product-moment correlation coefficient. r = correlation co-efficient, p = p-value and r^2 = the co-efficient of determination.

3.1.3. Correlations between sEMG Ratios and IV-RoMmax

The correlations between sEMG ratios and IV-RoMmax at all inter-vertebral levels are shown in (Table 5). The only significant relationship was found between the ratio of LES/TES and the IV-RoMmax at L4-5, and is demonstrated by the scatter plot in (Figure 5). This plot highlights the negative correlation between the LES/TES ratio and L4-L5 IV-RoMmax, and shows that when the muscle activity of the LES increases relative to that of the TES, there is a decrease in the IV-RoMmax at L4-L5. The only other correlation to approach significance was between LMU/LES ratio and the IV-RoMmax at L5-S1 (r = 0.37, p = 0.13).

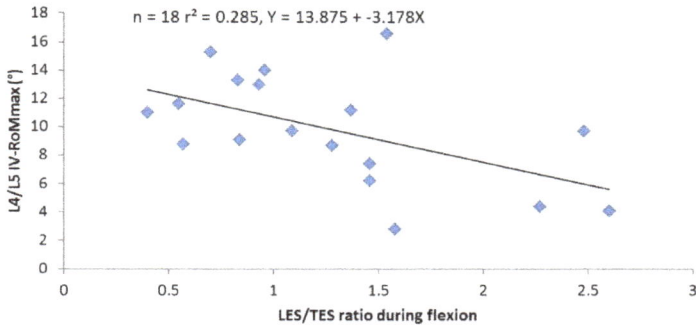

Figure 5. The relationship between the ratio of LES/TES and the IV-RoMmax at L4-5.

Table 5. Correlations between muscle activity ratios and IV-RoMmax at all inter-vertebral levels (n = 18).

Ratio		Inter-Vertebral Level			
		L2-L3	L3-L4	L4-L5	L5-S1
LMU/TES	r	0.046	−0.013	−0.236	0.152
	p	0.856	0.958	0.345	0.548
LMU/LES	r	−0.209	0.04	0.263	0.37
	p	0.405	0.875	0.292	0.13
LES/TES	r	0.095	−0.217	−0.533	−0.242
	p	0.708	0.387	0.023	0.333

r = the Pearson product-moment correlation coefficient, *p* = *p*-value.

3.2. Discussion

3.2.1. Reliability and Agreement

It is recommended that any procedures to be used in EMG studies should undergo reliability testing [43]. In this study, intra- and inter-session reliability and agreement was "substantial" for all muscle levels [40]. A common problem with sEMG studies is the great variability in their findings [44,45], therefore the high reliability shown in this study is reassuring. It is usual for a proportion of variability to be attributed to a lack of standardisation, and the method by which EMG variables are normalised [46]. The results however (Table 2) indicate that the standardisation of movement range, speed, and direction provided by the QF protocol may have played an important role in reducing the impact of variability resulting from these causes. It should be observed however that reliability and agreement was relatively poorer in the inter-session group, and of particular note was the increase in SEM for LES (3.9%). As muscle activity changes can be subtle during functional tasks, this may be a limitation for future inter-session studies.

3.2.2. Changes in sEMG Amplitudes at Different Stages of the Flexion Cycle

The results demonstrate that changes in activity of TES, LES, and LMU at various stages of the forward bending cycle, can all be to some degree related to the IV-RoMmax at lower lumbar levels (L4-5 and L5-S1). It has been suggested that intersegmental forces maintain or decrease inter-vertebral motions [47,48], it would seem logical then that if the role of the posterior muscles is to resist sagittal flexion, in order for inter-vertebral movement to occur, there must be a deactivation of this supporting musculature. Figure 6 shows an example of how the muscles most local to the L5-S1 inter-vertebral segment (LMU) demonstrate a significant decrease in activity during the final stage of flexion in a healthy control subject. This corresponds with the phase lag [49] in the initiation of movement at the adjacent inter-vertebral level from the motion graphs. The larger the change in activity between epochs, (in this case deactivation in the final stages of the flexion cycle) the larger the IV-RoMmax at L5-S1. This is suggestive of a degree of localised control, however, the stabilisation of the pelvis in order to keep the spine in the image frame and avoid hip joint contributions to motion cannot be ruled out as possible external influences. This direct relationship between corresponding levels was not apparent between the LES and the upper inter-vertebral lumbar motion segments (Table 5), and may be suggestive of anatomically specific control at this level. However, the potential importance of LES and TES was also highlighted.

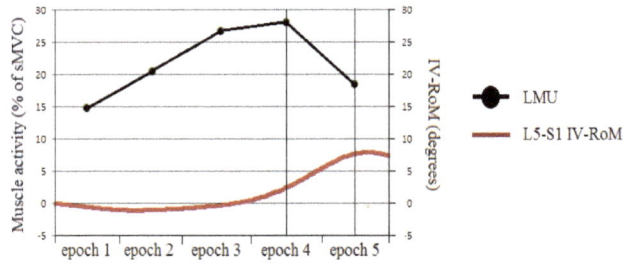

Figure 6. An example of LMU activity and lumbar IV-RoM during sagittal flexion.

Of particular interest is the apparent shift in effect between TES and LES on the IV-RoMmax of L5-S1 (Figure 7). As LES activity decreases between epochs 2 and 3 of the cycle (early mid stage) there is an associated increase in L5-S1 IV-RoMmax, whilst at the same stage of the cycle TES changes (decrease) are significantly associated with a decrease in L5-S1 IV-RoMmax (Figure 8). This indicates possible different roles for TES and LES in terms of the control of the range of motion at a distal motion segment. If there is more movement at L5-S1 there may be less activity of LES, more TES, and vice versa.

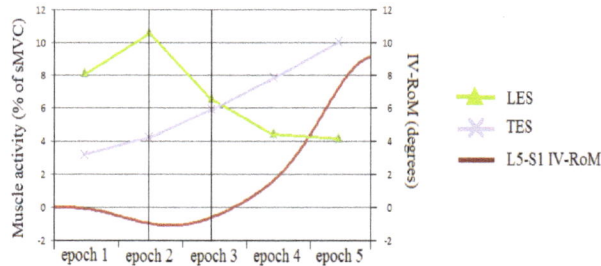

Figure 7. An example of LES and TES activity and L5-S1 IV-RoM during sagittal flexion (An example of a greater IV-RoMmax). Please note that the scales of both Y-axis are slightly different to those seen in Figure 8.

When considering the LES to be local (inter-segmental) and TES to be global (multi-segmental) [50], then these findings may have important clinical implications, as they raise the possibility of level specific stabilisation/control. Conflicting arguments have been put forward regarding the role of local and global muscles in spinal stability, Bergmark suggested that inter-segmental (local) muscles were the chief stabilisers [50], whereas Crisco and Panjabi concluded that the larger multi-segmental (global) muscles were more powerful [51]. In a study investigating the relative contribution of different trunk muscles to lumbar stability, Cholewicki and Van Vliet concluded that whilst inter-segmental and multi-segmental paraspinals had the greatest effect on stabilisation compared to other muscles (psoas and rectus abdominis), no distinction could be made between the two [52].

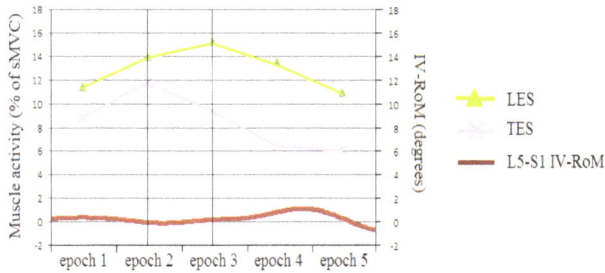

Figure 8. An example of LES and TES activity and L5-S1 IV-RoM during sagittal flexion (An example of a smaller IV-RoMmax). Please note that the scales of both Y-axis are slightly different to those seen in Figure 7.

There are many correlations that approach significance (Table 3), and therefore future studies with a larger sample size may well reveal more statistically important relationships, potentially with upper lumbar inter-vertebral levels.

3.2.3. The sEMG Ratios

Previous work has indicated a clear distinction between the kinematic behaviour of the upper and lower sections of the lumbar spine [53]. It was anticipated therefore that there may be relationships between the IV-RoMmax and the muscle activity ratio of LMU/LES. These were not evident, and suggest that the location of a motion segment within the spinal curvature, or the influence of passive structures (e.g., the strong iliolumbar ligament) may influence such interactions. The ratio of LES/TES however, did reveal a statistically significant negative relationship with the range of motion at L4-L5 (Figure 5 and Table 5).

The ratio of lumbar erector spinae over thoracic erector spinae activity has been investigated in several previous studies [38,39,54–56]. In a musculoskeletal trunk model based on the EMG data collected from two healthy participants, Cholewicki and McGill suggested that the preferential recruitment of the LES over the TES may be a strategy to increase spinal stiffness [54]. A further study comparing the muscle recruitment patterns in healthy controls to those of LBP patients, found higher LES/TES ratios in the latter [38]. These results led to the conclusion that the differences found between groups were likely to be an adaptation designed to enhance spinal stability. This theory was further supported by Van Den Hoorn *et al.* (2012), who also demonstrated a significantly higher LES/TES ratio in LBP patients during gait [55].

Reeves *et al.* also investigated this muscle activation imbalance in varsity athletes, and while maintaining that there was indeed a relationship between muscle imbalance between levels and LBP, the authors also found that in some individuals with a history of LBP, TES activity could be dominant [39]. The authors contend that this may be explained by pathology, e.g., the CNS optimising activation to minimise compression, or by a difference in muscle fibre types between groups in order to compensate for fatigue related pain [39]. Crucially however, there is also the mention of the possibility of the patterns being the result of different types of posture or lordosis, and that further studies may account for this effect.

The results of this study highlight that the ratio of LES/TES can vary in a population with no long term history of low back pain, and would appear to relate to variations in inter-vertebral mechanics in such a population. It has been proposed that lumbar inter-segmental movement is also influenced by spinal morphology [57], but these results provide more level-specific detailed information, and it is apparent that different recruitment strategies are required in accordance with inter-vertebral range changes. A question frequently asked in this field of research is whether these strategies are a cause or a consequence of the related kinematics.

It has been suggested that muscle imbalance between levels does not cause low back injury [39]. It is also suggested that imbalance is not necessarily tantamount to impairment. Therefore correcting muscle imbalance in patients should not be a priority. However if L4-L5 or L5-S1 are the segments of interest, or suspected levels of pain generation and movement at that level is considered to be part of the problem, then reducing the muscle imbalance may be of importance.

In a LBP free population sample, it might be assumed that variations in muscle activity patterns do not represent adaptations to pain. However, that is not to say that particular activity patterns and thus kinematic behaviours may not be risk factors for future LBP episodes. It also questions the conclusions of studies that compare LBP population groups with healthy pain free controls, as muscle activity patterns may not be adaptations to the episode.

It is suggested that achieving sufficient stability is a moving target, and that no single muscle can therefore be considered the best stabiliser, as the most important muscle is transient dependent on the task [58]. The results provide a demonstration of this concept in action during the task of forward bending. Whilst effect sizes are small, inter-vertebral movements have been shown here to be influenced by muscle activity. It would seem that IV-RoMmax depends not only on the relative activation of multiple trunk muscles, but also other biomechanical variables, therefore, the next logical step may be to assess the importance of each. This will require multivariate analysis of larger population samples. If the relative value of each factor can be determined, then better informed decisions regarding model types and inputs may be possible. The diversity of muscle activation patterns within a "normal" sample highlights the problem of using limited participant numbers as a basis for systems models, whereas reductionist approaches are typically weakened by the limitations of the size of the effects of the selected variables. If the variables with the greatest influence on kinematics can be found, then the selective use of these variables in models and LBP/control studies may be beneficial.

Finally, it is a limitation of this study that people with non-specific low back pain were not included, yet it would be important to know to what extent these relationships, which are consistent with maintaining appropriate restraint on vertebrae during bending, are disrupted in patients. If so, this would point to a potential route for patient stratification based on biomechanics. Such studies are now warranted. The study also only investigates a narrow population (*i.e.*, young healthy male adults) and so the results are not generalizable to other groups. It is anticipated that variations in kinematic and morphological parameters that are associated with age related change and gender would also affect IV-RoMmax, and therefore also warrant further investigation. Future investigators may also wish to incorporate measurements such as thoracic kyphosis and pelvic incidence in order to gain insight into changes in kinematic behaviour beyond the lumbar spine.

4. Conclusions

This study found weak to moderate but significant correlations between both muscle activity changes and ratios and IV-RoMmax at various inter-vertebral levels. Of particular interest was the correlation between decreased LMU and increased IV-RoMmax at L5-S1 in the latter stages of flexion, the apparent co-dependency between LES and TES during early to mid-flexion, and the effect of the LES/TES ratio on the IV-RoMmax at L4-L5. These relationships, when combined with other influencing factors, may be important when specific inter-vertebral levels are considered to be sources of pain generation and when considering rehabilitative or surgical planning. Multivariate investigations in larger samples are warranted, potentially leading to longitudinal outcome studies in LBP groups.

Acknowledgments: Acknowledgments: The study was funded by the EAC European Chiropractors Union Research Fund, and with contributions from the AECC Treatment-a-Month Club. We are also thankful for the assistance of Alex Breen, for measuring and analysing IV-RoMmax for the inter-observer study, and to Fiona Mellor for the image acquisitions. We are also grateful to Ian Swain and Mihai Dupac for their advice and suggestions and to Clive Osmond and Zoe Sheppard for their statistical guidance.

Author Contributions: Author Contributions: Alister du Rose served as project lead, performed the statistical analysis, operated the sEMG equipment, conducted the image analysis and wrote the first draft. Alan Breen operated the motion table. All authors contributed to the study design, procedural protocols, data acquisition, and the drafting of this paper. All authors read and approved the final manuscript.

Conflicts of Interest: Conflicts of Interest: The authors declare no conflict of interest.

Abbreviations

The following abbreviations are used in this manuscript:

AB	Alan Breen
ADR	Alister du Rose
AECC	Anglo-European College of Chiropractic
BMI	Body Mass Index
CI	Confidence Interval
CMRR	Common Mode Rejection Ratio
CNS	Central Nervous System
EAC	European Academy of Chiropractic
EMG	Electromyography
FRP	Flexion relaxation phenomenon
GP	General Practitioner
IAR	Instant axis of rotation
ICC	Intraclass Correlation Coefficient
IV-RoM	Inter-vertebral Range of Motion
IV-RoMmax	Maximum Inter-vertebral Range of Motion
LBP	Low Back Pain
LES	Lumbar erector spinae
LMU	Lumbar multifidus
NRES	National Research Ethics Service
QF	Quantitative Fluoroscopy
RMS	Root Mean Square
RoM	Range of Motion
SD	Standard Deviation
SEM	Standard error of measurement
TES	Thoracic erector spinae

References

1. Reeves, N.P.; Narendra, K.S.; Cholewicki, J. Spine stability: The six blind men and the elephant. *Clin. Biomech.* **2007**, *22*, 266–274. [CrossRef] [PubMed]
2. Panjabi, M.M. The stabilising system of the spine—Part 1: Function, dysfunction, adaptation and enhancement. *J. Spinal Disord.* **1992**, *5*, 383–389. [CrossRef] [PubMed]
3. Panjabi, M.M. The stabilising system of the spine—Part 2: Neutral zone and instability hypothesis. *J. Spinal Disord.* **1992**, *5*, 390–397. [CrossRef] [PubMed]
4. Sanchez-Zuriaga, D.; Lopez-Pascual, J.; Garrido-Jaen, D.; Garcia-Mas, M.A. A comparison of lumbopelvic motion patterns and erector spinae behavior between asymtomatic subjects and patients with recurrent low back pain during pain-free periods. *J. Manip. Physiol. Ther.* **2015**, *38*, 130–137. [CrossRef] [PubMed]
5. Kim, M.H.; Yoo, W.G.; Choi, B.R. Differences between two subgroups of low back pain patients in lumbopelvic rotation and symmetry in the erector spinae and hamstring muscles during trunk flexion when standing. *J. Electromyogr. Kinesiol.* **2013**, *23*, 387–393. [CrossRef] [PubMed]
6. Claus, A.P.; Hides, J.A.; Moseley, G.L.; Hodges, P.W. Different ways to balance the spine. *Spine* **2009**, *34*, E208–E214. [CrossRef] [PubMed]

7. Hashemirad, F.; Talebian, S.; Hatef, B.; Kahlaee, A.H. The relationship between flexibility and EMG activity pattern of the erector spinae muscles during trunk flexion-extension. *J. Electromyogr. Kinesiol.* **2009**, *19*, 746–753. [CrossRef] [PubMed]

8. Burnett, A.F.; Cornelius, M.W.; Dankaerts, W.; O'Sullivan, P.B. Spinal kinematics and trunk muscle activity in cyclists: A comparison between healthy controls and non-specific chronic low back pain subjects—A pilot investigation. *Man. Ther.* **2004**, *9*, 211–219. [CrossRef] [PubMed]

9. McGill, S.M.; Cholewicki, J.; Peach, J.P. Methodological considerations for using inductive sensors (3SPACE ISOTRAK) to monitor 3-D orthopaedic joint motion. *Clin. Biomech.* **1997**, *12*, 190–194. [CrossRef]

10. Kaigle, A.M.; Wesberg, P.; Hansson, T.H. Muscular and kinematic behavior of the lumbar spine during flexion-extension. *J. Spinal Disord.* **1998**, *11*, 163–174. [CrossRef] [PubMed]

11. Callaghan, J.P.; Gunning, J.L.; McGill, S.M. The relationship between lumbar spine load and muscle actitivity during extensor exercises. *Phys. Ther.* **1998**, *78*, 8–18. [PubMed]

12. Peach, J.P.; Sutarno, C.G.; McGill, S.M. Three-dimensional kinematics and trunk muscle myoelectric activity in the young lumbar spine: A database. *Arch. Phys. Med. Rehabil.* **1998**, *79*, 663–669. [CrossRef]

13. Dankaerts, W.; O'Sullivan, P.B.; Burnett, A.F.; Straker, L.M.; Davey, P.; Gupta, R. Discriminating healthy controls and two clinical subgroups of nonspecific chronic low back pain patients using trunk muscle activation and lumbosacral kinematics of postures and movements. *Spine* **2009**, *34*, 1610–1618. [CrossRef] [PubMed]

14. Breen, A.C.; Teyhan, D.S.; Mellor, F.E.; Breen, A.C.; Wong, K.W.N.; Deitz, A. Measurement of intervertebral motion using quantitative fluoroscopy: Report of an international forum and proposal for use in the assessment of degenerative disc disease in the lumbar spine. *Adv. Orthop.* **2012**. [CrossRef] [PubMed]

15. D'hooge, R.; Hodges, P.; Tsao, H.; Hall, L.; MacDonald, D.; Danneels, D. Altered trunk muscle coordination during rapid trunk flexion in people in remission of recurrent low back pain. *J. Electromyogr. Kinesiol.* **2013**, *23*, 173–181. [CrossRef] [PubMed]

16. Hodges, P.; van den Hoorn, W.; Dawson, A.; Cholewicki, J. Changes in the mechanical properties of the trunk in low back pain may be associated with recurrence. *J. Biomech.* **2009**, *42*, 61–65. [CrossRef] [PubMed]

17. Luhring, S.; Schinkel-Ivy, A.; Drake, J.D.M. Evaluation of the lumbar kinematic measures that most consistently characterize lumbar muscle activation patterns during trunk flexion: A cross-sectional study. *J. Manip. Physiol. Ther.* **2015**, *38*, 44–50. [CrossRef] [PubMed]

18. McGorry, R.W.; Lin, J.H. Flexion relaxation and its relation to pain and function over the duration of a back pain episode. *PLoS ONE* **2012**, *7*, e39207. [CrossRef] [PubMed]

19. Bogduk, N. *Clinical and Radiological Anatomy of the Lumbar Spine*, 5th ed.; Churchill Livingstone: London, UK, 2012.

20. Okawa, A.; Shiomiya, K.; Komori, H.; Muneta, T.; Arai, Y.; Nakai, O. Dynamic motion study of the whole lumbar spine by videofluoroscopy. *Spine* **1998**, *23*, 1743–1749. [CrossRef] [PubMed]

21. Teyhen, D.S.; Flynn, T.W.; Childs, J.D.; Abraham, L.D. Arthrokinematics in a subgroup of patients likely to benefit from a lumbar stabilization exercise program. *Phys. Ther.* **2007**, *87*, 313–325. [CrossRef] [PubMed]

22. Mellor, F.E.; Thomas, P.; Thompson, P.; Breen, A.C. Proportional lumbar spine inter-vertebral motion patterns: A comparison of patients with chronic non-specific low back pain and healthy controls. *Eur. Spine J.* **2014**, *23*, 2059–2067. [CrossRef] [PubMed]

23. Pearson, A.M.; Spratt, K.F.; Genuario, J.; McGough, W.; Kosman, K.; Lurie, J.; Sengupta, D.K. Precision of lumbar intervertebral measurements. *Spine* **2011**, *36*, 572–580. [CrossRef] [PubMed]

24. Teyhen, D.S.; Flynn, T.W.; Bovik, A.C.; Abraham, L.D. A new technique for digital fluoroscopic video assessment of sagittal plane lumbar spine motion. *Spine* **2005**, *30*, E406–E413. [CrossRef] [PubMed]

25. Yeager, M.S.; Cook, D.J.; Cheng, B.C. Reliability of computer-assisted lumbar intervertebral measurement using a novel vertebral motion analysis system. *Spine J.* **2014**, *14*, 274–281. [CrossRef] [PubMed]

26. Knutson, L.M.; Soderberg, G.L.; Ballantyne, B.T.; Clarke, W.R. A study of various normalization procedures for within day electromyographic data. *J. Electromyogr. Kinesiol.* **1994**, *4*, 47–59. [CrossRef]

27. Lehman, G.J.; McGill, S.M. The importance of normalization in the interpretation of surface electromyography: A proof of principle. *J. Manip. Physiol. Ther.* **1999**, *22*, 444–446. [CrossRef]

28. Dvorak, J.; Panjabi, M.M.; Chang, D.G.; Theiler, R.; Grob, D. Functional radiographic diagnosis of the lumbar spine. Flexion-extension and lateral bending. *Spine* **1991**, *16*, 562–571. [CrossRef] [PubMed]

29. Nelson-Wong, E.; Callaghan, J.P. Is muscle co-activation a predisposing factor for low back pain development during standing? A multifactorial approach for early identification of at-risk individuals. *J. Electromyogr. Kinesiol.* **2010**, *20*, 256–263. [CrossRef] [PubMed]

30. O'Shaughnessy, J.; Roy, J.F.; Descarreaux, M. Changes in flexion-relaxation phenomenon and lumbo-pelvic kinematics following lumbar disc replacement surgery. *J. Neuroeng. Rehabil.* **2013**. [CrossRef] [PubMed]

31. Anatomy.TV. Available online: https://anatomy.tv/new_home.aspx?startapp=&startres=&startstudyguide= &S=&ReturnUrl=&lpuserid=& (accessed on 2 December 2015).

32. Kim, H.W.; Ko, Y.J.; Rhee, W.I.; Lee, J.S.; Lim, J.E.; Lee, S.J.; Im, S.; Lee, J.I. Interexaminer reliability and accuracy of posterior superior iliac spine and iliac crest palpation for spinal level estimations. *J. Manip. Physiol. Therap.* **2007**, *30*, 386–389. [CrossRef] [PubMed]

33. Chin, K.R.; Kuntz, A.F.; Bohlman, H.H.; Emery, S.E. Changes in the iliac crest-lumbar relationship from standing to prone. *Spine J.* **2006**, *6*, 185–189. [CrossRef] [PubMed]

34. Billis, E.V.; Foster, N.E.; Wright, C.C. Reproducibility and repeatability: Errors of three groups of physiotherapists in locating spinal levels by palpation. *Man. Ther.* **2003**, *8*, 223–232. [CrossRef]

35. Chakraverty, R.; Pynsent, P.; Isaacs, K. Which spinal levels are identified by palpation of the iliac crests and the posterior superior iliac spines? *J. Anat.* **2007**, *210*, 232–236. [CrossRef] [PubMed]

36. Merz, O.; Wolf, U.; Robert, M.; Gesing, V.; Rominger, M. Validity of palpation techniques for the identification of the spinous process L5. *Man. Ther.* **2013**, *18*, 333–338. [CrossRef] [PubMed]

37. Demoulin, C.; Vanderthommen, M.; Duysens, C.; Crielaard, J.M. Spinal muscle evaluation using the Sorensen test: A critical appraisal of the literature. *Joint Bone Spine* **2006**, *73*, 43–50. [CrossRef] [PubMed]

38. Van Dieen, J.H.; Cholewicki, J.; Radebold, A. Trunk muscle recruitment patterns in patients with low back pain enhance the stability of the lumbar spine. *Spine* **2003**, *28*, 834–841. [CrossRef] [PubMed]

39. Reeves, N.P.; Cholewicki, J.; Silfies, S.P. Muscle activation imbalance and low-back injury in varsity athletes. *J. Electromyogr. Kinesiol.* **2006**, *16*, 264–272. [CrossRef] [PubMed]

40. Shrout, P.E. Measurement reliability and agreement in psychiatry. *Stat. Methods Med. Res.* **1998**, *7*, 301–317. [CrossRef] [PubMed]

41. De Vet, H.C.W.; Terwee, C.B.; Knol, D.L.; Bouter, L.M. When to use agreement *versus* reliability measures. *J. Clin. Epidemiol.* **2006**, *59*, 1033–1039. [CrossRef] [PubMed]

42. Mellor, F.E. An Evaluation of Passive Recumbent Quantitative Fluoroscopy to Measure Mid-Lumbar Intervertebral Motion in Patients with Chronic Non-Specific Low Back Pain and Healthy Volunteers. Ph.D. Thesis, Bournemouth University, Bournemouth, UK, 2014.

43. Soderberg, G.L.; Knutson, L.M. A guide for use and interpretation of kinesiologic electromyographic data. *Phys. Ther.* **2000**, *80*, 485–498. [PubMed]

44. Geisser, M.E.; Ranavaya, M.; Haig, A.J.; Roth, R.S.; Zucker, R.; Ambroz, C.; Caruso, M. A meta-analytic review of surface electromyography among persons with low back pain and normal, healthy controls. *J. Pain* **2005**, *6*, 711–726. [CrossRef] [PubMed]

45. Van Dieen, J.H.; Selen, L.P.J.; Cholewicki, J. Trunk muscle activation in low-back pain patients, an analysis of the literature. *J. Electromyogr. Kinesiol.* **2003**, *13*, 333–351. [CrossRef]

46. Lariviere, C.; Arsenault, A.B. On the use of EMG-ratios to assess the coordination of back muscles. *Clin. Biomech.* **2008**, *23*, 1209–1219. [CrossRef] [PubMed]

47. Panjabi, M.M.; Krag, M.H.; Dimnet, J.C.; Walter, S.D.; Brand, R.A. Thoracic spine centres of rotation in the sagittal plane. *J. Orthop. Res.* **1984**, *1*, 387–394. [CrossRef] [PubMed]

48. Kaigle, A.M.; Holm, S.H.; Hansson, T.H. Experimental instability in the lumbar spine. *Spine* **1995**, *20*, 421–430. [CrossRef] [PubMed]

49. Kanayama, M.; Abumi, K.; Kaneda, K.; Tadano, S.; Ukai, T. Phase lag of the intersegmental motion in flexion-extension of the lumbar and lumbosacral spine: An *in vivo* study. *Spine* **1996**, *21*, 1416–1422. [CrossRef] [PubMed]

50. Bergmark, A. Stability of the lumbar spine: A study in mechanical engineering. *Acta Orthop. Scand.* **1989**, *60*, 1–54. [CrossRef]

51. Crisco, J.J.; Panjabi, M.M. The intersegmental and multisegmental muscles of the lumbar spine: A biomechanical model comparing lateral stabilizing potential. *Spine* **1991**, *16*, 793–799. [CrossRef] [PubMed]

52. Cholewicki, J.; van Vliet, J.J., IV. Relative contribution of trunk muscles to the stability of the lumbar spine during isometric exertions. *Clin. Biomech.* **2002**, *17*, 99–105. [CrossRef]

53. Pavlova, A.V.; Cooper, K.; Meakin, J.R.; Barr, R.; Aspden, R. Internal lumbar spine motion during lifting. In Proceedings of the 21st Congress of the European Society of Biomechanics, Prague, Czech Republic, 5–8 July 2015.

54. Cholewicki, J.; McGill, S.M. Mechanical stability of the *in vivo* lumbar spine: Implications for injury and chronic low back pain. *Clin. Biomech.* **1996**, *11*, 1–15. [CrossRef]

55. Van den Hoorn, W.; Bruijn, S.M.; Meijer, O.G.; Hodges, P.W.; van Dieen, J.H. Mechanical coupling between transverse plane pelvis and thorax rotations during gait is higher in people with low back pain. *J. Biomech.* **2012**, *45*, 342–347. [CrossRef] [PubMed]

56. Willigenburg, N.W.; Kingma, I.; van Dieen, J.H. Center of pressure trajectories, trunk kinematics and trunk muscle activation during unstable sitting in low back pain patients. *Gait Posture* **2013**, *38*, 625–630. [CrossRef] [PubMed]

57. Pavlova, A.V.; Meakin, J.R.; Cooper, K.; Barr, R.J.; Aspden, R.M. The lumbar spine has an intrinsic shape specific to each individual that remains a characteristic throughout flexion and extension. *Eur. Spine J.* **2014**, *23*, S26–S32. [CrossRef] [PubMed]

58. McGill, S.M.; Grenier, S.; Kavcic, N.; Cholewicki, J. Coordination of muscle activity to assure stability of the lumbar spine. *J. Electromyogr. Kinesiol.* **2003**, *13*, 353–359. [CrossRef]

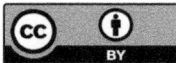

healthcare

Review

Demoralization, Patient Activation, and the Outcome of Spine Surgery

Andrew R Block

Texas Back Institute, Plano, TX 75093, USA; ablock@texasback.com; Tel.: +1-972-608-5000

Academic Editor: Robert J. Gatchel
Received: 25 November 2015; Accepted: 12 January 2016; Published: 19 January 2016

Abstract: It is now well established that psychosocial factors can adversely impact the outcome of spine surgery. This article discusses in detail one such recently-identified "risk" factor: demoralization. Several studies conducted by the author indicate that demoralization, an emotional construct distinct from depression, is associated with poorer pain reduction, less functional improvement and decreased satisfaction among spine surgery patients. However, there are indications that the adverse impact of risk factors such as demoralization can be mitigated by psychosocial "maximizing" factors—characteristics that propel the patient towards positive surgical results. One of these maximizing factors, patient activation, is discussed in depth. The patient activation measure (PAM), an inventory assessing the extent to which patients are active and engaged in their health care, is associated not only with improved spine surgery results, but with better outcomes across a broad range of medical conditions. Other maximizing factors are discussed in this article. The author concludes that the past research focus on psychosocial risk factors has limited the value of presurgical psychological screening, and that future research, as well as clinical assessment, should recognize that the importance of evaluating patients' strengths as well as their vulnerabilities.

Keywords: presurgical psychological screening; spine surgery; demoralization; patient activation; MMPI-2-RF; maximizing factors

1. Introduction

The use of surgery for protracted back and neck pain has increased rapidly over the past two decades, with spinal fusion accounting for a majority of this growth. For example, Rajaee *et al.* [1] examining the United States data set for the Healthcare Cost and Utilization Project (HCUP) for the years 1998 to 2008, found that spinal fusion increased 2.4 fold from 174,223 to 413,171. The average hospital costs associated with such surgeries have also increased significantly, as reported by Weinstein *et al.* [2] who found the hospital costs associated with spinal fusion averaged about $82,000 per patient, a 3.3 fold increase compared to 1998. By 2008 national hospital billing for spinal fusion alone was almost $34 billion.

Spine surgery can be, and often is, quite effective. For example, Weinstein *et al.* [3] in the Spine Patient Outcomes Research Trial (SPORT) study found that at both six months and two years post-op, patients undergoing laminectomy/discectomy obtained greater reductions in pain and improvements in functional ability than did patients treated non-surgically for herniated lumbar discs. Similarly, Mirza *et al.* [4] found that individual with back pain who underwent spine surgery (mostly spinal fusion) showed greater reduction in disability than did those who did not receive invasive treatment (see also Fritzell *et al.* [5]).

On the other hand, it is well established that spine surgery not infrequently fails to provide pain relief and improved functional ability. For example, a recent analysis of discectomy patients found 28% had unfavorable outcomes [6], with a 10% reoperation rate. In like fashion, Copay *et al.* [7] found that of patients who had undergone spine surgery (mostly spinal fusions) only 47% to 61% showed clinically significant improvement on any one of the outcome measures examined. Further, Brox *et al.* [8] found that long-term improvement after instrumented fusion was no better than treament with a combination of cognitive-behavioral intervention and exercise (see Mirza and Deyo [9] for a systematic review).

A large and growing body of research is finding that psychosocial risk factors can contribute significantly to the variability in spine surgery outcome (for reviews see Block [10]; Block, Gatchel, Deardorff and Guyer [11]. Research by our group (Block *et al.* [12]; Marek, Block and Ben-Porath [13]), and others (e.g., Edwards *et al.* [14]; Trief, Grant and Fredrickson [15]; Voohies, Jaing and Thomas [16]; Chiachana *et al.* [17]) demonstrate the adverse impact on surgery results of depression, elevated pain sensitivity, workers' compensation, somatic anxiety and poor pain coping, to name just a few. In one of our studies (Block *et al.* [18]) patients identified as having a high level of psychosocial risk had only about a 15% chance of obtaining good surgical outcome, as defined by reduction in pain and improvement in functional ability.

2. Demoralization

Until recently, much of the research on presurgical psychological screening (PPS), was based on the use of the original Minnesota Multiphasic Personality Inventory (Hathaway and McKinley [19]) or its first major revision, the MMPI-2. However, recent research by our group using the latest revision of this test, the MMPI-2-Restructured Form (MMPI-2-RF: Ben-Porath and Tellegan [20]) has identified another psychological factor, demoralization, that is powerfully associated with reduced outcome of both spine surgery (Marek, Block and Ben-Porath [13]) and spinal cord stimulation (Block, Marek and Ben-Porath [12]). Ben-Porath [21] defines demoralization as "a pervasive and affect-laden dimension of unhappiness and dissatisfaction with life". Demoralization, assessed by a 24-item scale exclusive to the MMPI-2-RF, scale RCd, includes items that "reflect the presence of dysphoric affect, distress, self-attributed inefficacy, low self-esteem and a sense of giving up" (p. 53). Such feelings appear to underlie a broad range of mental health disorders. For example, Simms *et al.* [22] found that among military veterans RCd elevations correlate strongly with both current and lifetime diagnosis of depressive and anxiety disorders, and with negative emotionality. Scale RCd, demonstrates desirable psychometric properties, including strong test-retest reliability $r^2 = 0.88$, and internal consistency (r^2 ranging from 0.87 to 0.93 depending on the population tested), with no significant differences between average scores of men and women (Tellegen and Ben-Porath [23], pp. 24–25).

Our research (Marek *et al.* [13]; Block, Marek, Ben-Porath and Ohnmeiss [24]) has found that elevated scores on the demoralization scale, RCd, are strongly correlated with poorer results at six months post spine surgery, including less improvement in pain and in self-reported physical disability, lower return to work rates, greater use of opioid medication, poorer satisfaction with surgical outcome, and worse overall outcome. Further, specific components of demoralization assessed by the MMPI-2-RF, including scales measuring Helplessness/Hopelessness, Self-Doubt and Inefficacy (a belief that one is incapable of making decisions and coping with difficulties), are significantly associated with poorer satisfaction and reduced results of both spine surgery (Block, Ben-Porath, Marek and Ohnmeiss [24]) and poorer results of spinal cord stimulation (Block, Marek, Ben-Porath and Kukal [12]). Further, scale RCd, is the only MMPI-2-RF scale associated with poor results in all the outcome areas assessed. For spinal cord stimulator candidates [12] T-scores of 60 (1 standard deviation above the mean) or greater on scale RCd significantly increased the relative risk ratio (RRR) for poor results on all measures utilized, including functional ability as assessed by the Oswestry Disability Index (RRR = 1.42), reported pain level (RRR = 1.47) and patient rating of dissatisfaction with outcome (RRR = 1.86). Unpublished data [25] by our group indicate similarly increased RRRs for poor outcome in spine surgery candidates.

Elevated scores on scale RCd have also been found to be associated with poorer conservative treatment outcomes in chronic low back pain. Tarescavage, Scheman and Ben-Porath [26] examining the effectiveness of an interdisciplinary treatment program for chronic low back pain, found significant correlations between scores on scale RCd with emotional distress and pain-related disability at the completion of the program.

A substantial literature exists on demoralization, especially in the context of other chronic medical conditions. Most of these studies use instruments other than the MMPI-2-RF, including the Diagnostic Criteria for Psychosomatic Research (DCPR: Fava *et al.* [27]) or the Demoralization Scale (DS: Kissane *et al.* [28]). A recent systematic review (Robinson *et al.* [29]) found that for individuals with a wide range of chronic illness and disease 13%–33% experience demoralization (depending on the measure utilized to assess this condition), and that demoralization is associated with poorly controlled physical symptoms, including fatigue, mobility constraints, breathing problems, constipation, memory and concentration problems. Further, for the medically ill patients studied there was also a strong negative association between activity level and demoralization.

Demoralization is distinct from depression, although both may include strong experience of negative emotions. Individuals who are depressed, in addition to displaying vegetative symptoms such as sleep disturbance, psychomotor retardation and lethargy, exhibit anhedonia, *i.e.*, inability to experience pleasure (de Figueiredo [30]). Demoralized individuals, on the other hand, can experience positive emotion, but are plagued by feelings of helplessness, loss of hope and meaninglessness (Sansone and Sansone [31]). Several studies have documented the divergence of demoralization and depression. Grandi, Sirri, Tossani and Fava [32] examining cardiac transplant patients, found that 71% of patients who were determined to be demoralized according to the DCPR did not fit the criteria for major depression. Similarly, Jacobsen *et al.* [33] found among patients with advanced cancer that, of those diagnosed with major depressive disorder, only 28.6% met the DCPR criteria for demoralization. While it is clear that spine surgery results are diminished in patients reporting high levels of depression (Chaichana *et al.* [17]; Adogwa *et al.* [34]), which is often assessed using the Zung depression inventory (Zung [35]), demoralization is a distinctive emotional state, and one which appears to exert particularly adverse effects on medical conditions in general, and spine surgery in particular.

3. Patient Activation

The feelings of ineffectiveness, helplessness and the sense of giving up that comprise the core of demoralization stand in sharp contrast to the behaviors and general health orientation that are associated with positive health outcomes. In order to achieve and maintain good health, individuals must be able take control over diet and exercise and seek out health information. Individuals also need to recognize when illness occurs, and be able to communicate with health care providers. They need to work with their physicians on plans to overcome or mitigate illness, and have the fortitude to follow through on these plans. Such an effective health orientation is captured by the Patient Activation Measure (PAM: Hibbard, Stockard, Mahoney and Tissler [36]).

The PAM is a 20-item questionnaire designed to assess the extent to which individuals are "engaged and active" in their own health care. The domains evaluated by the PAM include: (1). Belief that taking an active role in health is important; (2). Having the confidence and knowledge to take action; (3). Taking health-related action; (4). Staying the course under stress. In the original studies, PAM scores correlated significantly with the use of a glucose journal in diabetes, with following a low fat diet in patients with high cholesterol, with routinely exercising for patients with arthritis, and for seeking out information from health care providers. Further studies have found the PAM correlates significantly with both health outcomes and health care utilization. For example, in diabetics PAM scores predicted testing for, and control of Hemoglobin A_{1c}, and testing for low-density lipoprotein cholesterol, among others (Remmers, Hibbard, Mosen, Wagenfield, Hoye and Jones [37]). In an analysis of over 33,000 patients in a large health care delivery system in Minnesota, patients with the lowest scores on PAM (poorest patient activation as determined by their scores being in the lowest quartile) had much higher average health care costs than patients who displayed the highest levels of patient activation, a finding which held true not only for population as a whole, but for specific groups of patients, including those with hyperlipidemia, hypertension, and asthma (Hibbard, Green and Overton [38]).

Two previous studies have examined the role of patient activation in spine surgery patients. Skolasky, Mackenzie, Wegener and Riley [39] examined 65 patients who underwent surgery for degenerative lumbar stenosis, assessing the relationship of PAM scores to participation in post-operative physical therapy (PT). They found that PAM scores correlated strongly with both the number of PT sessions attended, and with patient "engagement" in PT, as assessed by the physical therapist using a standardized treatment engagement metric. Skolasky, Mackenzie, Wegener and Riley [40] went on to examine the relationship of patient activation to functional recovery in spine surgery patients. In this study, patients in the highest level (upper quartile) of PAM scores showed greater reduction in reported pain levels at post-op follow up than did patients with lower levels of patient activation, despite the fact that the patients with highest PAM levels reported less pain at baseline. Patients in the upper quartile of PAM scores also showed the greatest improvement in functional ability, as assessed by the Oswestry disability index (Fairbank [41]), and the greatest improvements in overall physical health as assessed by the SF-12 v 2 (Hurst, Duta and Kind [42]). The authors conclude that including interventions to improve patient activation, such as empowerment strategies, self-management strategies and education sessions, may lead to improvements in the outcome of spine surgery.

We have been examining the relationship of the PAM to the outcome of spine surgery. Thus far, we (Block, *et al.* Unpublished data [25]) have given the PAM, as well as the MMPI-2-RF to a group of patients prior to surgery (both spine surgery and spinal cord stimulator implantation), finding significant correlations of the PAM with improvements in functional ability as assessed by changes in scores on the Oswestry disability index ($r^2 = 0.33$, $p < 0.01$), reduction of negative affect as assessed by change scores on Likert-type emotion ratings ($r^2 = 0.26$, $p < 0.05$), and with patient satisfaction ($r^2 = 0.28$, $p < 0.05$) at an average of about 5 months post-op.

4. Psychological "Maximizing" Factors

Results with the PAM point to a very significant and long-neglected area in presurgical psychological screening of spine surgery candidates, *viz*, the assessment of patient characteristics that may militate towards improved outcomes. Certainly, my own research (see Block [10]) as well as that of others (Voorhies *et al.* [16]; denBoer *et al.* [43]), which has been focused on assessment of psychological "risk" factors, continues to demonstrate how specific psychological characteristics can undo even the most effective surgical intervention. We (Block, Marek, Ben-Porath and Ohnmeiss [24]) have found that, in addition to demoralization, several other characteristics assessed by the MMPI-2-RF are strongly correlated with reduced spine surgery results, including somatic sensitivity and malaise (Scales RC1 and MLS), low positive emotion (scale RC7), family problems (FML), social avoidance (SAV), and the PSY-5 scale negative emotionality/neuroticism (NEGE-r). However, the complexity of human nature is such that individuals may have strengths—traits, behaviors and emotional states–that can counteract more negative characteristics. Patient activation may be one such "maximizing factor"—one that could potentially reduce the adverse impact on some psychosocial risk factors, such as demoralization, on spine surgery results.

Other potential "maximizing factors" warrant exploration. Consider, for example, a patient who has a high level of family problems (elevated score on the MMPI-2-RF scale FML). Such a patient may simultaneously have a strong social support system outside the family, or even be satisfied with the level of support received by family members, despite the problems that exist within the family. Social support has been found to be an important predictor of improved health outcomes. For example, Mutran, Reitez, Mossey and Fernandez [44], examining recovery from hip surgery, found that patients with low levels of perceived support achieved less improvement in walking ability at 2 months post-op than did patients with higher level of support. In the case of spine surgery, Schade *et al.* [45] found that social support from the spouse was significantly related to greater pain relief in patients undergoing lumbar discectomy. Further, higher levels of perceived support have been found to be associated with less catastrophizing in patients who have longer pain durations (Cano [46]). Thus, it appears that the perception of satisfactory social support may be a factor that is associated with improved surgical outcome, and one which may mitigate some psychosocial risk factors, including catastrophizing and elevated levels of family problems.

A third potential characteristic that may help to maximize spine surgery results revolves around expectations for the outcome of spine surgery. Spine surgery has three major goals: reduce pain; improve functional ability; and correct the underlying physical pathology responsible for the pain and functional deficits. The extent to which these three goals are achieved, however, varies widely. Some patients coming to surgery expect total pain relief and a complete return to pre-morbid activity levels, while others may consent to surgery even though their expectation is that minimal improvements will occur. So, it is reasonable to consider whether patient expectations bear a relationship to surgical results. Although the results are not completely consistent, several studies show that greater expectations of improvement assessed pre-operatively are associated with more sanguine surgical results. For example, Yee *et al.* [47] examining spinal fusion patients, found that higher preoperative expectations were associated with greater improvement on the SF-36 physical domain score. Similarly, Soroceanu, Ching, Abdu and McGuire [48]) found higher outcome expectations to be associated with greater functional improvement (but not greater satisfaction) in a mixed group of patients undergoing lumbar and cervical spine surgery. Gepstein *et al.* [49] examining elderly patients who went decompression surgery for lumbar spinal stenosis found that positive outcome expectations were associated with greater outcome satisfaction. However, it is clear that having excessively optimistic expectations may work against surgical results and satisfaction. Patients whose high surgical expectations are not met report very low satisfaction with surgery outcome (Toyone *et al.* [50]). Thus, it appears that surgical success is more likely to be achieved when patients have expectations of significant, but not complete, pain relief and substantial, but not completely unrestricted, improvement in functional ability.

Patient activation, social support and positive outcome expectations are but three of a host of psychosocial factors that might potentially be associated with improved spine surgery results. Some other factors that have been found to correlate with improved outcome of treatment for pain, and may militate towards better spine surgery response include:

-- Positive pain coping strategies, such as optimism (Goodin and Bulls [51]; Bargiel-Matusicwicz and Kryzyskowska [52]), acceptance and mindfulness (McCracken and Vowels [53]);
-- Resilience (Sturgeon and Zaruta [54]; Ramirez-Maestre, *et al.* [55]) and Hardiness (Maddi [56]);
-- Spirituality and forgiveness (Rippentropp *et al.* [57]).

It would be of great value to explore these and other positive factors that may contribute to better spine surgery results.

5. Conclusions

A number of psychosocial risk factors for reduced spine surgery outcome are by now well established. Depression, somatic sensitivity, demoralization, substance abuse, vocational issues such as workers' compensation and litigation—all these are shown to have strong empirically-derived correlations with diminished results. However, the focus of PPS upon psychosocial risk factors has ignored much of the complexity of each case and provided limited insight into factors that may improve surgical outcomes. Research on patient activation, social support and surgical outcome expectations point to the importance of examining psychosocial "maximizing factors"—those patient characteristics that may mitigate the adverse impact of established risk factors, and may propel the patient towards good surgical response. In order to provide a full and effective picture of each patient's capacity for achieving reduction in pain and improvement in functional ability, the field of presurgical psychological screening must begin to focus as much on the patient's strengths as upon his or her vulnerabilities.

Acknowledgments: Acknowledgments: Some of the research reported in this paper was supported by a grant from The University of Minnesota Press, publisher of the MMPI-2-RF.

Conflicts of Interest: Conflicts of Interest: The author declares no conflict of interest.

References

1. Rajaee, S.S.; Bae, H.W.; Kanim, L.E.A.; Delamarter, R.B. Spinal fusion in the United States: Analysis of Trends from 1998 to 2008. *Spine* **2012**, *37*, 67–78. [CrossRef] [PubMed]
2. Weinstein, J.N.; Lurie, J.D.; Olson, P.R.; Bronner, K.K.; Fisher, E.S. United States' trends and regional variations in lumbar spine surgery: 1992–2003. *Spine* **2006**, *23*, 2707–2714. [CrossRef] [PubMed]
3. Weinstein, J.N.; Lurie, J.D.; Tosteson, T.D.; Lurie, J.D.; Tosteson, A.N.A.; Hanscom, B.; Skinner, J.S.; Abdu, W.A.; Hilibrand, A.S.; Boden, S.D.; *et al.* Surgical *vs* nonoperative treatment for lumbar disk herniation: The Spine Patient Outcomes Research Trial (SPORT). *J. Am. Med. Assoc.* **2006**, *296*, 2451–2459. [CrossRef] [PubMed]
4. Mirza, S.K.; Deyo, R.A.; Heagerty, P.J.; Turner, J.A.; Martin, B.I.; Comstock, B.A. One year outcomes of surgical *versus* non-surgical treatments for discogenic back pain: A community-based prospective cohort study. *Spine J.* **2013**, *13*, 1421–1433. [CrossRef] [PubMed]
5. Fritzell, P.; Hagg, O.; Wessberg, P.; Nordwall, A. Volvo Award Winner in Clinical Studies: Lumbar fusion *versus* nonsurgical treatment for chronic low back pain: A multicenter randomized controlled trial from the Swedish Lumbar Spine Study Group. *Spine* **2001**, *26*, 2521–2532. [CrossRef] [PubMed]
6. Sherman, J.; Cauthen, J.; Schoenberg, D.; Burns, M.; Reaven, N.L.; Griffith, S.L. Economic impact of improving outcomes of lumbar discectomy. *Spine J.* **2010**, *10*, 108–116. [CrossRef] [PubMed]
7. Copay, A.G.; Martin, M.M.; Subach, B.R.; Carreon, L.Y.; Glassman, S.D.; Schuler, T.C.; Berven, S. Assessment of spine surgery outcomes: Inconsistency of change amongst outcome measurements. *Spine J.* **2010**, *10*, 291–296. [CrossRef] [PubMed]
8. Brox, J.I.; Nygaard, O.P.; Holm, I.; Keller, A.; Ingebrigsten, T.; Reikeras, O. Four-year follow-up up of surgical *versus* non-surgical therapy for chronic low back pain. *Ann. Rheum. Dis.* **2010**, *69*, 1643–1648. [CrossRef] [PubMed]
9. Mirza, S.K.; Deyo, R.A. Systematic review of randomized trials comparing lumbar fusion surgery to nonoperative care for treatment of chronic back pain. *Spine* **2007**, *32*, 816–823. [CrossRef] [PubMed]
10. Block, A.R. Spine surgery. In *Presurgical Psychological Screening: Understanding Patients, Improving Outcomes*; Block, A.R., Sarwer, D.B., Eds.; American Psychological Association: Washington, DC, USA, 2013.
11. Block, A.R.; Gatchel, R.; Deardorff, W.; Guyer, R. *The Psychology of Spine Surgery*; American Psychological Association: Washington, DC, USA, 2003.
12. Block, A.R.; Marek, R.J.; Ben-Porath, Y.S.; Kukal, D. Associations between pre-implant psychosocial factors and spinal cord stimulation outcome: Evaluation using the MMPI-2-RF. *Assessment* **2015**. [CrossRef] [PubMed]
13. Marek, R.J.; Block, A.R.; Ben-Porath, Y.S. The Minnesota Multiphasic Personality Inventory-2-Restructured Form (MMPI-2-RF): Incremental validity in predicting early post-operative outcomes in spine surgery candidates. *Psychol. Assess.* **2015**, *27*, 114–124. [CrossRef] [PubMed]
14. Edwards, R.R.; Klick, B.; Buenaver, L.; Max, M.; Haythornthwaite, J.A.; Keller, R.B.; Altas, S.J. Symptoms of distress as predictors of pain-related sciatica treatment outcomes. *Pain* **2007**, *130*, 47–55. [CrossRef] [PubMed]
15. Trief, P.M.; Grant, W.; Fredrickson, B. A prospective study of psychological predictors of lumbar surgery outcome. *Spine* **2000**, *25*, 2616–2621. [CrossRef] [PubMed]
16. Voohies, R.; Jian, Z.; Thomas, N. Prediction outcome in the surgical treatment of lumbar radiculopathy using the Pain Drawing Score, McGill Short Form Pain Questionnaire and risk factors including psychosocial issues and axial joint pain. *Spine J.* **2007**, *7*, 516–524. [CrossRef] [PubMed]
17. Chaichana, K.L.; Mukherjee, D.; Adogwa, O.; Cheng, J.S.; McGirt, M.J. Correlation of preoperative depression and somatic perception scales with post-operative disability and quality of life after lumbar discectomy. *J. Neurosurg. Spine* **2011**, *14*, 261–267. [CrossRef] [PubMed]

18. Block, A.R.; Ohnmeiss, D.D.; Guyer, R.D.; Rashbaum, R.; Hochschuler, S.H. The use of presurgical psychological screening to predict the outcome of spine surgery. *Spine J.* **2001**, *1*, 274–282. [CrossRef]

19. Hathaway, S.R.; McKinely, H.C. *Manual for the Minnesota Multiphasic Personality Inventory*; Psychological Corporation: New York, NY, USA, 1951.

20. Ben-Porath, Y.S.; Tellegen, A. *MMPI-2-RF (Minnesota Multiphasic Personality Inventory-2-Restructured Form) Manual for Administration, Scoring and Interpretation*; University of Minnesota Press: Minneapolis, MN, USA, 2008.

21. Ben-Porath, Y.S. *Interpreting the MMPI-2-RF*; University of Minnesota Press: Minneapolis, MN, USA, 2012.

22. Simms, L.J.; Casilas, A.; Clark, L.A.; Watson, D.; Doebbeling, B.N. Psychometric evaluation of the restructured clinical scales of the MMPI-2. *Psychol. Assess.* **2005**, *17*, 345–358. [CrossRef] [PubMed]

23. Tellegen, A.; Ben-Porath, Y.S. *MMPI-2-RF Technical Manual*; University of Minnesota Press: Minneapolis, MN, USA, 2008.

24. Block, A.R.; Ben-Porath, Y.S.; Marek, R.J.; Ohnmeiss, D. Associations between MMPI-2-RF scores, workers' compensation status and spine surgery outcome. *J. Appl. Biobehav. Res.* **2014**, *19*, 248–267. [CrossRef]

25. Block, A.R.; Ben-Porath, Y.S.; Marek, R. Texas Back Institute, Plano, TX, USA. Psychological predictors of good and poor spine surgery outcome. Unpublished work, 2016.

26. Tarescavage, A.M.; Scheman, J.; Ben-Porath, Y.S. Reliability and validity of the Minnesota Multiphasic Personality Inventory-2-Restructured Form (MMPI-2-RF) in evaluations of low back pain patients. *Psychol. Assess.* **2014**, *27*, 443–446. [CrossRef] [PubMed]

27. Fava, G.A.; Freyberger, H.J.; Bech, P.; Christodoulou, G.; Sensky, T.; Theorell, T.; Wise, T.N. Diagnostic criteria for use in psychosomatic research. *Psychother. Psychosom.* **1995**, *63*, 1–8. [CrossRef] [PubMed]

28. Kissane, D.W.; Wein, S.; Love, A.; Lee, X.Q.; Kee, P.L.; Clarke, D.M. The Demoralization Scale: A report of its development and preliminary validation. *J. Palliat. Care* **2004**, *20*, 269–276. [PubMed]

29. Robinson, S.; Kissane, D.W.; Brooker, J.; Burney, S. A systematic review of the demoralization syndrome in individuals with progressive disease and cancer: A decade of research. *J. Pain and Symp. Manag.* **2015**, *49*, 595–610. [CrossRef] [PubMed]

30. Defiguiredo, J.M. Depression and demoralization: Phenomenologic differences and research perspectives. *Comp. Psychiatr.* **1993**, *34*, 308–311. [CrossRef]

31. Sansone, R.A.; Sansone, L.A. Demoralization in patients with medical illness. *Psychiatry* **2010**, *7*, 42–45. [PubMed]

32. Grandi, S.; Sirri, L.; Tossani, E.; Fava, G.A. Psychological characterization of demoralization in the setting of heart transplantation. *J. Clin. Psychiatry* **2011**, *72*, 648–654. [CrossRef] [PubMed]

33. Jacobsen, J.C.; Vanderwerker, L.C.; Block, S.D.; Friedlander, R.J.; Maciejewski, P.K.; Prigerson, G. Depression and demoralization as distinct syndromes: Preliminary data from a cohort of advanced cancer patients. *Indian J. Palliat. Care* **2006**, *12*, 8–15. [CrossRef]

34. Adogwa, O.; Parker, S.L.; Shau, D.N.; Mendenhall, S.K.; Aaronson, O.S.; Cheng, J.S.; Devin, C.J.; McGirt, M.J. Preoperative Zung depression scale predicts outcome after revision lumbar surgery for adjacent segment disease, recurrent stenosis and pseudoarthrosis. *Spine J.* **2012**, *12*, 179–185. [CrossRef] [PubMed]

35. Zung, W.W. A self-rating depression scale. *Arch. Gen. Psychiatry* **1965**, *12*, 63–70. [CrossRef] [PubMed]

36. Hibbard, J.H.; Stockard, J.; Mahoney, E.R.; Tusler, M. Development of the Patient Activation Measure (PAM): Conceptualizing and measuring activation in patients and consumers. *Health Serv. Res.* **2004**, *39*, 1005–1026. [CrossRef] [PubMed]

37. Remmers, C.; Hibbard, J.; Mosen, D.; Wagenfield, M.; Hoye, R.; Jones, C. Is patient activation associated with future health outcomes and healthcare utilization among patients with diabetes? *J. Ambul. Care* **2009**, *32*, 1–8. [CrossRef] [PubMed]

38. Hibbard, J.D.; Greene, G.; Overton, V. Patients with lower activation associated with high costs; delivery systems should know their patients' "scores". *Health Aff.* **2013**, *32*, 216–222. [CrossRef] [PubMed]

39. Skolasky, R.L.; Mackenzie, E.J.; Wegener, S.T.; Riley, L.H. Patient activation and adherence to physical therapy in persons undergoing spine surgery. *Spine* **2008**, *33*, E784–E791. [CrossRef] [PubMed]

40. Skolasky, R.L.; Mackenzie, E.J.; Wegener, S.T.; Riley, L.H. Patient activation and functional recovery in persons undergoing spine surgery. *J. Bone Joint Surg.* **2011**, *93*, 1665–1671. [CrossRef] [PubMed]

41. Fairbank, J. Use of the Oswestry Disability Index (ODI). *Spine* **1976**, *20*, 1535–1536. [CrossRef]

42. Hurst, M.P.; Duta, D.A.; Kind, P. Comparison of the MOS short form-2 (SF12) health status questionnaire with the SF 36 in patients with rheumatoid arthritis. *Br. J. Rheumatol.* **1998**, *37*, 862–869. [CrossRef] [PubMed]

43. Den Boer, J.J.; Oostendorp, R.A.B.; Beems, T.; Munneke, M.; Evers, A.W.M. Continued disability and pain after lumbar disc surgery: The role of cognitive-behavioral factors. *Pain* **2006**, *123*, 45–52. [CrossRef] [PubMed]

44. Mutran, E.J.; Reitzes, D.C.; Mossey, J.; Fernandez, M.E. Social support, depression and recovery of walking ability following hip fracture surgery. *J. Gernontol.* **1995**, *50*, 5354–5361. [CrossRef]

45. Schade, V.; Semmer, N.; Main, C.; Hora, J.; Boos, N. The impact of clinical, morphological, psychosocial and work-related factors on the outcome of lumbar discectomy. *Pain* **1999**, *80*, 239–249. [CrossRef]

46. Cano, A. Pain catastrophizing and social support in married couples with chronic pain: The moderating role of pain duration. *Pain* **2004**, *110*, 656–664. [CrossRef] [PubMed]

47. Yee, A.; Adjei, N.; Do, J.; Ford, M.; Finkelstein, J. Do patient expectations of spinal surgery relate to functional outcome? *Clin. Orthop. Relat. Res.* **2008**, *466*, 1154–1161. [CrossRef] [PubMed]

48. Soroceanu, A.; Ching, A.; Abdu, W.; McGuire, K. Relationship between preoperative expectations, satisfaction, and functional outcomes in patients undergoing lumbar and cervical spine surgery: A multicenter study. *Spine* **2012**, *37*, E103–E108. [CrossRef] [PubMed]

49. Gepstein, R.; Arinson, Z.; Adjunsky, A.; Folman, Y. Decompression surgery for lumbar spinal stenosis in the elderly: Preoperative expectations and postoperative satisfaction. *Spinal Cord* **2006**, *44*, 427–431. [CrossRef] [PubMed]

50. Toyone, T.; Tanaka, T.; Kato, D.; Kanayama, R.; Ostsuka, M. Patient expectations and satisfaction in lumbar spine surgery. *Spine* **2005**, *30*, 2689–2694. [CrossRef] [PubMed]

51. Goodin, B.R.; Bulls, H.W. Optimism and the experience of pain: Benefits of seeing the glass as half full. *Curr. Pain Headache Rep.* **2013**, *17*, 1–9. [CrossRef] [PubMed]

52. Bargiel-Matusicwicz, K.; Krzyszkowska, A. Dispositional optimism and coping with pain. *Eur. J. Med. Res.* **2009**, *14*, 271–274. [CrossRef]

53. McCracken, L.M.; Vowles, K.E. Acceptance and Commitment Therapy and Mindfull for chronic pain. *Am. Psychol.* **2014**, *69*, 178–185. [CrossRef] [PubMed]

54. Sturgeon, J.A.; Zaruta, A.J. Resilience: A new paradigm for adaptation to chronic pain. *Curr. Pain Headache Rep.* **2010**, *14*, 105–112. [CrossRef] [PubMed]

55. Ramirez-Maestre, C.; Esteve, R.; Lopez, A.E. The path to capacity: Resilience and chronic spinal pain. *Occup. Health Ergon.* **2012**, *37*, E251–E258. [CrossRef] [PubMed]

56. Maddi, S.R. The story of hardiness: Twenty years of theorizing, research and practice. *Consult. Psychol. J. Pract. Res.* **2002**, *54*, 173–185. [CrossRef]

57. Rippentropp, A.E.; Altmaier, E.M.; Chen, J.J.; Found, E.M.; Feffala, V.J. The relationship between religion/spirituality and physical, mental health and pain in a chronic pain population. *Pain* **2005**, *116*, 311–321. [CrossRef] [PubMed]

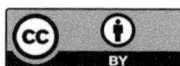

healthcare

MDPI

Review

Who Benefits from Chronic Opioid Therapy? Rethinking the Question of Opioid Misuse Risk

Elizabeth Huber [†], Richard C. Robinson *[,†], Carl E. Noe [†] and Olivia Van Ness [†]

The University of Texas Southwestern Medical Center at Dallas, 5323 Harry Hines Blvd., Dallas, TX 75390, USA; elizabeth.huber@utsouthwestern.edu (E.H.); carl.noe@utsouthwestern.edu (C.E.N.); Olivia.vanness@utsouthwestern.edu (O.V.N.)

* Correspondence: richard.robinson@utsouthwestern.edu; Tel.: +1-214-648-5277
† These authors contributed equally to this work.

Academic Editors: Robert J. Gatchel and Sampath Parthasarathy
Received: 24 February 2016; Accepted: 17 May 2016; Published: 25 May 2016

Abstract: Beginning in the late 1990s, a movement began within the pain management field focused upon the underutilization of opioids, thought to be a potentially safe and effective class of pain medication. Concern for addiction and misuse were present at the start of this shift within pain medicine, and an emphasis was placed on developing reliable and valid methods and measures of identifying those at risk for opioid misuse. Since that time, the evidence for the safety and effectiveness of chronic opioid therapy (COT) has not been established. Rather, the harmful, dose-dependent deleterious effects have become clearer, including addiction, increased risk of injuries, respiratory depression, opioid induced hyperalgesia, and death. Still, many individuals on low doses of opioids for long periods of time appear to have good pain control and retain social and occupational functioning. Therefore, we propose that the question, "Who is at risk of opioid misuse?" should evolve to, "Who may benefit from COT?" in light of the current evidence.

Keywords: chronic pain; chronic low back pain; opioids; chronic opioid therapy; biopsychosocial approach

1. Introduction

Beginning at the turn of the millennium, questions arose about the under-utilization of opioid pain medication to treat individuals suffering from chronic noncancer pain (CNCP) [1]. Terms such as "opiophobia" became used more widely and referenced a potentially irrational fear that providers had with regard to utilizing this class of medication [2]. With the support of pharmaceutical companies, many pain management physicians invested time and energy to educate the public and their peers that opioids could be used safely and effectively for CNCP, including chronic low back pain (CLBP) [1]. One focus that developed out of this movement was to identify those who were at risk for opioid misuse as well as to develop interventions for those who may have succumbed to addiction [3]. Measures such as the Pain Medication Questionnaire (PMQ) [4] and The Screener and Opioid Assessment for Patients with Pain (SOAPP) [5] were developed, as well as guidelines for urine drug testing, to identify those who were at risk of misusing their opioids or to determine who was engaging in aberrant, and potentially harmful, opioid use.

Since that time, the evidence for the efficacy of chronic opioid therapy has not grown in a substantial, or even discernible, manner [6,7]. Rather, evidence accumulated regarding the potential harmful effects of opioids, including substance use disorders, endocrinopathy, opioid-induced hyperalgesia, and death [7]. In fact, in a recent review of the use of chronic opioid therapy (COT) for chronic pain by Chou, Turner *et al.* [7] concluded, "Evidence is insufficient to determine the effectiveness of long-term opioid therapy for improving chronic pain and function. Evidence supports a dose-dependent risk for serious harms." (p. 276).

Despite these findings, opioids continue to be used for CNCP [8]. However, limited research has been conducted on those individuals who remain on low doses of opioids (e.g., 10–20 mg morphine equivalent) with adequate pain control and functioning. Therefore, we propose that the question should evolve from, "Who is at risk for opioid misuse?" to, "Who may benefit from COT?" given the current evidence for this intervention.

2. Chronic Pain

2.1. The Scope of the Problem

The International Association for the Study of Pain (IASP) [9] defines pain as "an unpleasant sensory and emotional experience associated with actual or potential tissue damage" and chronic pain as "pain persisting beyond the normal expected time of healing," which is typically considered pain that lasts for three to six months or more [10]. According to the Institute of Medicine (IOM) [11], approximately 100 million adults are afflicted by chronic pain in the United States. Gatchel, Peng, and colleagues [12] estimated that chronic pain accounts for more than 80% of physician visits. Furthermore, chronic low back pain (CLBP) is the most common chronic pain condition [11].

Pain is a costly condition, not only in terms of healthcare expenditures to treat chronic pain patients, but in terms of lost productivity and compensation for disability as well [13]. Furthermore, chronic pain is frequently associated with significant comorbid psychiatric conditions and emotional suffering [12]. It is difficult to measure the economic impact of chronic pain in the United States, as most studies focus on individual pain disorders rather than providing composite estimates across a broader range of common pain conditions [14]. Nonetheless, Gaskin and Richard [15] used the Medical Expenditure Panel Survey (MEPS) [16] to estimate the portion of U.S. health care costs attributable to pain, as well as the incremental annual costs associated with lower worker productivity as a result of pain. Their findings indicate that the annual costs of treating pain in the United States were greater than the costs of treating heart disease, cancer, and diabetes combined [15]. Gaskin and Richard [15] found that the total costs of treating pain annually fell somewhere between $560 and $635 billion in 2010 dollars, with additional health care costs due to pain ranging from $261 to $300 billion. They estimate the value of lost worker productivity due to pain ranged from $299 to $335 billion [15].

2.2. The Biopsychosocial Model

Given the high costs associated with treating chronic pain, it is not surprising that a significant amount of research has been conducted to better understand the causes and thus develop more effective methods to treat patients with pain. The biopsychosocial model is a theoretical approach that attempts to address health and illness based on a combination of biological, psychological, and social variables [17]. Underlying this model is the principal that all health-related issues, including pain, arise from a multifaceted interaction among these three factors. Research has demonstrated that it is not always possible to find a purely physiological cause in many cases of chronic pain; in particular, providers often struggle when reports of pain do not appear commensurate with identifiable physical pathology [18]. Prior to the development of the biopsychosocial model, physicians and researchers relied predominantly on a biomedical approach, which ascribes the etiology of disease, including pain, to biologic factors [17]. It was widely accepted among practitioners that the scope of the traditional biomedical model was too narrow to adequately address the complex processes that contribute to the condition of chronic pain [17]. A history of psycholosocial research has demonstrated the importance of emotional, behavioral, and cognitive factors that contribute to the perpetuation, and possibly the development, of chronic pain [19]. The authors propose that the biopsychosocial model represents the best current approach, one that is broader and better suited to address the multifaceted nature of pain, toward understanding and addressing chronic pain as an illness. The development of interdisciplinary pain management programs is largely attributable to the adoption by physicians of the biopsychosocial model to treat pain.

The evidence for the effectiveness of interdisciplinary pain management programs is substantial. For instance, Mayer, Gatchel *et al.* [20] conducted a two-year prospective study comparing participants of an interdisciplinary functional restoration group to a standard treatment group. At two years, 87% of participants in the treatment group had returned to work compared to 41% of the control group. Furthermore, individuals in the treatment group had twice as many surgeries and significantly more health care visits. Similar results on the effectiveness of interdisciplinary treatment have been found in the U.S. and abroad [21–25]. In an investigation of the efficacy of multidisciplinary pain centers (MPCs), Turk and Okifuji [26] concluded that, not only does the MPC approach yield better results for patients in terms of the reduction in pain, emotional distress, and the use of analgesic medication as compared to alternative medical and surgical treatment options, MPCs can also save billions of dollars in health care expenditures. From an intervention perspective, the biopsychosocial approach emphasizes the importance of treating the initiating and maintaining biological and psychosocial factors of chronic pain. From an assessment perspective, the biopsychosocial approach emphasizes the understanding of the biological, emotional, social, and cultural contributors to pain and defines success, broadly, as adequate functioning in these areas. Therefore, the authors propose that the biopsychosocial model represents the best theoretical framework for determining who benefits from COT.

3. Opioids to Treat Chronic Pain

According to the Centers for Disease Control and Prevention (CDC) [27], "In 2012, health care providers wrote 259 million prescriptions for opioid pain medication, enough for every adult in the United States to have a bottle of pills" (p. 1). Currently, evidence exists for pain relief from opioid therapy for short periods of time (approximately 16 weeks) [27]. For instance, Furlan, Sandoval *et al.* [28] evaluated 41 randomized control trials that investigated the effectiveness of opioids for a variety of pain conditions over a 5- to 16-week period and found that opioids outperformed placebos with regard to pain and functioning for individuals with neuropathic pain and fibromyalgia. Kalso, Edwards *et al.* [29] found similar results for the short-term use of opioids for musculoskeletal pain and neuropathic pain. More recently, Sander-Kiesling [30] followed 379 participants for one year in an open-label study after the conclusion of a randomized control trial and reported continued effectiveness of the combination of prolonged release oxycodone and naloxone.

With regard to the development of addiction, Noble, Treadwell *et al.* [31] reviewed 26 studies, which consisted of a single randomized controlled trial and 25 long-term, uncontrolled trials. The authors noted that only 0.27% of the participants demonstrated evidence of addiction. Although the evidence was rated as "weak," individuals who tolerated opioids showed clinically significant pain relief [31]. In a comprehensive review of the literature, only 3.27% of individuals with chronic pain were reported as developing abuse or addiction after exposures to COT, and approximately 12% of the studies reviewed found aberrant drug related behavior with regard to prescribed opioids [32]. However, limited research has been conducted to examine which individuals are likely to benefit from COT with more attention being given to who is at risk for addiction or pain medication misuse.

Opioid prescription use has grown more controversial among physicians, elected officials, and the public in light of potentially harmful effects, primarily including physical dependence and psychological addiction [1]. Furthermore, there has been a rise in recent years in opioid abuse, between 1999 and 2012, the CDC estimates there was a 300% increase in overdose deaths related to opioids [8]. The CDC estimates that for every death in 2010 resulting from opioid overdose, there were: 733 nonmedical users of opioids, 108 people with abuse/dependence on opioids, 26 emergency room visits related to opioid misuse or abuse and 10 opioid abuse treatment admissions [8].

In addition to the risk of abuse, other common side effects of opioid use include sedation, dizziness, nausea, vomiting, constipation, physical dependence, tolerance, and respiratory depression [33]. Factors that have been shown to put patients at a higher risk for opioid abuse include being under

65 years of age, having a previous history of opioid abuse, people taking high daily doses of opioids, low socioeconomic status and those living in rural areas, Medicaid populations, patients with a history of depression, anxiety, posttraumatic stress disorder or childhood sexual abuse, and those taking psychotropic medications, other central nervous system depressants, or illicit drugs [8,34].

Beyond addiction, COT has been associated with unintentional overdose, fractures, myocardial infraction, endocrinological changes, and motor vehicle accidents [7]. For instance, a cohort study of 9940 individuals receiving COT for CNCP identified 51 opioid overdoses and six deaths [35]. Risk of overdose increased by prescribed dose, with individuals on greater than 100 mg morphine equivalent having a 1.8% annual overdose rate. Increased risk of fractures was found to be greater for individuals prescribed opioids [36], and individuals prescribed 20 mg morphine equivalent or greater were at higher risk of motor vehicle accidents [37]. Despite these findings, the question remains as to who may benefit from COT.

3.1. Does Anyone Benefit from Chronic Opioid Therapy?

Although research citing the risks associated with COT is abundant, there is also a consensus that opioids may be a beneficial aspect of treatment for some individuals with chronic pain [6]. Studies have indicated that patients with specific types of pain, including osteoarthritis pain, diabetic neuropathy pain, and low back pain, may benefit from controlled COT [38]. Several factors have been identified as contributing to the success of long-term opioid use for this select group of chronic pain patients, including appropriate informed consent and development of an individualized opioid management plan, proper initiation and titration of medication, careful monitoring throughout treatment including dose escalations, and management of breakthrough pain [6,39]. Indeed, the American Pain Society has issued clinical guidelines to assist physicians in prescribing chronic opioid therapy for CNCP [6]. Although the guidelines are useful once a physician has decided upon opioid use as an appropriate treatment method, limited evidence exists to pre-identify which particular chronic pain patients may benefit from COT.

3.2. The Case for Inclusive Screening Measures

As a result of the increasing prevalence of opioid abuse and related complications and deaths, a number of measures have been developed to assist providers in identifying those chronic pain patients at a higher risk for opioid abuse or misuse. Such measures include the Screening Instrument for Substance Abuse Potential [40], the Prescription Abuse Checklist [41], the Prescription Drug Use Questionnaire [42], the Pain Assessment and Documentation Tool [43], and the Pain Medication Questionnaire [4]. The Screener and Opioid Assessment for Patients with Pain (SOAPP) and its revised version, the SOAPP-R, were developed to assess suitability of COT for patients with chronic pain based on the similar goal of identifying and excluding those patients most at risk for substance abuse [5]. Although all of these instruments may be effective to varying degrees at identifying which patients have a higher likelihood of abusing opioids, they all may be viewed as exclusion measures such that they are meant to identify those patients who should be excluded from opioid treatment. One of the inherent limitations of these measures is that, while they identify (with varying degrees of accuracy) those patients that should be excluded from opioid therapy, the implicit conclusion is that any patients not at risk for abuse are equally suitable candidates for this form of treatment. The authors argue, based on the review of the literature and clinical observations by those in the pain management field, that individuals who benefit physically, emotionally, and socially from COT can be identified. Furthermore, we propose that identification of these individuals goes beyond excluding those who are at risk for opioid misuse. We propose that an ideal candidate for COT would present with no evidence of aberrant opioid use, maintain good social and occupational functioning, experience manageable levels of pain, and engage in adaptive emotional regulation. Exclusion screening measures, while useful, are insufficient to differentiate among chronic pain patients. Currently, there does not exist an inclusion measure, or cohesive set of predictive factors, meant to identify patients who would likely benefit from COT.

Operationalizing what is considered a positive outcome for any intervention for chronic pain is complicated. Pain is not only a sensory experience, but also impacts physical, emotional, and social functioning. The Initiative on Methods, Measurement and Pain Assessment in Clinical Trials (IMMPACT) has attempted to address this issue. Six core domains were identified: (a) pain; (b) physical functioning; (c) emotional functioning; (d) self-report ratings of improvement and satisfaction; (e) symptoms and adverse events; and (f) participant disposition [44]. The first five domains appear to be directly applicable to the determining success of COT. Although the extent of improvements needed in each domain is beyond the scope of this article, IMMPACT recommendations recommend improvements of at least 30% in pain and improvements, or return to normative levels, in physical and emotional functioning [45]. In general, individuals with chronic pain on opioids for long-term use would ideally have lower levels of pain as well as intact physical, emotional, social, and occupational functioning.

3.3. Developing Inclusion Measures: The Biopsychosocial Approach as a Foundation

As the biopsychosocial approach is considered to be an effective model for the treatment of chronic pain [12], it represents the most comprehensive foundation from which to design screening tools [12]. The goal of such a measure would be to obtain, from multiple sources (*i.e.*, patients, laboratory tests, *etc.*), the biological, psychological, and social factors that we hypothesize might contribute to successful long-term opioid therapy. We define "successful" long-term opioid therapy to include the following: a reduction in perceived pain level and associated physical symptoms (biological); improved, or maintained, social or occupational functioning (social); and active coping and adaptive emotional regulation (psychological).

4. Potential Inclusion Factors

Although one factor may not capture those who may benefit, a combination of factors may be useful. Furthermore, inclusion screening tools are not suggested to be used in place of exclusion tools, but rather as a complement. Another potential shift may need to occur with regard to the development of inclusion screening tools, namely, a shift from more "state"-like factors to those that are more "trait"-like in nature. State-like factors by definition are transitory and heavily influenced by changes in the environment, such as a shift in affect after a positive experience. Trait-like factors, although modifiable, remain relatively more stable over time, such as a tendency to work diligently in many areas of one's life [46]. Early in the development of exclusion screening tools, an emphasis was placed on current and past substance use, current and past depressive and anxiety symptoms, and legal history, along with other state and trait factors [3,4]. States and traits were often conflated in these measures. Problems arose, as depression and anxiety are often natural consequences of pain, even in individuals without a previous history of these difficulties [47,48]. For an inclusion measure, an emphasis on trait-like characteristics may help to ameliorate the concern for fluctuating mental and emotional states.

Below is an initial attempt to describe some of the potential factors for future research into who may benefit from COT.

4.1. Biological

Unlike the measures designed to detect opioid misuse, biological factors may outweigh psychosocial factors in determining who may benefit from opioids. For instance, identifying those individuals who are at low risk of opioid abuse or who develop tolerance more slowly may best be determined under the biological heading of the biopsychosocial approach.

4.1.1. Pain Condition

Previous evidence suggests that individuals who have failed non-opioid interventions and experience moderate to severe pain may be appropriate for long-term opioid use [6,29,30,49]. Individuals with arthritic, musculoskeletal, and neuropathic chronic pain, with limited psychosocial overlay, and in the absence of established opioid misuse risk factors, may constitute a minimal threshold that could be combined with remaining factors to determine who may benefit from COT [6].

4.1.2. Genetic Factors

With the advent of more sophisticated and cost-effective techniques for genetic testing, the potential for identifying those who may benefit from COT has increased. Evidence from twin and adoption research points to a heritable vulnerability for opioid dependence [50]. For instance, Tsuang, Bar *et al.* [51] concluded that genetic factors accounted for 34% of the variance of drug use with a moderate contribution (43%) to opioid dependence.

Evidence for the role of genetic polymorphisms is still in the early, but expanding, stages of investigation. Several potential polymorphisms have been identified that are related to opioids, including A118G, DRD2, DRD4, OPRM1, OPRD1, OPRK1, and BDNF, to name only a few [51,52]. For example, the single nucleotide polymorphism (SNP) A118G, associated with the μ opioid receptor, appears to decrease the effectiveness of morphine [52]; genes related to the cytochrome P450 (CYP450) system of the liver, CYP2D6 polymorphisms, impact metabolization of codeine [53]; and the SNP UGT2B7, associated with UDP-glucuronosyltransferases, has been found to correlate with morphine metabolization [54].

Along with the study of genetic polymorphisms, genome-wide linkage studies provide another opportunity to examine the genetics of opioid use. Gelernter, Panhuysen *et al.* [54] evaluated 393 related individuals with a minimum of one family member who met criteria for opioid dependence. The investigators concluded that the evidence "strongly supports a risk locus for a trait defined by symptoms related to heavy opioid use on chromosome 17" (p. 764).

4.2. Psychological

Potential psychological and social factors that could be examined have been explored in other populations and serve as protective factors against the impact of stress on physical, emotional, and social functioning. The authors do not propose that these factors would improve the efficacy of COT, but rather would decrease the chances of engaging in maladapative coping, such as aberrant drug behavior, avoidance of social activity, and a limiting of self-care activities (e.g., exercise). As COT has the potential to negatively impact mood and cognition [55,56], identifying and studying protective factors against such outcomes is warranted.

4.2.1. Resiliency

Resiliency has been defined as a "dynamic process encompassing positive adaptation within the context of significant adversity" [57] (p. 543), and it represents an ideal candidate factor for who may benefit from COT. The research on resiliency spans over 40 years, and the validity of this construct serving as a protective factor in the face of stress or adversity is well established [58]. For example, resiliency was found to relate to lower pain and lower negative affect over time among individuals with chronic pain [59]. Although more research is needed, resiliency within the context of chronic pain may be one factor to be considered regarding whom may benefit from COT.

4.2.2. Personality

The Big Five personality traits offer another area of potential variables that point to who may benefit from COT. The Big Five traits have a strong evidence basis with regard to the validity of the constructs and continued predictive value of individuals' behavior over time [46].

For instance, higher levels of neuroticism have been associated with higher levels of pain and lower levels of functioning [60]. Furthermore, higher scores on extraversion [61], openness [62], and conscientiousness [63] have been found to be related to more active coping among individuals with chronic pain. With the exception of neuroticism, which could be seen as an exclusion factor, extraversion, openness, and conscientiousness represent potential inclusion factors.

4.3. Social

4.3.1. Social Support

The concept of social support is a widely recognized mediating factor with regard to stress [64] and represents another potential inclusive factor regarding who may benefit from COT. An intact social support system, as well as an ability to make use of that support system, decreases the negative impact of stress, both physically and emotionally [65]. In a study with 78 rheumatoid arthritis patients who were followed for five years, the authors concluded that low levels of social support impacted disability and pain levels over the course of a five-year period [66]. However, social support should be considered one factor, and it is quite possible that individuals with limited social support could benefit from COT.

4.3.2. Employment

The nature and context of employment may also play a role in the determination of who benefits from COT. Employment serves as a stabilizing force with regard to identity and socioeconomic stress [67]. Although much has been written about the negative impact of the loss of one's job or the potentially damaging effects of the workers' compensation or disability systems [67], a relevant construct in this area relates to "secondary loss" [68]. Specifically, this concept refers to the types of losses that occur when employment is lost or significantly diminished. Furthermore, research provides evidence for the health benefits of employment [69], and this broad area provides several potential inclusion factors concerning who may benefit from COT, including job satisfaction and stability of employment. As with social support, this area requires further research and individuals who are unemployed after a work-related injury may benefit from COT.

5. Directions for Future Research and Conclusions

This review article has attempted to present an alternative perspective on the question of opioid misuse risk with the goal of spurring additional research into who may benefit from COT. We propose that focusing on opioid misuse risk may inadvertently lead to the assumption that individuals who are not at high risk of misusing opioids would therefore benefit from COT. Identifying those at risk and those who benefit can be seen as complementary areas of inquiry. Additional research is needed to: (a) operationalize what constitutes a positive outcome for individuals on COT; (b) identify and evaluate those who have been maintained on low doses of opioids with good pain control and functioning; and (c) prospectively evaluate potential biological, psychological, and social factors that may predict who benefits from COT. Although qualitative research is often disparaged by those engaged in quantitative research efforts, the importance of qualitative research cannot be understated in a nascent area of study with regard to generating a hypothesis for future quantitative evaluation. We argue that this line of investigation would benefit from both qualitative and quantitative research endeavors in the future.

Acknowledgments: The Eugene McDermott Center for Pain Management was endowed in 1993 at the University of Texas Southwestern Medical Center through a gift from the Biological Humanics Foundation. The staff at the center are grateful for the continued generosity and support from Mrs. Eugene McDermott and Mary McDermott Cook.

Author Contributions: Elizabeth Huber engaged in the majority of manuscript preparation, including researching chronic opioid therapy and potential factors that may guide selection of who benefits from long-term opioid therapy. Richard C. Robinson reviewed, edited and expanded upon the research discussed in this manuscript by the first author. Carl E. Noe originally developed the idea regarding who may benefit from chronic opioid therapy and was instrumental in the review and preparation of the manuscript. Olivia Van Ness reviewed, edited and expanded upon the essential elements of the manuscript.

Conflicts of Interest: The authors declare no conflict of interest.

References

1. Catan, T.; Perez, E. A Pain-Drug Champion Has Second Thoughts. Available online: http://www.thblack.com/links/RSD/A%20Pain-Drug%20Champion%20Has%20Second%20Thoughts%20-%20WSJ.pdf (accessed on 17 December 2012).
2. Bennett, D.S.; Carr, D.B. Opiophobia as a barrier to the treatment of pain. *J. Pain Palliat. Care Pharmacother.* **2002**, *16*, 105–109. [CrossRef] [PubMed]
3. Robinson, R.C.; Gatchel, R.J.; Polatin, P.B.; Deschner, M.; Gajraj, N.; Noe, C. Screening for problematic opioid behavior. *Clin. J. Pain* **2001**, *17*, 220–228. [CrossRef] [PubMed]
4. Adams, L.L.; Gatchel, R.J.; Robinson, R.C.; Polatin, P.; Gajraj, N.; Deschner, M.; Noe, C. Development of a self-report screening instrument for assessing potential opioid medication misuse in chronic pain patients. *J. Pain Symptom Manag.* **2004**, *27*, 440–459. [CrossRef] [PubMed]
5. Butler, S.F.; Fernandez, K.; Benoit, C.; Budman, S.H.; Jamison, R.N. Validation of the revised screener and opioid assessment for patients with pain (SOAPP-R). *Pain* **2008**, *9*, 360–372. [CrossRef] [PubMed]
6. Chou, R.; Fanciullo, G.J.; Fine, P.G.; Adler, J.A.; Ballantyne, J.C.; Davies, P.; Donovan, M.I.; Fishbain, D.A.; Foley, K.M.; Fudin, J. Clinical guidelines for the use of chronic opioid therapy in chronic noncancer pain. *Pain* **2009**, *10*, 113–130. [CrossRef] [PubMed]
7. Chou, R.; Turner, J.A.; Devine, E.B.; Hansen, R.N.; Sullivan, S.D.; Blazina, I.; Dana, T.; Bougatsos, C.; Deyo, R.A. The effectiveness and risks of long-term opioid therapy for chronic pain: A systematic review for a national institutes of health pathways to prevention workshop. *Ann. Intern. Med.* **2015**, *162*, 276–286. [CrossRef] [PubMed]
8. CDC (Center for Disease Control and Prevention). Opioid Painkiller Prescribing. Available online: http://www.cdc.gov/vitalsigns/opioid-prescribing/ (accessed on 17 July 2015).
9. IASP (International Association for the Study of Pain). Part III: Pain terms, a current list with defitions and notes on usage. In *Classifications of Chronic Pain*; Merskey, H., Bogduk, N., Eds.; IASP Press: Seattle, WA, USA, 1994; pp. 209–214.
10. Turk, D.C. IASP taxonomy of chronic pain syndromes: Preliminary assessment of reliability. *Pain* **1987**, *30*, 177–189. [CrossRef]
11. Institute of Medicine of the National Academy of Science. *Relieving Pain in America: A Blueprint for Transforming Prevention, Care, Education, and Research*; National Academies Press: Washington, DC, USA, 2011.
12. Gatchel, R.J.; Peng, Y.B.; Peters, M.L.; Fuchs, P.N.; Turk, D.C. The biopsychosocial approach to chronic pain: Scientific advances and future directions. *Psychol. Bull.* **2007**, *133*, 581–624. [CrossRef] [PubMed]
13. Gatchel, R.J. *Clinical Essentials of Pain Management*; American Psychological Association: Washington, DC, USA, 2005.
14. Stewart, W.F.; Ricci, J.A.; Chee, E.; Morganstein, D.; Lipton, R. Lost productive time and cost due to common pain conditions in the us workforce. *JAMA* **2003**, *290*, 2443–2454. [CrossRef] [PubMed]
15. Gaskin, D.J.; Richard, P. The economic costs of pain in the United States. *Pain* **2012**, *13*, 715–724. [CrossRef] [PubMed]
16. Cohen, J.W.; Monheit, A.C.; Beauregard, K.M.; Cohen, S.B.; Lefkowitz, D.C.; Potter, D.E.; Sommers, J.P.; Taylor, A.K.; Arnett, R.H., 3rd. The medical expenditure panel survey: A national health information resource. *Inquiry* **1996**, *33*, 373–389. [PubMed]
17. Gatchel, R.J.; Turk, D.C. Criticisms of the biopsychosocial model in spine care: Creating and then attacking a straw person. *Spine* **2008**, *33*, 2831–2836. [CrossRef] [PubMed]
18. Gatchel, R.J.; Turk, D.C. *Psychological Approaches to Pain Management: A Practitioner's Handbook*; The Guilford Press: New York, NY, USA, 1996.
19. Kerns, R.D.; Sellinger, J.; Goodin, B.R. Psychological treatment of chronic pain. *Ann. Rev. Clin. Psychol.* **2011**, *7*, 411–434. [CrossRef] [PubMed]

20. Mayer, T.G.; Gatchel, R.J.; Mayer, H.; Kishino, N.; Kelley, J.; Mooney, V.A. Prospective two-year study of functional restoration in industrial low back pain. *J. Am. Med. Assoc.* **1987**, *258*, 1181–1182. [CrossRef]

21. Hazard, R.G.; Fenwick, J.W.; Kalisch, S.M.; Redmond, J.; Reeves, V.; Frymoyer, J.W. Functional restoration: A one-year prospective study of patients with low back pain. *Spine* **1989**, *14*, 157–161. [CrossRef] [PubMed]

22. Patrick, L.; Altmaier, E.; Found, E. Long-term outcomes in multidisciplinary treatmetn of chronic low back pain: Results of a 13-year follow-up. *Spine* **2004**, *29*, 850–855. [CrossRef] [PubMed]

23. Bendix, A.E.; Bendix, T.; Vaegter, K.; Lund, C.; Frolund, L.; Holm, L. Multidisciplinary intensive treatment for chronic low back pain: A randomized, prospective study. *Clevel. Clin. J. Med.* **1996**, *63*, 62–69. [CrossRef]

24. Hildebrandt, J.; Pfingsten, M.; Saur, P.; Jansen, J. Prediction of success from a multidisciplinary treatment program for chronic low back pain. *Pain* **1997**, *22*, 990–1001. [CrossRef]

25. Oslund, S.; Robinson, R.C.; Clark, T.C.; Garofalo, J.P.; Behnk, P.; Walker, B.; Walker, K.E.; Gatchel, R.J.; Mahaney, M.; Noe, C.E. Long-term effectiveness of a comprehensive pain management program: Strengthening the case for interdisciplinary care. *Proc. Bayl. Univ. Med. Cent.* **2011**, *22*, 211–214.

26. Turk, D.C.; Okifuji, A. Treatment of chronic pain patients: Clinical outcomes, cost-effectiveness, and cost-benefits of multidisciplinary pain centers. *Crit. Rev. Phys. Rehabil. Med.* **1998**, *10*, 181–208. [CrossRef]

27. Manchikanti, L.; Vallejo, R.; Manchikanti, K.N.; Benyamin, R.M.; Datta, S.; Christo, P.J. Effectiveness of long-term opioid therapy for chronic non-cancer pain. *Pain Phys.* **2011**, *14*, E133–E156.

28. Furlan, A.; Chaparro, L.E.; Irvin, E.; Mailis-Gagnon, A. A comparison between enriched and nonenriched enrollment randomized withdrawal trials of opioids for chronic noncancer pain. *Pain Res. Manag.* **2011**, *16*, 337–351. [CrossRef] [PubMed]

29. Kalso, E.; Edwards, J.E.; Moore, R.A.; McQuay, H.J. Opioids in chronic non-cancer pain: Systematic review of efficacy and safety. *Pain* **2004**, *112*, 372–380. [CrossRef] [PubMed]

30. Sandner-Kiesling, A.; Leyendecker, P.; Hopp, M.; Tarau, L.; Lejcko, J.; Meissner, W.; Sevcik, P.; Hakl, M.; Hrib, R.; Uhl, R.; *et al.* Long-term efficacy and safety of combined prolonged-release oxycodone and naloxone in the management of non-cancer chronic pain. *Int. J. Clin. Pract.* **2010**, *64*, 763–774. [CrossRef] [PubMed]

31. Noble, M.; Treadwell, J.R.; Tregear, S.J.; Coates, V.H.; Wiffen, P.J.; Akafomo, C.; Schoelles, K.M. Long-term opioid management for chronic noncancer pain. *Cochrane Database Syst. Rev.* **2010**. [CrossRef]

32. Fishbain, D.A.; Cole, B.; Lewis, J.; Rosomoff, H.L.; Rosomoff, R.S. What percentage of chronic nonmalignant pain patients exposed to chronic opioid analgesic therapy develop abuse/addiction and/or aberrant drug-related behaviors? A structured evidence-based review. *Pain Med.* **2008**, *9*, 444–459. [CrossRef] [PubMed]

33. Ricardo Buenaventura, M.; Rajive Adlaka, M.; Nalini Sehgal, M. Opioid complications and side effects. *Pain Physician* **2008**, *11*, S105–S120.

34. Boscarino, J.A.; Rukstalis, M.; Hoffman, S.N.; Han, J.J.; Erlich, P.M.; Gerhard, G.S.; Stewart, W.F. Risk factors for drug dependence among out-patients on opioid therapy in a large us health-care system. *Addiction* **2010**, *105*, 1776–1782. [CrossRef] [PubMed]

35. Dunn, K.M.; Saunders, K.W.; Rutter, C.M.; Banta-Green, C.J.; Merrill, J.O.; Sullivan, M.D.; Weisner, C.M.; Silverberg, M.J.; Campbell, C.I.; Psaty, B.M.; *et al.* Opioid prescriptions for chronic pain and overdose: A cohort study. *Ann. Intern. Med.* **2010**, *152*, 85–92. [CrossRef] [PubMed]

36. Li, L.; Setoguchi, S.; Cabral, H.; Jick, S. Opioid use for noncancer pain and risk of fracture in adults: A nested case-control study using the general practice research database. *Am. J. Epidemiol.* **2013**, *178*, 559–569. [CrossRef] [PubMed]

37. Gomes, T.; Redelmeier, D.A.; Juurlink, D.N.; Dhalla, I.A.; Camacho, X.; Mamdani, M.M. Opioid dose and risk of road trauma in canada: A population-based study. *JAMA Intern. Med.* **2013**, *173*, 196–201. [CrossRef] [PubMed]

38. Portenoy, R.K.; Farrar, J.T.; Backonja, M.-M.; Cleeland, C.S.; Yang, K.; Friedman, M.; Colucci, S.V.; Richards, P. Long-term use of controlled-release oxycodone for noncancer pain: Results of a 3-year registry study. *Clin. J. Pain* **2007**, *23*, 287–299. [CrossRef] [PubMed]

39. Ashburn, M.A.; Staats, P.S. Management of chronic pain. *Lancet* **1999**, *353*, 1865–1869. [CrossRef]

40. Coambs, R.; Jarry, J.; Santhiapillai, A.; Abrahamsohn, R.; Atance, C. The sisap: A new screening instrument for identifying potential opioid abusers in the management of chronic nonmalignant pain within general medical practice. *Pain Res. Manag.* **1996**, *1*, 155–162. [CrossRef]

41. Chabal, C.; Erjavec, M.K.; Jacobson, L.; Mariano, A.; Chaney, E. Prescription opiate abuse in chronic pain patients: Clinical criteria, incidence, and predictors. *Clin. J. Pain* **1997**, *13*, 150–155. [CrossRef] [PubMed]

42. Compton, P.; Darakjian, J.; Miotto, K. Screening for addiction in patients with chronic pain and "problematic" substance use: Evaluation of a pilot assessment tool. *J. Pain Symptom Manag.* **1998**, *16*, 355–363. [CrossRef]

43. Passik, S.D.; Kirsh, K.L.; Whitcomb, L.; Portenoy, R.K.; Katz, N.P.; Kleinman, L.; Dodd, S.L.; Schein, J.R. A new tool to assess and document pain outcomes in chronic pain patients receiving opioid therapy. *Clin. Ther.* **2004**, *26*, 552–561. [CrossRef]

44. Turk, D.C.; Dworkin, R.H.; Allen, R.R.; Bellamy, N.; Brandenburg, N.; Carr, D.B.; Cleeland, C.; Dionne, R.; Farrar, J.T.; Galer, B.S.; *et al.* Core outcome domains for chronic pain clinical trials: Immpact recommendations. *Pain* **2003**, *106*, 337–345. [CrossRef] [PubMed]

45. Dworkin, R.H.; Turk, D.C.; Farrar, J.T.; Haythornthwaite, J.A.; Jensen, M.P.; Katz, N.P.; Kerns, R.D.; Stucki, G.; Allen, R.R.; Bellamy, N.; *et al.* Core outcome measures for chronic pain clinical trials: Immpact recommendations. *Pain* **2005**, *113*, 9–19. [CrossRef] [PubMed]

46. John, O.P.; Robins, R.W.; Pervin, L.A. *Handbook of Personality, Third Edition: Theory and Research*, 3rd ed.; The Guilford Press: New York, NY, USA, 2008.

47. Fishbain, D.A.; Cutler, R.B.; Rosomoff, H.L.; Rosomoff, R.S. Chronic-pain associated depressions: Antecedt or consequence of chronic pain? *Clin. J. Pain* **1997**, *13*, 116–137. [CrossRef] [PubMed]

48. Staats, P.S. Pain, depression and survival. *Am. Fam. Physician* **1999**, *60*, 42–43. [PubMed]

49. Furlan, A.D.; Reardon, R.; Weppler, C. Opioids for chronic noncancer pain: A new canadian practice guideline. *CMAJ* **2010**, *182*, 923–930. [CrossRef] [PubMed]

50. Mistry, C.J.; Bawor, M.; Desai, D.; Marsh, D.C.; Samaan, Z. Genetics of opioid dependence: A review of the genetic contribution to opioid dependence. *Curr. Psychiatry Rev.* **2014**, *10*, 156–167. [CrossRef] [PubMed]

51. Tsuang, M.T.; Bar, J.L.; Harley, R.M.; Lyons, M.J. The harvard twin study of substance abuse: What we have learned. *Harv. Rev. Psychiatry* **2001**, *9*, 267–279. [CrossRef] [PubMed]

52. Lotsch, J.; Oertel, B.G.; Ultsch, A. Human models of pain for the prediction of clinical analgesia. *Pain* **2014**, *155*, 2014–2021. [CrossRef] [PubMed]

53. Sadhasivam, S.; Chidambaran, V. Pharmacogenomics of opioids and perioperative pain management. *Pharmacogenomics* **2012**, *13*, 1719–1740. [CrossRef] [PubMed]

54. Gelernter, J.; Panhuysen, C.; Wilcox, M.; Hesselbrock, V.; Rounsaville, B.; Poling, J.; Weiss, R.; Sonne, S.; Zhao, H.; Farrer, L.; *et al.* Genomewide linkage scan for opioid dependence and related traits. *Am. J. Hum. Genet.* **2006**, *78*, 759–769. [CrossRef] [PubMed]

55. Merrill, J.O.; Von Korff, M.; Banta-Green, C.J.; Sullivan, M.D.; Saunders, K.W.; Campbell, C.I.; Weisner, C. Prescribed opioid difficulties, depression and opioid dose among chronic opioid therapy patients. *Gen. Hosp. Psychiatry* **2012**, *34*, 581–587. [CrossRef] [PubMed]

56. Sjogren, P.; Thomsen, A.B.; Olsen, A.K. Impaired neuropsychological performance in chronic nonmalignant pain patients receiving long-term oral opioid therapy. *J. Pain Symptom Manag.* **2000**, *19*, 100–108. [CrossRef]

57. Luthar, S.S.; Cicchetti, D.; Becker, B. The construct of resilience: A critical evaluation and guidelines for future work. *Child Dev.* **2000**, *71*, 543–562. [CrossRef] [PubMed]

58. Slepian, P.M.; Ankawi, B.; Himawan, L.K.; France, C.R. Development and initial validation of the pain reslience scale. *J. Pain* **2016**, *17*, 462–472. [CrossRef] [PubMed]

59. Zautra, A.J.; Johnson, L.M.; Davis, M.C. Positive affect as a source of resilience for women in chronic pain. *J. Consult. Clin. Psychol.* **2005**, *73*, 212–220. [CrossRef] [PubMed]

60. Goodwin, R.D.; Cox, B.J.; Clara, I. Neuroticism and physical disorders among adults in the community: Results from the national comorbidity survey. *J. Behav. Med.* **2006**, *29*, 229–238. [CrossRef] [PubMed]

61. Ramirez-Maestre, C.; Lopez Martinez, A.E.; Zarazaga, R.E. Personality characteristics as differential variables of the pain experience. *J. Behav. Med.* **2004**, *27*, 147–165. [CrossRef] [PubMed]

62. Nitch, S.R.; Boone, K.B. Normal personality correlates of chronic pain subgroups. *J. Clin. Psychol. Med. Settings* **2004**, *11*, 203–209. [CrossRef]

63. Bolger, N. Coping as a personality process: A prospective study. *J. Pers. Soc. Psychol.* **1990**, *59*, 525–537. [CrossRef] [PubMed]

64. Cohen, S.; Wills, T.A. Stress, social support, and the buffering hypothesis. *Psychol. Bull.* **1985**, *98*, 310–357. [CrossRef] [PubMed]

65. Field, R.J.; Schuldberg, D. Social-support moderated stress: A nonlinear dynamical model and the stress-buffering hypothesis. *Nonlinear Dyn. Psychol. Life Sci.* **2011**, *15*, 53–85.

66. Evers, A.W.M.; Kraaimaat, F.W.; Geenen, R.; Jacobs, J.W.G.; Bijlsma, J.W.J. Pain coping and social support as predictors of long-term functional disability and pain in early rheumatoid arthritis. *Behav. Res. Threapy* **2003**, *41*, 1295–1310. [CrossRef]

67. Robinson, R.C.; Garofalo, J.P. Workers' compensation and other disability insurance systems involved in occupational musculoskeletal disorders. In *Handbook of Musculoskeletal Pain and Disability Disorders in the Workplace*; Gatchel, R.J., Schultz, I.S., Eds.; Springer-Verlag: New York, NY, USA, 2014.

68. Gatchel, R.J.; Adams, L.; Polatin, P.B.; Kishino, N.D. Secondary loss and pain-associated disability: Theoretical overview and treatment implications. *J. Occup. Rehabil.* **2002**, *12*, 99–110. [CrossRef] [PubMed]

69. Modini, M.; Joyce, S.; Mykletun, A.; Christensen, H.; Bryant, R.A.; Mitchell, P.B.; Harvey, S.B. The mental health benefits of employment: Results of a systematic meta-review. *Australas. Psychiatry* **2016**. [CrossRef] [PubMed]

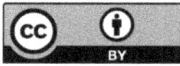

healthcare

MDPI

Article

Military Chronic Musculoskeletal Pain and Psychiatric Comorbidity: Is Better Pain Management the Answer?

Cindy A. McGeary [1], Donald D. McGeary [1,*], Jose Moreno [1] and Robert J. Gatchel [2]

[1] Department of Psychiatry, The University of Texas Health Science Center at San Antonio, San Antonio, TX 78229, USA; mcgearyc@uthscsa.edu (C.A.M.); morenojl@uthscsa.edu (J.M.)
[2] Department of Psychology, The University of Texas at Arlington, Arlington, TX 76019, USA; gatchel@uta.edu
*   Correspondence: mcgeary@uthscsa.edu; Tel.: +1-210-562-6700

Academic Editor: Sampath Parthasarathy
Received: 4 March 2016; Accepted: 27 June 2016; Published: 30 June 2016

Abstract: Chronic musculoskeletal pain, such as low back pain, often appears in the presence of psychiatric comorbidities (e.g., depression, posttraumatic stress disorder (PTSD)), especially among U.S. military service members serving in the post-9/11 combat era. Although there has been much speculation about how to best address pain/trauma psychiatric symptom comorbidities, there are little available data to guide practice. The present study sought to examine how pre-treatment depression and PTSD influence outcomes in a functional restoration pain management program using secondary analysis of data from the Department of Defense-funded Functional and Orthopedic Rehabilitation Treatment (FORT) trial. Twenty-eight FORT completers were analyzed using a general linear model exploring how well depression and PTSD symptoms predict post-treatment pain (Visual Analog Scale (VAS) pain rating), disability (Oswestry Disability Index; Million Visual Analog Scale), and functional capacity (Floor-to-Waist and Waist-to-Eye Level progressive isoinertial lifting evaluation scores) in a sample of active duty military members with chronic musculoskeletal pain and comorbid depression or PTSD symptoms. Analysis revealed that pre-treatment depression and PTSD symptoms did not significantly predict rehabilitation outcomes from program completers. Implications of these findings for future research on trauma-related pain comorbidities are discussed.

Keywords: chronic musculoskeletal pain; low back pain; psychiatric comorbidities; PTSD; depression; military service members

1. Introduction

The comorbidity between chronic musculoskeletal pain conditions (such as low back pain) and psychiatric conditions (like depression and posttraumatic stress disorder (PTSD)) has been well documented in the extant research literature; this is especially salient in studies of U.S. military service members who are at increased risk of developing both musculoskeletal pain and psychiatric trauma symptoms during post-9/11 military service [1,2]. Studies of United States military service members have found rates of depression disorders ranging from 10% to 46% [3,4], and PTSD from 2% to 60% [4]. Psychiatric disorder prevalence has been found to be similar between both active duty and reserve military components [5]. Service members with a chronic musculoskeletal pain condition are likely to develop more than one psychiatric comorbidity, and there is good reason to believe that military members with either PTSD or depression develop a vulnerability to the other condition. For example, a 2007 study of military veterans found that 36% of veterans with depression also screened positive for PTSD [6]. This comorbidity may be due to the overlapping symptoms found in both depression and

PTSD. Comorbid depression and PTSD can result in significantly increased risk of suicide in service members with traumatic injuries [7].

Posttraumatic stress disorder and depression are particularly common among individuals with chronic pain conditions. Patients have been found to develop depression secondary to chronic pain [8]. One study of Australian military members found that service members with musculoskeletal pain disorders were at increased risk of mental health-related quality of life (including diagnoses of depression and PTSD) problems [9]. Conversely, individuals with either depression or PTSD are more likely to report severe problems with pain and lower quality-of-life than those without psychiatric conditions [10]. Both PTSD and depression can affect pain in myriad ways. In a randomized controlled trial of 250 veterans, it was found that depression and PTSD had significant independent influence over quality-of-life, psychosocial well-being, and disability in veterans with chronic pain [11]. Some suggest that the comorbidity of PTSD and chronic pain may actually be mediated by depression and facets of anxiety [12] and through feelings of sadness and fear [13], although others suggest that the pain-PTSD comorbidity is mediated through avoidance [14].

Individual treatments for military PTSD, depression, and chronic musculoskeletal pain are well-documented (cf [15]), but there are still fundamental questions about how to best address comorbid pain and psychiatric trauma symptoms. Numerous theories of these comorbidities have been postulated [16], but there is not much evidence to support any of them based on the extant research. Thus, there is little guidance on the best treatment approaches to comorbid trauma pain, and most studies of pain and psychiatric comorbidity emphasize a need for integrated pain and psychosocial intervention to address the complexity of the problem [14,16]. Some small, randomized studies have found promising pain-related outcomes from integrated cognitive and behavioral therapy programs designed to actively address both chronic pain and PTSD [17,18], but there is still not enough evidence to fully support an integrated approach. More information is needed about how PTSD and depression affect functional outcomes in programs designed to specifically address chronic pain (with little to no emphasis on psychiatric comorbidity). Unfortunately, few clinical trials have been developed specifically to meet this purpose, and extant guidance describing the integration between interventions for chronic pain and psychiatric comorbidities are limited "recommendations" without much justification or description for how these services could or should be integrated [16].

The present study is a preliminary attempt to explore the contribution of psychiatric comorbidities to functional pain management outcomes, accomplished through a secondary analysis of the data from the Functional and Orthopedic Rehabilitation Treatment (FORT) pain management program, a randomized clinical trial of military pain management funded by the Department of Defense [19]. The FORT trial was designed to assess the efficacy of a functional restoration pain management program for military service members with chronic pain, but was not designed or powered to specifically assess how psychiatric comorbidities impacted treatment outcomes. However, FORT participants presented with a range of psychiatric comorbidities that were measured as part of the trial and may shed preliminary light on the question of pain and psychiatric comorbidity. In the FORT study, participants were either randomized to treatment-as-usual (TAU) or the FORT program. FORT participants completed a three-week functional restoration based program. Functional restoration programs focus on improving physical functioning through physical reconditioning, psychosocial interventions, and coping skills training. FORT included an interdisciplinary team approach to pain management that included a group-based psychosocial intervention for pain management and coping skills training and a group-based physical therapy program for reconditioning. Over the course of the three weeks, participants attended 12 psychosocial/coping skills group sessions and 12 physical therapy reconditioning group sessions. Treatment-as-usual participants continued to receive military standard of care through their Military Treatment Facility. Participants included U.S. active duty service members with service-related chronic orthopedic pain from all military branches. Basic demographics and outcomes from the FORT study can be found in Gatchel et al. [19]. In preparation for the present secondary analysis, the study team considered the inclusion of both FORT and TAU participant data.

The TAU participants demonstrated little significant change in functional outcomes or psychiatric variables from pre- to post-treatment (or in longer-term follow-up; [19]), but the FORT participants demonstrated significant variability. Because the primary aim of this secondary analysis was to assess systematic change in pain outcomes possibly attributable to pre-treatment psychiatric comorbidity, the study team chose to isolate this preliminary analysis to the participants showing the most change in their outcome data: the FORT participants (all of whom completed the FORT program and are hereafter referred to as FORT completers). Furthermore, because the FORT study was not specifically designed to assess the primary aim of this secondary analysis, the study team chose to limit the preliminary analysis to the pre-treatment to post-treatment interval, forgoing analysis of longer-term outcomes that are more likely to be confounded by unforeseen or unassessed variables influencing the contribution of psychiatric comorbidity to long-term outcomes. FORT completer data were analyzed to address the following hypotheses:

H1: Pre-treatment pain severity (based on visual analog pain ratings) and disability (based on functional capacity evaluation and self-report measure of disability) will be significantly related to pre-treatment depression and PTSD symptoms.

H2: Pre-treatment PTSD will have a significant effect on pre- to post-treatment pain and disability outcomes among FORT completers.

H3: Pre-treatment depression will have a significant effect on pre- to post-treatment pain and disability outcomes among FORT completers.

H4: Depression, but not PTSD symptoms will significantly predict post-treatment pain and disability outcomes among FORT completers.

2. Materials and Methods

2.1. Subjects

This study included a total of 50 active duty military participants spread across all four branches of the military, with a sub-analysis of 28 FORT completers who reported depression and PTSD symptoms at pre-treatment. Details on the FORT intervention can be found in Gatchel et al. [19]. FORT completers were assessed for numerous pain-related psychosocial and physical outcomes. Self-report measures and a functional capacity evaluation were completed at pre-treatment, post-treatment, and 12-month follow-up (although only pre- and post-treatment data are used in the present analysis). Once enrolled, study participants were assigned to one of two treatment groups randomly using a dynamic urn randomization strategy that balanced the groups on age, gender, race/ethnicity, injury site, and time since pain onset. One treatment group received Functional Restoration (FR, $n = 28$) and the other group received treatment-as-usual (TAU, $n = 22$). Review Gatchel et al. for a more in-depth discussion of patient demographics [19].

2.2. Measures

Demographic data, including sex, age, branch of service, race/ethnicity, and duration of pain, were collected. Psychosocial and pain measures selected for this study are commonly used psychosocial assessments with strong validity and reliability. The following measures were administered:

Oswestry Disability Inventory (ODI). The ODI is a 10-item self-report questionnaire that measures the degree of experienced functional impairment due to low back pain an individual is experiencing the day of administration [20]. This measure is considered the gold standard for measuring low back pain related disability, with higher scores indicating greater functional impairment.

Million Visual Analog Scale (MVAS). This measure is a 15-item visual analog measure of pain intensity and disability related to low back pain [21]. The MVAS measures current functioning. This instrument produces a total functional disability score ranging from 0 to 150, with higher scores indicating greater pain intensity and disability. The MVAS assesses body functions, daily activities, and social life.

Beck Depression Inventory (BDI-II). The BDI-II is a widely used self-report inventory used to measure depression symptom severity. The BDI-II consists of 21 items assessing symptoms of depression over a two-week period [22].

PTSD CheckList-Military (PCL-M). Since this paper is based on a secondary analysis of the FORT study, the PCL-M was administered rather than the updated PCL-5. The PCL is a 17-question checklist in which participants are asked to endorse symptoms of PTSD commensurate with those listed in the DSM-IV on a Likert-scale, ranging from 1 to 5. The PCL-M has been supported in the literature as a solid PTSD screening instrument, with good correlation of the overall PCL score to the Clinician-Administered PTSD Scale (CAPS) [23].

36-Item Short Form Health Survey Summary (SF-36). The SF-36 is a 36-item self-report questionnaire measuring 8 dimensions (physical functioning, role limitations due to physical problems, pain, general health perceptions, social functioning, vitality, role limits due to emotional health, and mental health) over a four-week period that contribute to 2 summary scales—the Physical Component and Mental Component Summary Scales [24]. It is a measure of health-related quality-of-life, with higher scores indicating greater functioning.

Visual Analog Scale (VAS). The VAS is a nonverbal self-report assessment of pain severity on a 10-cm line [25]. Each end of the line is anchored by an extreme (i.e., no pain or worst imaginable pain). Participants are asked to report how much pain they are experiencing at the time of administration. Higher scores on the line indicate greater pain severity.

Physical Measures. A modified version of the California Functional Capacity Protocol [26] was used to evaluate human performance, including functional strength using a progressive isoinertial lifting evaluation [27]. This protocol was administered by a physical therapist using standardized tasks. Lifting measures included a weighted box lift from Floor to Waist (FW) and Waist to Eye-Level (WEL).

2.3. Procedures

The FORT study obtained IRB approval from the University of Texas at Arlington and Wilford Hall Medical Center located on Lackland Air Force Base. All applicable ethical standards were followed in accordance with the 1964 Helsinki declaration. The FORT program was a Department of Defense (DoD)-funded study that included an intensive three-week interdisciplinary chronic pain management intervention based on a functional restoration pain model (described above). The intervention included group-based physical therapy, and cognitive-behavioral group therapy focused on increasing overall functioning. Once consent was obtained, participants were randomly assigned to one of two conditions. The treatment conditions consisted of FR treatment or TAU. Study participants were assessed for physical and psychosocial variables associated with chronic pain experience at pretreatment, post-treatment, and one-year follow-up, although only the pre- and post-treatment assessments for FORT completers who reported pre-treatment depression and PTSD symptoms were used in the present analysis.

2.4. Data Analysis

The contribution of psychiatric conditions (depression and PTSD) to post-treatment pain and disability were assessed using general linear models (GLM). To prepare for GLM, pain, disability and psychiatric data were scrutinized for normality to ensure that underlying assumptions of GLM were met. Assessment of linear relationship between the criterion (pain VAS, ODI, MVAS, Lifting) and predictor (depression, PTSD) variables was assessed using a zero-order Pearson product-moment correlation matrix. Relevant demographic variables (gender, age, service branch) were analyzed using ANOVA and correlation (based on data structure) to detect systematic differences in criterion variables that would require inclusion of these variables in GLM as covariates. Pre-treatment scores for the criterion variables were included in all GLM models as covariates.

3. Results

The sample included 28 successful completers of the FORT pain management program who also reported pre-treatment depression and PTSD symptoms. FORT completers were 57% male, and all of the completers were serving in either the United States Air Force (USAF; 82%) or the United States Army (USA; 18%). Approximately 80% of the FORT completers presented with spinal pain as their primary complaint, with low back pain representing the majority of spinal pain cases. Over half of the sample self-identified as Caucasian, non-Hispanic. The average age of the sample was 36 years old, with an average time in pain of 61 months. There were no significant differences on any demographic or pain outcome variables between the 28 FORT completers and TAU participants, although FORT completers did report significantly lower depression symptoms at pre-treatment than TAU participants (see Table 1).

Table 1. Comparison of pre-treatment demographic, pain and psychiatric variables between Functional and Orthopedic Rehabilitation Treatment (FORT) completers and non-completers (who were given treatment as usual).

Variable	Assessment	FORT Completers $N = 28$	TAU $N = 22$	p-Value
	Age (yrs)	36.3	35.8	0.780
	Time in Pain (mos)	61.5	64.1	0.879
Demographics	Sex (% male)	57	43	0.890
	Service Branch (% USAF)	82	55	0.064
	Race (% Caucasian, non-Hispanic)	64	64	0.587
	Self-Report Disability (Mean (SD))			
	MVAS	74.1 (25.3)	78.0 (20.8)	0.586
	ODI	17.2 (8.9)	18.7 (6.1)	0.488
	Functional Capacity (Mean (SD))			
	Floor-to-Waist Lift (lbs)	49.3 (36.5)	46.7 (20.8)	0.779
Pain Characteristics	Waist-to-Eye Lift (lbs)	42.4 (15.9)	36.0 (14.3)	0.144
	Health-Related Quality of Life (Mean (SD))			
	SF-36 Physical	34.4 (10.4)	35.8 (6.9)	0.555
	SF-36 Mental	51.0 (8.7)	50.7 (8.8)	0.887
	Pain Intensity (Mean (SD))			
	VAS	5.6 (3.6)	4.8 (4.8)	0.498
	Depression (Mean (SD))			
Psychiatric Symptoms	BDI-2	9.5 (6.9)	14.9 (10.2)	0.034
	PTSD (Mean (SD))			
	PCL-M	27.9 (8.3)	31.9 (11.6)	0.164

As shown in Table 2, FORT completers demonstrated a significant correlation between PTSD symptom scores, and both self-report disability and a measure of functional capacity at pre-treatment. Self-report disability was positively correlated with PTSD on the ODI and MVAS measures, accounting for 11% to 28% of the variance in these measures. PTSD symptoms were negatively correlated with waist-to-eye level lifting, but did not demonstrate a significant relationship with floor-to-waist lifting. Depression scores demonstrated a similar pattern. Pre-treatment BDI scores were significantly and positively related to pre-treatment ODI and MVAS scores, accounting for 8% to 26% of the variance based on the coefficient of determination. Once again, depression symptoms were negatively correlated with pre-treatment waist-to-eye level lifting, but were not significantly related to floor-to-waist level lifting. Neither psychiatric symptom was significantly correlated with pain intensity rating.

Table 2. Correlation of Posttraumatic stress disorder CheckList-Military (PCL-M) and Beck Depression Inventory (BDI) scores to self-report measures of disability (Oswestry Disability Inventory (ODI), Million Visual Analog Scale (MVAS)) and lifting scores (Floor-to-Waist (FW), Waist-to-Eye Level (WEL)) among FORT completers.

r (On-Tailed) p-Value	ODI	MVAS	FW	WEL	VAS
PCL-M	0.527	0.326	−0.083	−0.324	0.226
	<0.001	0.011	0.284	0.011	0.057
BDI	0.513	0.278	−0.058	−0.323	−0.048
	<0.001	0.025	0.345	0.011	0.371

PTSD and depression scores were entered into a general linear model (GLM) to examine the extent to which pre-treatment psychiatric symptom scores predict pain management outcomes (including self-report disability, functional capacity, and pain severity). One-way ANOVA and Pearson product-moment correlation were used to identify potential covariates for entry into the GLM. There was a significant difference between the sexes on floor-to-waist and waist-to-eye level lifting at post-treatment (with males lifting more than females), and a significant difference between the military services on ODI score (with US Army members reporting more disability than Air Force personnel). Sex was entered as a covariate in analysis of functional capacity variables, and service branch was entered as a covariate in analysis of ODI scores. As shown in Table 3, there were no significant effects of depression and PTSD symptoms on any of the criterion variables after controlling for pre-treatment scores and identified covariates, although psychiatric symptoms reached near-significance on a few criteria. PTSD symptoms (as measured by the PCL-M) had a near-significant association with post-treatment MVAS self-report disability scores after controlling for pre-treatment MVAS scores ($p = 0.058$) and depression symptoms, and PTSD symptoms had a near-significant association with post-treatment waist-to-eye level lifting ($p = 0.077$) after controlling for pre-treatment lifting capacity and gender.

Table 3. General linear model (GLM) of PTSD predicting post-treatment self-report disability (controlling for pre-treatment disability scores).

Predictor	Assessment	F-Test	p-Value
Pre-Treatment BDI	ODI	1.375	0.264
	MVAS	0.056	0.814
	FW	0.810	0.452
	WEL	1.310	0.281
	VAS	1.210	0.277
Pre-Treatment PCL-M	ODI	1.943	0.137
	MVAS	3.770	0.058
	FW	0.326	0.724
	WEL	2.732	0.077
	VAS	0.186	0.669

Because neither psychiatric symptom variable was able to significantly predict posttreatment pain outcomes on its own, analyses of Hypothesis 4 (evaluating an interaction between the two symptoms) were not conducted.

4. Discussion

The present study is the first to explore the effect of common comorbid psychiatric symptoms on post-treatment outcomes for chronic musculoskeletal active duty pain patients who completed a functional restoration program. As expected, this secondary analysis revealed that pre-treatment scores of pain severity and disability were found to be related to pre-treatment depression and PTSD symptoms. This echoes numerous extant findings emphasizing the significant relationship between chronic pain symptoms and psychiatric comorbidities. Surprisingly, despite of the significant pre-treatment correlations between depression and PTSD symptoms with pain-related objective and subjective disability measures, neither had a significant influence on post-treatment functional outcomes in this military cohort. Although there have been numerous recommendations for integrating pain management and psychosocial management of comorbid pain and depression/PTSD to effectively address the comorbidity, the present findings suggest that it may be possible to effectively address comorbid chronic pain without specifically attending to the psychiatric symptoms (at least for those with subsyndromal psychiatric symptoms). One potential explanation for the present finding is that the FORT program led to a reduction in psychiatric symptoms, lessening their effect on post-treatment functional outcomes. This hypothesis makes sense in light of the significant correlations between depression/PTSD symptoms and functional/disability measures at pre-treatment, as well as evidence from previously published findings from this cohort showing a significant improvement in psychiatric symptoms from pre- to post-treatment among treatment completers [19]. It is also possible, however, that effectively reducing pain-related disability and functional capacity improved depression and PTSD symptoms based on links between these symptoms and chronic pain that are mediated by disability and functional incapacity. Indeed, depression and PTSD have been shown in prior studies to have a strong influence on disability and functioning that lead to a more intense pain experience [28], although other studies have shown that pain outcomes can improve even when psychiatric symptoms do not. For example, a study of 142 non-severe head-injured trauma patients found that those who completed a multidimensional pain management program reported no improvement in their psychiatric symptoms, but did report significant pain relief at post-treatment [29]. This aligns with other evidence in the extant literature showing that the presence of chronic pain does little to predict treatment outcomes in psychosocial interventions targeting PTSD [30]. Clearly, more work is needed to explore the relationship between these conditions.

There were several limitations of this research study. First, the present re-analysis examined a small small sub-sample ($n = 28$) of FORT data over a brief time (3 weeks). This was done to focus the analysis on a more variable data sub-sample most likely to illuminate the influence of pre-treatment psychiatric symptoms on functional rehabilitation outcomes, but the narrow sample likely diminished statistical power and obscured some significant findings (although some near-significant relationships were still uncovered). A large majority of the sample was Air Force (77%); therefore, results may not be generalizable to the other services. It would be beneficial in the future to have a broader representation of the services included in the FORT program. This study was conducted prior to military members returning from Operation Enduring Freedom (OEF) and Operation Iraqi Freedom (OIF), so reported psychiatric comorbidities for the present sample were likely milder than those of more recent veterans. However, the preliminary data generated by this research offers a good foundation for future research because musculoskeletal injuries increase among military service members and veterans due to injuries related to OEF/OIF. In fact, 47% of OEF/OIF returning deployers are reporting chronic pain [5], and chronic pain is likely to continue to grow even as rates of PTSD and traumatic brain injury stabilize in the U.S. military and Veterans Affairs [31]. Further research in functional restoration is needed with returning deployers based on increased musculoskeletal pain disorders in the military.

5. Conclusions

This study raises continued questions regarding the best treatment for complex chronic musculoskeletal pain in military and veteran populations, and gives some rise to questions about the need for integrated psychiatric and pain management interventions to adequately address complex polymorbid pain. Although this preliminary re-analysis did not definitively answer the research question, it did offer an early finding supporting the potential of functional improvements alone as adequate for good pain management is this complex population. Despite multiple calls for integrated treatment programs (which can be expensive and difficult to implement due to the specialty resources required [32]), it is possible that the emphasis of future study and research should be on finding effective pain management interventions for this complex population, ignoring interventions that are effective for the amelioration of comorbid psychiatric symptoms. Future studies should also explore the long-term socioeconomic and quality-of-life implications of improved function and disability outcomes in complex comorbid pain patients. If improvements in function and disability lead to decreased healthcare utilization and increased quality-of-life in military comorbid pain patients (as has already been demonstrated in some preliminary studies [33–35]), then better pain management strategies should certainly receive greater attention.

Acknowledgments: The writing of this manuscript was supported by Robert Gatchel's Department of Defense (DoD) grant from the Congressionally Directed Medical Research Program's Peer Review Medical Research Program (DAMD 17-03-1-055). No funds were obtained to cover the cost to publish in open access.

Author Contributions: Cindy A. McGeary and Donald D. McGeary developed the research questions for the paper and analyzed data from an existing dataset that belongs to Robert J. Gatchel. Robert J. Gatchel developed this dataset from previous DoD grant funding (Congressionally Directed Medical Research Program's Peer Review Medical Research Program; DAMD 17-03-1-0055). Cindy A. McGeary and Donald D. McGeary analyzed the data. Cindy A. McGeary, Donald D. McGeary, Robert J. Gatchel and Jose Moreno wrote the paper. All authors had final approval on the version to be submitted for publication.

Conflicts of Interest: The authors declare no conflicts of interest. The views expressed in this article are those of the authors and are not the official policy of the Department of Defense or the United States Air Force.

References

1. Geisser, M.E.; Roth, R.S.; Bachman, J.E.; Eckert, T.A. The relationship between symptoms of post-traumatic stress disorder and pain, affective disturbance and disability among patients with accident and non-accident related pain. *Pain* **1996**, *66*, 2017–2214. [CrossRef]

2. Bryant, R.A.; O'Donnell, M.L.; Creamer, M.; McFarlane, A.C.; Clark, C.R.; Silove, D.S. The psychiatric sequelae of traumatic injury. *Am. J. Psychiatry* **2010**, *167*, 312–320. [CrossRef] [PubMed]

3. Gadermann, A.M.; Engel, C.C.; Naifeh, J.A.; Nock, M.K.; Petukhova, M.; Santiago, P.N.; Wu, B.; Zaslavsky, A.M.; Kessler, R.C. Prevalence of DSM-IV major depression among US military personnel: Meta-analysis and simulation. *Mil. Med.* **2012**, *177*, 47–59. [CrossRef] [PubMed]

4. Stevelink, S.A.; Malcolm, E.M.; Mason, C.; Jenkins, S.; Sundin, J.; Fear, N.T. The prevalence of mental health disorders in (ex-) military personnel with a physical impairment: A systematic review. *Occup. Environ. Med.* **2015**, *72*, 243–251. [CrossRef] [PubMed]

5. Cohen, G.H.; Fink, D.S.; Sampson, L.; Galea, S. Mental health among reserve component military service members and veterans. *Epidemiol. Rev.* **2015**, *37*, 7–22. [CrossRef] [PubMed]

6. Campbell, D.G.; Felker, B.L.; Liu, C.F.; Yano, E.M.; Kirchner, J.E.; Chan, D.; Rubenstein, L.V.; Chaney, E.F. Prevalence of depression-PTSD comorbidity: Implications for clinical practice guidelines and primary care-based interventions. *J. Gen. Intern. Med.* **2007**, *22*, 711–718. [CrossRef] [PubMed]

7. Bryan, C.J.; Clemans, T.A.; Hernandez, A.M.; Rudd, M.D. Loss of consciousness, depression, posttraumatic stress disorder, and suicide risk among deployed military personnel with mild traumatic brain injury. *J. Head Trauma Rehabil.* **2013**, *28*, 13–20. [CrossRef] [PubMed]

8. Rudy, T.E.; Kerns, R.D.; Turk, D.C. Chronic pain and depression: Toward a cognitive-behavioral mediation model. *Pain* **1988**, *35*, 129–140. [CrossRef]

9. Kelsall, H.L.; McKenzie, D.P.; Forbes, A.B.; Roberts, M.H.; Urquhart, D.M.; Sim, M.R. Pain-related musculoskeletal disorders, psychological comorbidity, and the relationship with physical and mental well-being in Gulf War veterans. *Pain* **2014**, *155*, 685–692. [CrossRef] [PubMed]

10. Morasco, B.J.; Lovejoy, T.I.; Lu, M.; Turk, D.C.; Lewis, L.; Dobscha, S.K. The relationship between PTSD and chronic pain: Mediating role of coping strategies and depression. *Pain* **2013**, *154*, 609–616. [CrossRef] [PubMed]

11. Outcalt, S.D.; Kroenke, K.; Krebs, E.E.; Chumbler, N.R.; Wu, J.; Yu, Z.; Bair, M.J. Chronic pain and comorbid mental health conditions: Independent associations of posttraumatic stress disorder and depression with pain, disability, and quality of life. *J. Behav. Med.* **2015**, *38*, 535–543. [CrossRef] [PubMed]

12. Teo, I.; Jensen, M.P.; Tan, G. Anxiety Sensitivity and Depression: Explaining Posttraumatic Stress Disorder Symptoms in Female Veterans with Chronic Pain. *Mil. Behav. Health* **2014**, *2*, 173–179. [CrossRef]

13. Finucane, A.M.; Dima, A.; Ferreira, N.; Halvorsen, M. Basic emotion profiles in healthy, chronic pain, depressed and PTSD individuals. *Clin. Psychol. Psychother.* **2012**, *19*, 14–24. [CrossRef] [PubMed]

14. Bosco, M.A.; Gallinati, J.L.; Clark, M.E. Conceptualizing and treating comorbid chronic pain and PTSD. *Pain Res. Treat.* **2013**. [CrossRef] [PubMed]

15. Committee on the Assessment of Ongoing Effects in the Treatment of Posttraumatic Stress Disorder; Institute of Medicine. *Treatment for Posttraumatic Stress Disorder in Military and Veteran Populations: Initial Assessment*; National Academy Press: Washington, DC, USA, 2014.

16. McGeary, D.; Moore, M.; Vriend, C.A.; Peterson, A.L.; Gatchel, R.J. The evaluation and treatment of comorbid pain and PTSD in a military setting: An overview. *J. Clin. Psychol. Med. Settings* **2011**, *18*, 155–163. [CrossRef] [PubMed]

17. Vranceanu, A.M.; Hageman, M.; Strooker, J.; ter Meulen, D.; Vrahas, M.; Ring, D. A preliminary RCT of a mind body skills based intervention addressing mood and coping strategies in patients with acute orthopaedic trauma. *Injury* **2015**, *46*, 552–557. [CrossRef] [PubMed]

18. Andersen, T.E.; Andersen, L.A.; Andersen, P.G. Chronic pain patients with possible co-morbid post-traumatic stress disorder admitted to multidisciplinary pain rehabilitation—A 1-year cohort study. *Eur. J. Psychotraumatol.* **2014**. [CrossRef] [PubMed]

19. Gatchel, R.J.; McGeary, D.D.; Peterson, A.; Moore, M.; LeRoy, K.; Isler, W.C.; Hryshko-Mullen, A.S.; Edell, T. Preliminary findings of a randomized controlled trial of an interdisciplinary military pain program. *Mil. Med.* **2009**, *174*, 270–277. [CrossRef] [PubMed]

20. Fairbanks, J.C.; Couper, J.; Davies, J.B.; O'Brien, J.P. The Oswestry low back pain disability questionnaire. *Physiotherapy* **1980**, *66*, 271–273.

21. Million, R.; Hall, W.; Nilsen, K.H.; Baker, R.D.; Jayson, M.I.V. Assessment of the progress of the back pain patient. *Spine* **1982**, *7*, 204–212. [CrossRef] [PubMed]

22. Beck, A.T.; Steer, R.A.; Brown, G.K. *Beck Depression Inventory Manual*, 2nd ed.; Psychological Corporation: San Antonio, TX, USA, 1996.

23. Blanchard, E.B.; Jones-Alexander, J.; Buckley, T.C.; Forneris, C.A. Psychometric properties of the PTSD Checklist (PCL). *Behav. Res. Ther.* **1996**, *34*, 669–673. [CrossRef]

24. Ware, J.E.; Sherbourne, C.D. The MOS 36-Item Short-Form Health Survey (SF-36): I. Conceptual framework and item selection. *Med. Care* **1992**, *30*, 473–483. [CrossRef] [PubMed]

25. Mooney, V.; Cairns, D.; Robertson, J. A system for evaluating and treating chronic back disability. *West. J. Med.* **1976**, *124*, 370–376. [PubMed]

26. Matheson, L.N.; Mooney, V.A.; Grant, V.; Leggett, S.; Kenny, K. Standardized evaluation of work capacity. *J. Back Musculoskelet. Rehabil.* **1996**, *6*, 249–264. [CrossRef]

27. Mayer, T.G.; Barnes, D.; Nichols, G.; Kishino, N.D.; Coval, K.; Piel, B.; Hoshino, D.; Gatchel, R.J. Progressive Isoinertial Lifting Evaluation: II. A Comparison with Isokinetic Lifting in a Disabled Chronic Low-Back Pain Industrial Population. *Spine* **1988**, *13*, 998–1002. [CrossRef] [PubMed]

28. Roth, R.S.; Geisser, M.E.; Bates, R. The relation of post-traumatic stress symptoms to depression and pain in patients with accident-related chronic pain. *J. Pain* **2008**, *9*, 588–596. [CrossRef] [PubMed]

29. Browne, A.L.; Appleton, S.; Fong, K.; Wood, F.; Coll, F.; de Munck, S.; Newnham, E.; Schug, S.A. A pilot randomized controlled trial of an early multidisciplinary model to prevent disability following traumatic injury. *Disabil. Rehabil.* **2013**, *35*, 1149–1163. [CrossRef] [PubMed]

30. Goodson, J.T.; Lefkowitz, C.M.; Helstrom, A.W.; Gawrysiak, M.J. Outcomes of prolonged exposure therapy for veterans with posttraumatic stress disorder. *J. Trauma. Stress* **2013**, *26*, 419–425. [CrossRef] [PubMed]

31. Lew, H.L.; Cifu, D.X.; Crowder, T.; Hinds, S.R. National prevalence of traumatic brain injury, posttraumatic stress disorder, and pain diagnoses in OIF/OEF/OND Veterans from 2009 to 2011. *J. Rehabil. Res. Dev.* **2013**. [CrossRef] [PubMed]

32. Gatchel, R.J.; McGeary, D.D.; McGeary, C.A.; Lippe, B. Interdisciplinary chronic pain management: Past, present, and future. *Am. Psychol.* **2014**, *69*, 119–130. [CrossRef] [PubMed]

33. Luo, X.; Pietrobon, R.; Sun, S.X.; Liu, G.G.; Hey, L. Estimates and patterns of direct health care expenditures among individuals with back pain in the United States. *Spine* **2004**, *29*, 79–86. [CrossRef] [PubMed]

34. Walker, B.F.; Muller, R.; Grant, W.D. Low back pain in Australian adults. Health provider utilization and care seeking. *J. Manip. Physiol. Ther.* **2004**, *27*, 327–335. [CrossRef] [PubMed]
35. McGeary, D.D.; Seech, T.; Peterson, A.L.; McGeary, C.A.; Gatchel, R.J.; Vriend, C. Health Care Utilization After Interdisciplinary Chronic Pain Treatment: Part I. Description of Utilization of Costly Health Care Interventions. *J. Appl. Biobehav. Res.* **2012**, *17*, 215–228. [CrossRef]

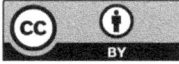

MDPI AG

St. Alban-Anlage 66

4052 Basel, Switzerland

Tel. +41 61 683 77 34

Fax +41 61 302 89 18

http://www.mdpi.com

Healthcare Editorial Office

E-mail: healthcare@mdpi.com

http://www.mdpi.com/journal/healthcare